Physical evaluation
of the dental patient

Physical evaluation of the dental patient

CHARLES L. HALSTEAD, D.D.S., M.S.D.

Professor and Chairman,
Department of Oral Medicine,
Professor, Department of Oral Pathology,
Emory University School of Dentistry,
Atlanta, Georgia

GEORGE G. BLOZIS, D.D.S., M.S.

Professor and Chairman,
Section of Oral Pathology,
Oral Diagnosis, and Oral Medicine,
The Ohio State University
College of Dentistry,
Columbus, Ohio

ALAN J. DRINNAN, D.D.S., M.B., Ch.B., B.D.S.

Professor and Chairman,
Department of Oral Medicine,
State University of New York at Buffalo
School of Dentistry,
Buffalo, New York

RONALD E. GIER, D.M.D., M.S.D.

Professor and Chairman,
Department of Oral Diagnosis,
University of Missouri, Kansas City,
School of Dentistry,
Kansas City, Missouri

The C. V. Mosby Company

ST. LOUIS • TORONTO • LONDON   1982

MOSBY

A TRADITION OF PUBLISHING EXCELLENCE

Editor: Darlene B. Warfel
Assistant editor: Melba J. Steube
Book design: Nancy Steinmeyer
Cover design: Diane Beasley
Production: Jeanne A. Gulledge

The C.V. Mosby Company
11830 Westline Industrial Drive, St. Louis, Missouri 63141

Library of Congress Cataloging in Publication Data

Main entry under title:

Physical evaluation of the dental patient.

    Bibliography: p.
    Includes index.
    1. Mouth—Examination. 2. Oral manifestations
of general diseases. 3. Physical diagnosis.
I. Halstead, Charles L. [DNLM: 1. Dentistry.
2. Diagnosis. WB 141 P578]
RK308.P47   616.07′5′0246176   81-18676
ISBN 0-8016-0887-2   AACR2

C/CB/B 9 8 7 6 5 4 3 2 1   01/A/044

Foreword

The need for a well-prepared and clearly written book on the physical evaluation of dental patients is self-evident. Dentistry has advanced from its early concerns with relief of pain, repair and replacement, and biomedical aspects, to its present interests in prevention of disease and provision of service to the public, who make up the total patient population. Dentistry has accepted its increasing responsibilities without abandoning its primary function of providing dental health services. This is a source book for the dentist with broadened perspectives.

Diagnosis as a discipline of dentistry has moved beyond detection of cavities, periodontal disease, and lesions of the soft tissues and bone, to evaluation of the total patient. It is true that dental education expounded the importance of medical evaluation even before the turn of the century, but for too many years it was a sterile pedagogic exercise, teaching something in which the dentist was rarely a participant. The Joint Commission on the Accreditation of Hospitals, in which the American Dental Association is now a corporate partner with the American Medical Association, the American Hospital Association, the American College of Surgeons, and the American College of Physicians, now permits qualified oral and maxillofacial surgeons to be authorized to perform admitting history and physical examinations for hospitalized patients. It did not extend this privilege to all dentists, because it did not believe their predoctoral education to be sufficient in scope or duration. There can be no question, however, of the "right" or "responsibility" of dentists to conduct physical examinations of the patients in their practices. The simple fact is that *dentists should perform physical examinations of their patients* regardless of the semantics of authorization versus responsibility.

Dentists examine and treat most patients more frequently than do their physicians. The dentist may be the first to detect early signs of extraoral disease. Not only are hypertension, anemia, and diabetes likely to be detected by the dentist, but blood dyscrasias, nutritional deficiencies, metabolic imbalances, neurologic and psychiatric problems, extraoral neoplasms, and other abnormal conditions may first be apparent to the dentist who makes physical evaluations of his or her patients. The dentist is not usurping the role of the physician in performing these examinations but is accepting an obligation as a primary health provider. Perhaps *primum non nocere* (in the first place do no harm) should be broadened to include "and do not overlook potential harm."

In carrying out the physical evaluation of the patient, one should not let the details of examination and testing preclude viewing the total patient. I am reminded of the tale of two sons whose father gave them both horses that were almost identical. Since they wished to be able to tell their horses apart when they were pastured in the same field, they had a veterinarian make complete physical examinations in an attempt to identify any differences. He reported that the height, weight, length, tail length, mane, teeth, and eyes, as well as laboratory findings, were identical for both the brown horse and the white horse. Don't become lost in detail while overlooking the obvious.

The authors of *Physical Evaluation of the Dental Patient* present the rationale and methods of physical evaluation. The ability to effectively evaluate the physical condition of any patient requires basic knowledge that the dentist gains through predoctoral, postdoctoral, and continuing education, an appreciation of the importance of careful, thoughtful, and detailed examination of the patient, and a source of current information for use by the examining dentist. It is more important to know where to find information than to attempt to store all the data in one's brain. At some future time such information may be stored in and retrieved from computers, but a well-planned text and the dentist's brain now serve those functions very well. Here is that text.

Accept your responsibility, and give your patients the benefit of complete health care to the very limit of your ability.

Hamilton B. G. Robinson, D.D.S., M.S., Sc.D.

Dean Emeritus and Professor Emeritus, University of Missouri, Kansas City, School of Dentistry

Preface

This book is a comprehensive discussion of a thorough physical evaluation of the dental patient appearing for routine dental treatments. Such terms as *diagnosis, diagnostic work-up, medical-dental history,* and others have been used to describe this process, which has been emphasized in the modern practice of dentistry for many years.

The presentation of this material in the dental school curriculum varies widely in the depth of presentation and the particular departments responsible for such material. We represent departments of oral medicine, oral pathology, and oral diagnosis, and believe that the material as presented in this book is appropriately suited for any of these areas, according to the individual school's philosophy and faculty personnel.

We have combined and organized material, some of which may be found in various textbooks on such subjects as oral diagnosis, oral medicine, and internal medicine for dentists, and also in physical diagnosis and physical evaluation textbooks written for medical students. We believe that the subject material is organized in a logical manner and reaches the appropriate depth for the undergraduate dental student, the general practitioner, and most specialty practitioners of dentistry. Some dental specialists, particularly oral and maxillofacial surgeons and hospital-based practitioners, may require more depth of knowledge in some of the systemic evaluation.

Where it is appropriate, each chapter follows a format that divides the subject into (1) introductory material, (2) anatomy and physiology, (3) technique of examination, and (4) the more common abnormalities that may be encountered during a physical evaluation.

Few dental educators would quarrel with the suggestion that every graduating dental student of the 1980s should be able to determine which patients can receive routine dental care without any special considerations and with no risks of complications. It is generally agreed that the dentist should be able to obtain an appropriate medical history, but beyond this point consensus ceases. Some feel that the dentist should be able to measure vital signs, and evaluate hearts, lungs, and neurologic systems. However, the suggested depths of such "hands-on" evaluations vary considerably.

In an already overcrowded dental curriculum, it would seem inappropriate to suggest that every graduating dentist be trained to become proficient to any significant degree in physical diagnosis. However, we believe that a graduating dental student and practitioner should be able to understand the reasons why physical evaluations of dental patients are necessary and should be able to establish rapport with patients to obtain medical information. In addition, the dentist should know how to examine in detail the face, neck, and oral cavity, and should be familiar with the principles and the common language of physical examination techniques used for evaluating the cardiovascular, respiratory, gastrointestinal, genitourinary, and neurologic systems.

We believe that this book, which, no doubt, in the minds of some will be considered "too much" for a dental professional, and by others as "far too brief," offers a reasonable and attainable level of understanding about an important area in dental practice.

We wish to acknowledge the valuable contributions of Dr. Frank M. Beck for his efforts in writing the chapter on patient interviewing and psychologic assessment, Dr. Dwight R. Weathers for the in-depth chapter on the skin, and Dr. Norman D. Mohl for his invaluable assistance in the chapters discussing the temporomandibular joint and occlusion.

We are greatly indebted to the audiovisual departments of Emory University School of Dentistry, Ohio State College of Dentistry, State University of New York at Buffalo, and University of Missouri, Kansas City, School of Dentistry. They have provided the many photographs and other illustrations.

Last, but certainly not least, we wish to express our gratitude to our wives, who have patiently endured the many months of the combined efforts represented by this book.

Charles L. Halstead
George G. Blozis
Alan J. Drinnan
Ronald E. Gier

Contents

1 Introduction

Primum non nocere (in the first place do no harm) is an important axiom that should always be remembered by those who profess to treat patients. The treatment provided for any condition, whether it be surgical or medical, must not "harm" the patient. There is not only an ethical but also a legal responsibility to consider a patient's well-being. The dentist must be constantly aware that routine dental procedures in certain patients might lead to serious outcomes, including death.

The need to consider the medical health of dental patients before beginning dental treatment has been recognized for many years, and dental curricula have devoted time to such subjects as clinical medicine, patient evaluation, and physical diagnosis. The National Association of Dental Faculties (NADF), established in the United States in 1884, made recommendations about the contents of acceptable dental curricula. For a Class A dental school rating, it was necessary that a school devote certain minimal hours to particular subjects. The importance of medical evaluation by dentists was recognized, and in 1899 the NADF required that there be at least 84 hours of instruction in clinical medicine, to be given during the last year of the 3-year dental curriculum.

The need for pretreatment physical evaluation of dental patients has never been more important than it is today. The great advances in modern medicine and therapeutics have resulted in more and more people surviving previously fatal or severely debilitating diseases. These people now live longer and more productive lives and, of course, can be expected to seek dental treatment. The dentist clearly needs to know, for example, whether a patient is being treated with anticoagulation drugs or antiinflammatory medications and must be aware of the possibilities of interactions occurring between drugs that he or she may prescribe and those that a patient may already be taking for another condition. A dental patient should never receive any medication, including local anesthetic agents, until the dentist is satisfied that the patient neither has a history of drug allergy nor is taking any medications that could deleteriously interact with those the dentist is intending to use.

In 1976 the Council on Dental Education of the American Dental Association, recognizing the importance of pretreatment physical evaluations, approved "Guidelines for Teaching Physical Evaluation in Dental Education." The purpose of these guidelines was "to delineate the scope of an acceptable course in physical evaluation at the predoctoral level and to present methods for achieving this objective." Because of the importance of this subject area and the need for the reader to appreciate the scope of the American Dental Association's recommended program, the guidelines are reproduced in toto at the end of this chapter.

1

LEGAL RESPONSIBILITIES FOR PHYSICAL EVALUATION

Apart from any ethical considerations, the dentist has an important legal obligation to evaluate all patients carefully and could be held liable if a patient were to suffer injury or death following dental treatment that had been provided without a proper consideration of the patient's overall health. Conway[2] published an excellent essay in 1974 on the dentist's legal responsibility for physical evaluation, and much of the following is derived from his paper.

The legal responsibility for the physical evaluation of a dental patient arises from the dental law of the state in which the dentist practices and from court decisions and doctrines that develop from malpractice litigation.

State dental laws

Some states (including California, Maine, Michigan, and Pennsylvania) specifically authorize dentists to conduct physical evaluations. For example, in California the definition of dental practice indicates that dentists may diagnose and treat diseases of the oral anatomy and states that "diagnosis and treatment may involve the use of physical evaluation." Even if no reference to the conduct of a physical evaluation by a dentist is made in a state's dental practice regulations, however, it does not follow that a dentist is *not* authorized to perform one. In New York State the dental practice act indicates that a dentist "undertakes to diagnose by any means or methods." This certainly suggests that a physical examination might be one of those "means or methods" by which a dentist diagnoses a patient's condition.

Conway points out the need to differentiate "authorization" from responsibility. The states' dental laws authorize those things a dentist may do but do not necessarily concern themselves with a dentist's responsibilities. The dentist's legal responsibility for the physical evaluation of patients develops from decisions made in the various courts of law.

Court decisions indicating the responsibilities of the dentist

Malpractice has been defined as negligence that causes an injury. This negligence may be an error of omission or of commission. Several court case examples will illustrate acts of omission of physical evaluation procedures that have been offered in testimony in dental malpractice cases. In Connecticut a middle-aged woman died after having a general anesthetic administered to her in a dental office before multiple dental extractions. The patient suffered several episodes of cyanosis, and the anesthetic lasted longer than was expected. Unfortunately the patient died. A malpractice suit was instituted against the dentist, and at the trial expert testimony revealed that the patient had a history of circulatory problems and that "the dentist's preoperatory examination of the patient was perfunctory"—*no medical history had been recorded by the dentist.**

A similar case occurred in New Jersey. A 65-year-old woman collapsed in the dental office after a dental appointment during which she had a local anesthetic for a single filling. She apparently suffered a stroke at that time and died a few days later. Legal action was instituted against the dentist. It was alleged that the dentist had failed to take a medical history before administering the local anesthetic. The jury found the dentist guilty of malpractice, a decision upheld by the New Jersey Supreme Court.†

---

*Cited as 429 F. 2d 117. The reader may not be familiar with legal citations. The first figure (429) refers to the volume of the F (federal) second series, page 117.

†Cited as 167 A. 2d 625. This citation refers to volume 167, Atlantic Second Series, page 625. The reference indicates that the case was heard in a state court in one of the group of states that are reported in the "Atlantic" series.

The dentist had used a local anesthetic, Xylocaine with epinephrine. The jury heard that Xylocaine containing epinephrine was contraindicated for patients with a history of circulatory problems, a contraindication printed on the label of the Xylocaine container. No history had been taken. The jury apparently concluded that, if the dentist had taken a history and been told by the patient about circulatory problems, he would not have used a local anesthetic containing epinephrine. This conclusion would not *necessarily* have been correct.

It should be remembered that there is no consensus about whether local anesthetics containing epinephrine are *always* contraindicated in patients with a history of cardiovascular problems. Many dentists think that the advantage of the vasoconstrictive action of the epinephrine, which prolongs the effect of the anesthetic, may outweigh any possible systemic effects of the epinephrine. Even if aware that the patient had a history of circulatory problems, the dentist may still have elected to use a local anesthetic containing epinephrine. However, this issue was not the important one. The dentist failed to evaluate his patient.

The previous two cases are examples of problems arising because adequate medical histories were not taken. The following case*, which at the time of this writing (1981) is not yet settled, indicates that a good medical history alone may not be sufficient.

A man went to the office of an oral surgeon in Washington State for the removal of an impacted wisdom tooth. He had been suffering from severe headaches before his visit and in fact had a severe headache the day he went to the surgeon's office. Before extraction of the tooth, the patient

---

*Cited as Wash. App., 594 P. 2d 923. The reference indicates that this case was heard in the Court of Appeals of Washington State. The P refers to the "Pacific" series of law reports.

completed a medical history questionnaire. He indicated that he did not know if he had high blood pressure, but that it had never been diagnosed for him before. The oral surgeon injected the patient with a local anesthetic containing epinephrine and performed the oral surgery. Following the surgery the patient was taken to a recovery room, during which time it was noted by his wife that he was suffering from fever and chills and that he appeared disoriented. He had to be assisted to his car by his wife and the oral surgeon, and he became ill, vomiting on several occasions. The following day his condition worsened, and he was admitted to a hospital with a preliminary diagnosis of cerebral hemorrhage. The dentist was sued for damages by the patient, who alleged malpractice on the oral surgeon's part, in that he failed to determine whether the patient was in fact suffering from hypertension. The patient contended that the oral surgeon knew, or should have known, of the risks involved in injecting the local anesthetic into a patient suffering from hypertension, and that he failed to inform the patient of these risks before treatment. When the case was first heard in the county superior court, judgment was made for the oral surgeon. The patient appealed to the court of appeals, where the justices reversed the judgment (2 for—1 dissenting) and remanded the case back for retrial. Subsequent appeal of this decision to the Washington State Supreme Court resulted in further consideration by the court of appeals and a decision of 3:0 was made that the case be returned for judgment in the county superior court.

During the case it was noted that there was nothing in the medical history questionnaire that would protect a person who was unaware that he was suffering from high blood pressure. It was also noted that the oral surgeon did *not* check the blood pressure, a procedure of a few minutes' duration, to determine whether the patient suffered from hypertension, and

in that respect the preanesthetic evaluation could be considered inadequate.

There were other issues involved in this case, particularly concerning the question of informed consent, but the case illustrates well the dangers that could result if adequate pretreatment physical evaluations are not performed.

It should be remembered that the physical evaluation procedure includes not only the history but also an examination of the patient. This examination may be straightforward, involving such relatively easy procedures as blood pressure determination, which can be accomplished by the dentist, or it may require a referral for detailed studies involving sophisticated tests; for example, a radionuclear scan of an organ system. The degree to which a physical examination should be conducted by the dentist will naturally depend on the dentist's own training, on the nature of the dental procedures planned, and, to some extent, on the facts about the patient's health that are obtained from the medical history and preliminary examination of the patient. Conway made a very important reference to the fact that the American Dental Association's Council on Dental Therapeutics has published a book, *Accepted Dental Therapeutics,* that devotes a complete chapter to history taking. He wrote: "The fact that the national organization of dentists chooses to put into one of its prime publications a recommendation that dentists engage in history-taking and routinely include some kind of physical evaluation of their patients does have legal effect." He believed that this emphasis on physical evaluation, including history taking, might well be cited by expert witnesses as a criterion of professional standards in dentistry. In his judgment "there is no question that the dentist has a legal responsibility to undertake some kind of history-taking of his patient as the minimum physical evaluation."

CURRENT TRENDS

The whole question of physical evaluation by the dentist is undergoing close study at this time, not only by the dental profession but by others with a special interest in the health care provided by dentists. The Joint Commission on the Accreditation of Hospitals, which includes representatives from such organizations as the American Hospital Association, the American Medical Association, the American College of Surgeons, and the American Dental Association, is interested in the physical evaluation of patients admitted to hospitals for dental care. For many years it was a requirement in nearly all hospitals that a licensed physician conduct a physical evaluation of every patient who enters the hospital. The possible future role of the dentist in conducting these examinations in place of the physician's examination is unknown, although it has been suggested that the dentist assume this responsibility.

In December 1980 the Joint Commission on the Accreditation of Hospitals approved revisions to its accreditation manual that permit qualified oral surgeons to take responsibility for the admission history and physical examination required of patients admitted to a hospital. It is obvious that there will be changing responsibilities for the dentist during the 1980s.

HEALTH SCREENING BY THE DENTIST

The primary reason for performing a pretreatment physical evaluation of each dental patient is to be certain that the patient is not suffering from any condition that could be aggravated by the provision of dental treatment. However, there is another important reason for performing a physical evaluation, a reason that is becoming more and more significant as the need for detecting diseases in their early stages and instituting appropriate therapy immediately is recognized.

Detection of early disease of which the patient may be unaware can frequently be made by a dentist during his physical evaluation. Since many patients see their dentists more frequently than they see their physicians, the dentist may be the first professional counselor to learn about their early signs and symptoms. Many diseases in their first stages might not require any special modification of dental treatment; nevertheless, it is often to the patient's benefit that such diseases be recognized and treated. There are several common medical conditions that, with a minimum of time and equipment, might be recognized by the dentist early in their development. These conditions include hypertension, diabetes mellitus, and anemia. The value of recording the blood pressure in dental practice has been claimed in several papers. The techniques for measuring blood pressure are reviewed in Chapter 7.

In the very early stages of hypertension, since there may be no signs or symptoms other than the elevated blood pressure, a patient may not be aware that there is a problem. It has been estimated that some 23 million Americans, about 10% of the adult population, have diastolic blood pressures of 95 mm Hg or greater. Only about half these people realize that they have the disease. Untreated hypertension can lead to cardiovascular problems, including heart failure, atherosclerosis, cerebral vascular accidents (strokes), and renal failure.

Several authors have reported the results of their studies on the incidence of undetected hypertension in groups of patients visiting dental offices and clinics for treatment. The importance of determining which people have elevated blood pressures and, just as important, seeing that those who require treatment receive it have been reviewed by many authors (for example, Berman and others).[1]

In early diabetes and anemia there are few symptoms, and a patient may ignore the significance of, say, urinary frequency (suggesting diabetes) or a tendency to tire easily (anemia).

Some authors have suggested that the dentist, as a routine part of the physical evaluation procedure, not only determine blood pressure but also take blood and urine samples to determine any abnormality in the blood and urine. There is no doubt that in some patient populations these tests would reveal a relatively high incidence of previously undetected disease. Whether the costs of performing blood and urine examinations on *all* dental patients would be justified remains to be determined.

The whole question of health screening in medical practice is under intense scrutiny at this time, particularly in regard to its cost and effectiveness. There are those who question the value of conducting multiple tests on apparently healthy people. The development of modern medical diagnostic techniques has meant that there are more and more sophisticated and expensive tests available, and at some point a decision must be made as to when to stop ordering tests as screening instruments. Attention has been drawn to a not uncommon situation, aptly called the "Ulysses syndrome."*[3] The characteristic features are the mental and physical disorders that follow the discovery of a "false positive" result. Otherwise healthy patients who are subjected to screening tests may be found to have an "abnormal" value (subsequently found to be a "false positive"). They are then investigated further and "make a long journey through the investigative arts and experience a number of adventures before reaching their point of departure once again." The Ulysses syndrome is a side effect of investigations rather than of therapy. Rang[3] has reviewed this and

pointed out that the normal range of values for most laboratory investigations excludes the upper and lower 2.5% of the results.

The normal bell-shaped distribution curve applies to most biologic variables. Most laboratory normal ranges cover two standard deviations from the mean value, that is, 95% of the population. The upper and lower 2.5% of the normal results would therefore be regarded as outside the laboratory's normal range. Thus, some 5% of a normal population would be labeled abnormal according to laboratory tests, even though there is nothing wrong with them. If it is assumed that, say, 100 healthy people have 20 tests performed on each one of them, it can be expected that 100 abnormal results will be found. Of course, this problem must be kept in perspective, and as Rang concludes, the syndrome "can be prevented if the clinician views with suspicion the unexpected abnormal result." He points out that the cause of the syndrome is attributable "to a meritorious desire to investigate a patient fully, the pathogenesis to gullibility!"

In concluding this introductory chapter to a book on physical evaluation, the following points are emphasized:

1. The physical evaluation of a dental patient before the provision of dental treatment, either in the office or hospital setting, is a legal responsibility of the dentist.
2. Some form of pretreatment medical history is essential for all patients.
3. A physical evaluation should be developed to the depth necessary. The degree of history taking and examination will depend on the answers to the initial questions concerning the patient's health status; for example, a patient with a history of some chronic debilitating disease who is taking multiple medications will clearly need a

---

*Ulysses, the Greek hero, after fighting in the Trojan War, returned home. It took him 20 years, during which he was involved in a series of needless encounters, some pleasurable, some dangerous. The Ulysses syndrome applies to patients who start healthy enough but make a long journey involving many tests before returning home!

much more detailed medical history and evaluation than a person with no history of any medical disorder.

4. The dentist is in a very favorable position to detect early disease of which the patient may be unaware by simple screening measures, such as blood pressure determination and blood and urine tests. He or she should remember that any abnormality should be investigated further, although not every abnormal finding will necessarily contraindicate the provision of routine dental treatment.

It has been said the dentist should "never treat a stranger." The objective of the physical evaluation is for dentists to "know" their patients to assure that they will always satisfy the maxim *primum non nocere*.

Guidelines for teaching physical evaluation in dental education*

In an effort to improve dental education, the Council on Dental Education recognizes that it has the responsibility for developing instructional guidelines in specific subject areas when significant problems exist. In approving the principle for developing instructional guidelines, the Council's intent is to provide guidance to educational institutions in establishing an adequate and appropriate level of instruction, as well as scope and depth of content in the specific subject area. Therefore, such guidelines should be viewed as a means of assisting educational institutions in upgrading instruction. Council approved subject area guidelines should not be construed as rigid requirements nor should they be interpreted as challenging the academic freedom of faculty or an institution in fulfilling its own stated educational goals.

INTRODUCTION

Because of the effects of systemic diseases and medications on dental procedures, as well as the possible effect of dental treatment on systemic health problems, there is an obvious need for the dentist to be properly trained in the physical evaluation of patients. The term "physical evaluation," as used in this document, refers to obtaining the medical history, appropriate aspects of performing a physical examination, and interpreting the laboratory tests necessary to obtain a sufficient data base to responsibly plan and carry out dental therapy and enhance the patient's health care.

The purpose of the *Guidelines* is to delineate the scope of an acceptable course in physical evaluation at the predoctoral level and to present methods for achieving this objective. They are not intended to expand dental practice into primary-care medicine but rather to produce a dental graduate who delivers comprehensive dental care in a superior fashion. These *Guidelines* include a general description of acceptable didactic and clinical course content, curricular sequence, faculty qual-

*As approved by the Council on Dental Education, American Dental Association, December 1976.

ifications and suggestions for implementation of continuing clinical applications.

While the *Guidelines* represent an acceptable model, it is understood that the course structure may be varied commensurate with teaching methodologies and resources of each institution. However, the objectives, as outlined in this document, should be achieved.

A. Educational goal

Instruction in physical evaluation should provide sufficient knowledge to permit the student to recognize normal physical findings, as well as significant deviations. This will enable the student to modify or defer dental treatment, if indicated, or refer patients to appropriate medical sources for evaluation.

To achieve this educational goal, the course in physical evaluation should provide the dental student with the knowledge, judgment and skill to assess a patient's health status. Upon completion of the course, the student will:

1. Perform and record a complete medical history
2. Perform and record appropriate aspects of a physical examination
3. Order and interpret appropriate laboratory tests
4. Initiate an appropriate medical consultation or referral for the suspected problem
5. Evaluate the data base obtained and make appropriate decisions on modification of dental treatment
6. Interpret the results of the physical evaluation to the patient and explain how these factors will influence dental treatment

B. Prerequisites

The course in physical evaluation should be incorporated into the curriculum either during or as soon as possible after completion of the core basic science instructional program so that correlation of the basic sciences and this subject area can be achieved. It is also important that instruction in physical evaluation be provided early enough so that the students can gain adequate clinical reinforcement during their clinical experiences.

C. Course content

The course must include both a didactic and a clinical component. It is the responsibility of the coordinator to carefully review the total curriculum for dental students and exclude unnecessary repetition of course content.

The following outline presents major subject categories that should be included in the didactic portion. The examples of disease states cited under the various sections should serve as a base for course content. Major emphasis should be placed on evaluation and management of acute and chronic disease states which may be observed in dental practice.

Laboratory tests, when appropriate, should be used for basic diagnostic evaluation. Laboratory tests should not be repeated if available from other sources and are current.

Didactic component

1. *Past medical history:* Instruction in obtaining facts of past medical history should emphasize areas which may alter, influence or be altered by dental therapy.
   a. Chief complaint
   b. Past illness
   c. Past hospitalization
   d. Allergy
   e. Present medical care
   f. Medications
   g. Social history
   h. Family history
2. *Psychological and attitudinal evaluation:* Assessment of patient behavior and emotional status.
3. *System evaluation:* Symptomatology, physical examination and laboratory tests used to evaluate specific disease states of special interest to the dentist (including concepts of medical management and suggested dental modifications).
   a. Head and neck
      It is assumed that the dental student has attained skill on the examination not only of the teeth and oral cavity, but also of the head and neck. As a result, the *Guidelines* make no reference to eye, ear, nose and throat examination.
   b. Respiratory
      1) Pertinent symptoms
      2) Physical signs
      3) Laboratory tests
      4) Disease states of special interest
         a) Chronic: e.g., diminished respiratory reserve, asthma
         b) Acute: e.g., acute respiratory distress, obstruction, trauma
      5) Management
         a) Principles of medical management
         b) Dental treatment modification

c. Cardiovascular
   1) Pertinent symptoms
   2) Physical signs
   3) Laboratory tests
   4) Disease states of special interest
      a) Chronic: e.g., hypertension, congestive heart failure, angina and myocardial infarction, coronary artery disease, rheumatic heart disease, congenital heart disease and prosthetic valves
      b) Acute: e.g., hypertension, arrhythmias, angina, myocardial infarction, shock
   5) Management
      a) Principles of medical management
      b) Dental treatment modification
d. Gastrointestinal
   1) Pertinent symptoms
   2) Physical signs
   3) Laboratory tests
   4) Disease states of special interest
      a) Chronic: e.g., hepatic failure, malabsorption syndromes, hepatitis
      b) Acute: e.g., acute abdomen
   5) Management
      a) Principles of medical management
      b) Dental treatment modification
e. Genitourinary
   1) Pertinent symptoms
   2) Physical signs
   3) Laboratory tests
   4) Disease states of special interest
      a) Chronic: e.g., renal failure, transplant and dialysis patient
      b) Acute: e.g., acute tubular necrosis, obstruction
   5) Management
      a) Principles of medical management
      b) Dental treatment modification
f. Neurologic
   1) Pertinent symptoms
   2) Physical signs
   3) Laboratory tests
   4) Disease states of special interest
      a) Chronic: e.g., cerebral vascular disease
      b) Acute: e.g., seizure disorder, stroke, head injury
   5) Management
      a) Principles of medical management
      b) Dental treatment modification
g. Hematopoietic
   1) Pertinent symptoms
   2) Physical signs
   3) Laboratory tests
   4) Disease states of special interest
      a) Chronic: e.g., anemia, leukemia, bleeding and clotting problems
      b) Acute: e.g., bleeding, oral ulceration, septicemia
   5) Management
      a) Principles of medical management
      b) Dental treatment modification

h. Endocrine
   Pertinent symptoms, physical signs and laboratory tests for evaluation of the following organ systems:
   1) Pituitary gland
      a) Disease states of special interest: e.g., hyperpituitarism, hypopituitarism
      b) Management
         1. Principles of medical management
         2. Dental treatment modification
   2) Adrenal glands
      a) Disease states of special interest: e.g., Addison's disease, Cushing's disease, pheochromocytoma
      b) Management
         1. Principles of medical management
         2. Dental treatment modification
   3) Pancreas
      a) Disease states of special interest: e.g., diabetes
      b) Management
         1. Principles of medical management
         2. Dental treatment modification
   4) Parathyroid glands
      a) Disease states of special interest: e.g., hyperparathyroidism, hypoparathyroidism
      b) Management
         1. Principles of medical management
         2. Dental treatment modification
   5) Thyroid gland
      a) Disease states of special interest: e.g., hyperthyroidism, hypothyroidism
      b) Management
         1. Principles of medical management
         2. Dental treatment modification

Clinical component

The purpose of the clinical component of the course is to provide the dental student with practical experience in taking complete medical histories and performing appropriate aspects of physical examinations.

This practical experience should emphasize normal findings and instill awareness of deviations from normal. Teaching aids may be used to supplement and complement this basic instruction. It is understood that the extent of clinical experience for students in such a course will depend upon the resources of the various institutions. A wide variety of methods of implementation are available, including integration with medical school courses, hospital clerkships, preceptorships, etc.

The practical aspect of this course may best begin as supervised medical history taking and physical examination sessions with students assuming the patient role. Each student should then complete a medical history and physical examination on a number of patients with a variety of disease states likely to be encountered in a dental practice and record pertinent physical findings. The patients should have been examined previously by a faculty member so that students may be evaluated in terms of performance and competency. These experiences should occur in the dental clinic, medical outpatient clinic or hospital.

D. Length of course

It is expected that appropriate curriculum time will be made available to achieve the objectives of the didactic course and clinical experiences in physical evaluation. It is recognized that because various mechanisms will have to be employed to achieve the objectives of the clinical component of this course, the time devoted to this aspect will vary.

E. Faculty

One individual should be designated as the coordinator with the responsibility for organizing the physical evaluation course and integrating the program within the various departments and clinics of the school and extramural facilities. This individual should have a qualified staff to assist in teaching the course.

The course should be taught by both physicians and dentists and other faculty having appropriate backgrounds. In the event the course is integrated into the combined medical-dental curriculum, there should be enrichment by dental faculty. It is suggested that, ideally, the basic didactic information on the various systems be provided by health specialists.

F. Continuing clinical application

In an effort to provide continuing clinical application, it will be expected that as an integral part of a pre-admission profile, an appropriate medical history and physical evaluation to include, at least, vital signs, and examination of head and neck, respiratory and cardiovascular systems will be performed on patients admitted to the dental school clinic for treatment. To accomplish this end, it is also necessary that a mechanism be developed so that appropriate laboratory tests can be ordered. The dental school should, also, have a clinical laboratory available where students can perform simple laboratory tests similar to those which can be done by a dentist in practice.

All clinical patients should have histories and physical examinations updated on a periodic basic.

It is suggested that the clinical dental faculty will complete the basic physical evaluation course through the mechanism of in-service training, or continuing education so that they will understand the objectives of the course and will provide the necessary reinforcement in the clinics. Success of this program is dependent upon such clinical reinforcement.

REFERENCES

1. Berman, C.L., Guarino, M.A., and Giovannoli, S.M.: High blood pressure detection by dentists, J. Am. Dent. Assoc. **87**:359, 1973.
2. Conway, B.J.: The dentist's legal responsibility for physical evaluation, J. Hosp. Dent. Prac. **8**:111, 1974.
3. Rang, M.: The Ulysses syndrome, Can. Med. Assoc. J. **106**:122, 1972.

2 Diagnostic process

When the word *diagnosis* is used, it invariably conjures up the thought of serious illness, doctors, and lifesaving decisions. The process of establishing a diagnosis is almost always associated with the health professions, tending to create the impression that it is unique to them. The process in fact is a part of everyday life and is used by almost everyone at one time or another with varying degrees of sophistication.[4] Problems such as a malfunctioning appliance, a jammed door, or a wilting leaf on a plant are resolved by the same diagnostic process. Information pertinent to the problem is accumulated and analyzed, and the specific nature of the problem is usually identified.

The word diagnosis is derived from the Greek words *dia* (through) and *gnosis* (knowledge) and is defined as to know apart or to distinguish. For our purposes, diagnosis can be defined as the process of determining the nature of an abnormality or disease that is producing signs or symptoms, or both.

The ability to make a diagnosis is predicated on several different factors. The knowledge of how to conduct a careful and thorough investigation of a problem is important, but still more important is a knowledge of the diseases that might be causing the problem. Being able to distinguish between health and disease frequently is not difficult. In the examples of the malfunctioning appliance, jammed door, or wilting leaf, the fact that something is wrong is not difficult to determine. This is usually also true with patients. Determining the specific cause that is producing the problem is the challenge, and resolving it requires a basic knowledge of the system and the problems that might afflict it. An important point that becomes apparent now is that it is difficult to make a diagnosis of a disease without knowing that the disease exists. This point is made poignantly in a statement attributed to Goethe: "We see only what we know."

A correct diagnosis is the basis for the appropriate and adequate treatment of a patient with disease. By knowing the diagnosis the clinician will know the natural history of the disease (what to expect) and the most effective form of therapy (what to do). This information in turn provides the basis for a prognosis, which is a forecast of the probable course of the disease with or without treatment. Often this is the type of information that is of immediate concern to patients.

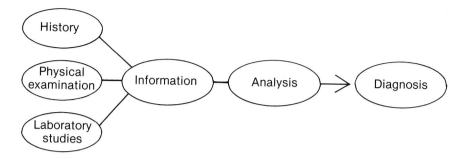

Fig. 2-1. Outline of components of diagnostic process.

DIAGNOSTIC PROCESS

Usually the diagnostic process begins as the effect of one of two different causes. A patient may seek help as a result of identifying something that is perceived as disease, or because some evidence of disease has been detected during a routine examination. Regardless of the cause that initiates the diagnostic process, the clinician must proceed in the same systematic fashion and be thorough and complete in the assessment of the problem. The same format should always be followed whether the problem appears trivial or catastrophic. However, the apparent nature of the problem will tend to influence the time and effort required to establish the diagnosis. Also, not all the information offered by a patient may be essential. The experienced clinician knows that a diagnosis depends not on all the facts, but on crucial facts, and will sort the relevant from the irrelevant.

In pursuing a diagnosis the clinician must be alert to the influence of bias. During the initial stages of the investigation, a feature of the problem that suggests a specific diagnosis may be noted. This observation can help narrow the range of the investigation, but it can also reduce the objectivity with which the investigation is pursued. The clinician must be alert to this pitfall and guard against it.

The diagnostic process consists of three distinct functions that usually are not apparent because they are performed as a continuum. The initial step in this process is *accumulation of information.* The subsequent steps are *analysis of information* and *making the diagnosis* (Fig. 2-1).

Accumulation of information

Information regarding a disease can be obtained by history, examination, and various laboratory studies. One of these procedures or any combination of them may be essential in making a diagnosis. Their specific contributions will vary with the nature of the disease. The clinical appearance of a lesion alone may provide sufficient information to make a diagnosis, whereas in some cases the full gamut of the investigation may not provide sufficient information for an answer.

The *history* (Chapter 5) is obtained from the patient by careful questioning. Essentially it should provide a narrative of the patient's problem in chronologic order from the onset to the present time. Though the history deals with all the events that relate to the patient's disease, much of it usually pertains to abnormal sensations that are perceived by the patient and referred to as symptoms (for example, pain, burning, and weakness—Chapter 20). At times the history may be an invaluable and the sole source of information, as would be the situation for a patient with a mild case of tic douloureux. Conversely, the history may be of limited value, as would be the case with a patient who has an asymptomatic lesion that is an incidental finding during a routine examination. Generally, the history is more valuable in providing information for a diagnosis than either the physical examination or laboratory investigations.[2] Bird[1] made the following observation:

Of all the technical aids which increase the doctor's power of observation, none comes even close in value to the skillful use of spoken words—the words of the doctor and the words of the patient. Throughout all of medicine, use of words is still the main diagnostic technic, and while in therapy many mechanical and chemical aids are truly miraculous in their effectiveness, words continue to play a tremendous role.

The *physical examination* is the technique used to identify changes produced by disease that can be seen or palpated. These changes are objective evidence of disease and are referred to as signs. Signs must be evaluated as to their character, distribution, and location so that distinctive features that might be of diagnostic significance can be identified (Chapters 3, 5, and 20). Subtle changes become more apparent with experience, and the habit of careful observation enhances the ability to note these changes. The importance of a sound knowledge of normal and the appearance of its variations becomes apparent now. If the clinician does not have this background, disease may be overlooked or normal interpreted as disease. The slightest deviation from normal should arouse suspicion and requires an assessment of its significance. While performing the examination, the clinician must be purpose-

9

fully looking for something and not just looking at the tissues.

The *laboratory examination* of a patient is usually conducted to gain supporting data for a diagnosis or to rule out the possibility of other diseases. When laboratory investigations are requested, the disease possibilities have frequently been considerably narrowed by information obtained through the history and physical examination. Some concept of the problem has been formulated, and the laboratory investigation proceeds on this basis. Laboratory studies should not be ordered routinely except when they are used for health-screening programs to detect unsuspected disease. They should be selected for the specific information that they will provide. For some diseases laboratory studies are the ultimate source for the diagnosis, such as a biopsy for cancer. In other situations, for instance aphthous ulcers, laboratory studies that help establish a diagnosis are not available. In these situations laboratory studies can be used to rule out similar diseases, but ultimately a diagnosis must be made on the basis of the information obtained from the history and physical examination.

Analysis of information

After the data have been collected, some time will be spent on organizing and evaluating this information. The amount of time spent is variable and obviously is related to the complexity of the problem. This data "processing" is frequently an ongoing procedure and begins with the initial collection of information. With simple or routine problems it may appear that the diagnosis was made instantaneously and as if little or no effort had been devoted to organization and evaluation of the information. This merely reflects the fact that it is an ongoing procedure and that a few distinctive features were sufficient to identify the problem. To completely separate the analysis of information from diagnosis making is virtually im-

possible. As soon as the initial bits of information are gathered, general diagnostic categories are formulated (for example, neoplastic, infectious, or allergic). This tends to limit the number of diseases that must be considered, which in turn will narrow the scope of information gathering. As information is obtained, it must be evaluated for relevance and validity. Some patients tend to be superfluous, and others are inclined to embellish the information that they provide. This segment of the diagnostic process essentially involves the sorting and categorizing of information.

Making the diagnosis

Some have likened the process of making a diagnosis to that of developing a hypothesis. Though the clinician must hypothesize to establish a basis for proceeding with a diagnostic investigation, he or she primarily uses deductive reasoning to sort the facts and work toward a known goal, a specific disease. Each bit of information that is obtained should help narrow the number of diseases that can be considered. Eventually a diagnosis is made through a process of elimination on the basis of the specific changes produced by the problem. This diagnosis may be either clear-cut or provisional, requiring verification either by additional laboratory studies or by clinical observation.

For example, if an area of discoloration is noted on a tooth, problems such as fluorosis, enamel hypomaturation, Turner's tooth, and caries would have to be considered. As additional information, such as the presence of surface cavitation and decalcification, is obtained, the diagnosis becomes apparent: caries. The concept of diagnosis is stated well in a general but somewhat detailed definition provided by Jevons[3] in 1873.

Diagnosis consists in comparing the qualities of a certain object with the definitions of a series of classes; the absence in the object of any one quality stated in the definition excludes it from the class thus de-

fined; whereas, if we find every point of a definition exactly fulfilled in the specimen, we may at once assign it to the class in question.

Pathology establishes a foundation for making a diagnosis by its listing and classification of diseases. This foundation, plus information pertaining to the clinical features and laboratory investigations unique to the various diseases, allows for their compartmentalization, which facilitates a systematic review while a diagnosis is being made. Infrequently there is a mild or incomplete expression of disease so that typical or diagnostic features are not present. This may pose a perplexing and at times insolvable problem. In such cases the diagnostician should rule out serious disease, if possible, and provide symptomatic relief until more information is available or until there is a remission of disease. Diseases that have similar clinical features and do not have a specific diagnostic laboratory test present another diagnostic problem. At times these problems may be resolved by noting the response of the patient to a trial course of therapy that is specific for a certain disease.

As with almost everything else, experience enhances the ability to make a diagnosis. This reflects both the increased awareness of the subtle changes in the clinical features of disease and the knowledge gained from the repetitive observations of the slight variations that occur in the same diseases. The value of experience is most apparent when a dental student begins working in the clinic. At the onset a diagnosis of caries can be difficult, but after a few years of practice one can make this diagnosis without apparent thought or effort.

At times it appears as if a clinician has special intuitive qualities that enable him to make a rapid or "snap" diagnosis. On the basis of apparently limited information, a diagnosis is made that is not readily apparent to others. This clinician is not intuitive, but essentially an individual who is a meticulous and critical observer and who has the capacity to identify and interrelate both the obvious and subtle changes of disease. These are attributes that all clinicians should strive to attain.

TYPES OF DIAGNOSES

Occasionally an adjective is used with the word *diagnosis* to qualify its meaning. It is a relatively infrequent but useful practice. At the onset of a diagnostic investigation, the term *working* or *tentative* diagnosis may be used. This implies that the available information favors a certain diagnosis but that additional diagnostic studies will be conducted to substantiate this impression. A *clinical* diagnosis is one that is based solely on information obtained through the history and physical examination. In these situations specific laboratory studies that would help establish a diagnosis are usually not available. If a diagnosis is made solely on specific changes seen in x-ray films without the benefit of other studies, it is referred to as a *radiographic* diagnosis. When several different diseases can reasonably be held responsible for the patient's signs and symptoms, a differential diagnosis is proposed. A *differential* diagnosis is a list, in order or probability beginning with the most likely, of all the possible diseases that should be considered. Evidence for (pro) and against (con) each diagnosis should be listed in the diagnosis. It essentially represents an expanded working diagnosis. The term *final diagnosis* indicates that a definitive diagnosis has been made on the basis of all necessary observations and laboratory investigations.

A patient with rather nonspecific oral lesions is shown in Fig. 2-2, and following is an example of a case summary and a possible differential diagnosis for this patient.

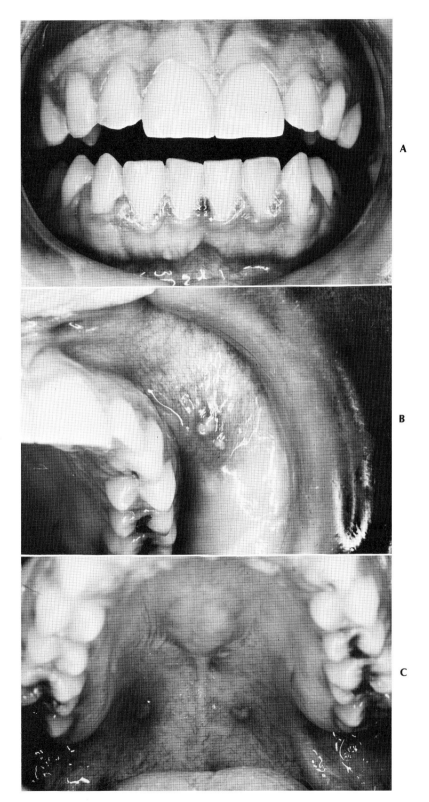

Fig. 2-2. A, Inflamed and edematous interdental papillae and marginal gingiva. **B,** Cluster of superficial ulcers with surrounding erythema on buccal mucosa. **C,** Two isolated ulcers on soft palate.

CASE SUMMARY

A 21-year-old white female complains of a sore mouth and throat that has been present for the past 4 days. There was a rapid onset of symptoms that are becoming more severe. The patient has been in good general health and still feels relatively well except for the soreness. There is no history of a previous similar problem. The patient denies the presence of lesions on other mucous membranes or on the skin. Oral temperature is 37.2° C. Shallow ulcers are present on the left buccal mucosa and soft palate. The palatal ulcers have a membranous surface. Segments of the gingiva are slightly enlarged and erythematous. Both the submandibular and cervical lymph nodes are enlarged and tender bilaterally.

DIFFERENTIAL DIAGNOSIS

1. Primary herpetic gingivostomatitis
   Pro: Gingival involvement
   Bilaterally enlarged and tender lymph nodes
   Sore throat
   Con: Occurs primarily in children
   Usually see more ulcers
   Expect more systemic symptoms
2. Hand, foot, and mouth disease
   Pro: Lesions may be limited to oral cavity
   Con: Occurs in younger individuals
   Usually has skin lesions (85%)
   Marked lymphadenitis infrequent
   Systemic symptoms relatively common
3. Minor aphthous ulcers
   Pro: Number of ulcers usually limited to 4 to 6
   Minimal systemic symptoms
   Occurs in females more often
   Con: Gingiva should not be involved
   Lymphadenitis less marked and localized
   No history of previous episodes (? initial attack)
4. Behçet's syndrome
   Pro: Oral lesions may appear as incomplete disease complex
   Appropriate age range
   Con: No ocular, genital, or skin lesions
   Marked lymphadenitis infrequent
   Occurs in males more often

A differential diagnosis should list all the diseases that could reasonably produce similar lesions. After each disease the information that either supports or rejects the diagnosis should be outlined. Appropriate laboratory studies should be ordered to substantiate or exclude each disease. In this case both the oral cytologic findings and a viral culture were positive for the herpes simplex virus and supported the diagnosis of primary herpetic gingivostomatitis.

The ability to make a diagnosis by the application of scientific knowledge and to recommend treatment on the basis of this diagnosis makes dentistry a profession instead of a craft. This ability of making a diagnosis must be practiced carefully and not abused, since without it dentists are nothing more than technicians. Langmuir[5] made a succinct but complete statement as to the character of the practice of clinical medicine. This statement is equally apropos of the character of the practice of clinical dentistry.

The clinician takes a history, performs a physical examination, orders appropriate laboratory tests and observes the clinical course. All along, he is endeavoring to synthesize his findings into a coherent hypothesis. At some point he begins to recognize a clinical syndrome and proceeds to make a diagnosis. Only then can he set a prognosis and prescribe a treatment. Although much is said about the art of medicine, this process of arriving at a diagnosis in actuality is a consummate scientific achievement.*

---

*Reprinted by permission of N. Engl. J. Med. **271:**772, 1964.

REFERENCES

1. Bird, B.: Talking with patients, ed. 2, Philadelphia, 1973, J.B. Lippincott Co.
2. Hampton, J.R., and others: Relative contributions of history-taking, physical examination, and laboratory investigation to diagnosis and management of medical outpatients, Br. Med. J. **2:**486, 1975.
3. Jevons, W.S.: The principles of science: a treatise in logic and scientific method, London, 1873, Macmillan Publishers, Ltd.
4. King, L.S.: What is a diagnosis? J.A.M.A. **202:**714, 1967.
5. Langmuir, A.D.: The training of the physician, N. Engl. J. Med., **271:**772, 1964.

3 Principles and techniques of physical examination

The educational goal in teaching clinical examination to dental students is to permit the student to recognize normal anatomy and physiology, normal variations, and early signs and symptoms of disease. This will readily lead to a diagnosis that will enable the student to prepare and render an intelligent plan of dental treatment for the patient. A thorough, comprehensive examination also allows intelligent modification or possible deferment of treatment when indicated. In other instances, it enables the dentist to refer patients to appropriate health practitioners for further evaluation and consultation.

The student and especially the experienced dental practitioner must always guard against the examination process's becoming too routine. The dentist will see many normal and healthy patients in the average general practice. The relatively low yield of significant pathosis may tend to lull the practitioner into taking shortcuts and developing a false sense of security that could be disastrous to the patient with a significant disease problem.

As the dental student acquires more knowledge, particularly of pathology, and consistently performs more thorough clinical examinations, the yield of significant findings will increase.

A CLINICIAN

The primary purpose of this text is to prepare the dental student to become a clinician. Judge and Zuidema point out that "the word clinician comes from the Greek word meaning bed and the clinician is the doctor at the patient's bedside."[1] The dental corollary to this would imply that the clinician is the doctor at the patient's chairside. The clinician is the doctor who accepts responsibility for the patient's health care by planning the strategy and executing the tactics of therapeutic care. The clinician does not treat a disease but treats patients who are ill. The term *disease* is an impersonal one that describes a cluster of interrelated phenomena as discussed in any pathology textbook. *Illness,* on the other hand, results from the interaction between a disease and a specific patient. The clinical phenomena caused by an illness include subjective sensations called *symptoms* and objective changes called *signs* (Chapters 2 and 20). Symptoms must be deduced from the verbal information given by the patient. Signs indicate anatomic and physiologic changes that the clinician must learn to recognize.

One important requirement for the effectiveness of the clinician is *empathy* (Chapter 5). Empathy requires sensitivity; it has been defined as appreciative perception or the ability to feel as another is feeling. The patient almost always brings to the examination certain degrees of anxiety either about his or her chief complaint or about the examination itself. These feelings impair the accuracy of findings and doctor-patient rapport. The examiner's demeanor should demonstrate self-confidence, patience, courtesy, consideration, and gentleness. All procedures should be explained without conveying surprise, alarm, worry, distaste, or annoyance to the patient. When pain or discomfort is necessary to assess or treat the condition, the examiner should advise the patient and proceed with care. The development or lack of development of empathy and diagnostic skills differentiates the outstanding from the average clinician.

BASIC PRINCIPLES AND TECHNIQUES

The basic principles of clinical examination are essentially the same for medicine and for dentistry. The four classical techniques of physical examination are *inspection, palpation,* *percussion,* and *auscultation.* The physician who performs general physical examinations uses each of these techniques routinely, whereas various medical specialists will vary a great deal as to which of these techniques they will use most frequently. For example, the cardiologist will probably use auscultation as much as or perhaps more than percussion or palpation. The dermatologist will use inspection and palpation more routinely. So it is with the dentist; all four techniques may be used from time to time, but inspection and palpation are perhaps the most useful on a routine basis. In certain clinical situations, however, percussion and auscultation, modified for the dentist's needs, are invaluable techniques.

An underlying principle or general guideline for the dentist's approach to clinical examination is to (1) examine each patient as if the patient had an early stage of cancer and (2) advise and treat each patient as if the patient were your closest friend or relative.

APPLICATION OF BASIC TECHNIQUES

Apart from the many systemic diseases, there are approximately 200 diseases or disorders of the oral and paraoral soft tissues and approximately 300 diseases of osseous tissues of the skull and jaws. The dentist may be the first clinician to suspect or diagnose any of these diseases. Careful clinical inspection, including radiographs, and palpation are sufficient diagnostic techniques to detect most of these conditions.

Inspection

Inspection is perhaps the most productive and frequently used examina-

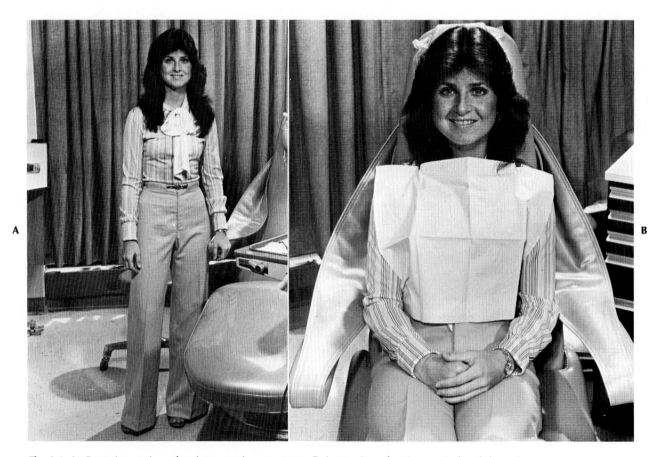

Fig. 3-1. A, Gross inspection of patient entering operatory. **B,** Inspection of patient seated and draped.

tion technique. Inspection may be defined as observation with the unaided eye. Observation of a patient needs to be distinguished and separated from evaluation. Observation is the visual recognition of physical characteristics and actions. Evaluation is the determination of the cause and effect of the observations. Observation is a complex process that allows the examiner to perceive physical signs and relate the observations to relevant knowledge or to past experience. The only requirements for inspection are adequate lighting and adequate exposure of the area to be examined.

Inspection is the least mechanical of the basic examination techniques. It can yield the most information, but it may be the most difficult to learn. Some abnormalities are obvious to even the untrained eye, but many changes that may be significant may not be obvious without knowledge, training, experience, and practice. The major effort, therefore, in becoming a diagnostician is acquiring the background knowledge to make one's observations meaningful. This in turn requires practice and study.

To become an effective observer the examiner must be deliberate and systematic and must maintain concentration. A slight oversight may mean a missed diagnosis. An orderly, systematic approach should make one less susceptible to errors of omission. This principle applies to the entire examination process. The sequence in which the examination proceeds is usually not as important as being systematic and comprehensive.

Judge and Zuidema state that "there are at least three major sources of inaccurate observation." These can be categorized as (1) oversight, (2) forgetting, and (3) bias. One can minimize oversight by repetition or habituation of technique. Forgetting may be minimized by recording notes and observations as soon as possible. Bias is a lifelong challenge that requires one to constantly guard against prejudices.

Inspection may be considered in two broad categories: (1) general observation or gross inspection of the patient, and (2) close, detailed inspection at close range in the dental chair (Fig. 3-1). This chapter deals primarily with gross inspection. Inspection that is done at close range when the patient is seated in the dental chair reveals more localized findings regarding surface contours and textural and color change. These changes are discussed in detail in Chapter 6 and in the site-by-site examination chapters. The purpose of general observation of a patient is to get an insight into his general state of health. By watching a patient, the clinician may readily identify the very sick; but it must also be recognized that many patients who have systemic diseases for which they are being treated may not show obvious signs of the diseases.

There are several reasons for the dentist's attempting to evaluate the patient's general state of health. Foremost is the protection of the patient from harm that might be caused by dental treatment. The second reason is to protect the dentist and auxiliary staff from possible contagious diseases, such as hepatitis or venereal disease. In addition, the dentist can serve as a case finder in suspecting early systemic disease problems, since many patients see dentists periodically but may visit their physicians only sporadically.

General observation should begin upon the first visit of the patient to the office and should continue at every opportunity. Auxiliary personnel can be trained to watch for significant features and greatly assist the dentist in this portion of the examination.

General observations may yield information specifically in regard to:

1. Stature
2. Body type
3. Posture
4. Gait
5. Mobility
6. Symmetry
7. Sex
8. Color
9. Skin
10. Head, face, and neck
11. Hair
12. Hands
13. Responses and function
14. Dress
15. Cleanliness

Stature. Stature is strictly defined as the patient's height. Observations are made as to the patient's height, either through measurement or through estimation. The extremes are relatively easy to estimate; the very tall person is defined as a giant, the short as a

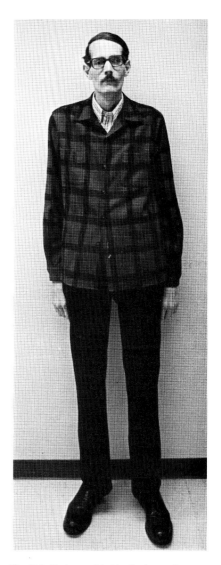

Fig. 3-2. Patient with Marfan's syndrome. Patients with this syndrome may show clefting of lip and palate, bifid uvula, and long, narrow teeth.

15

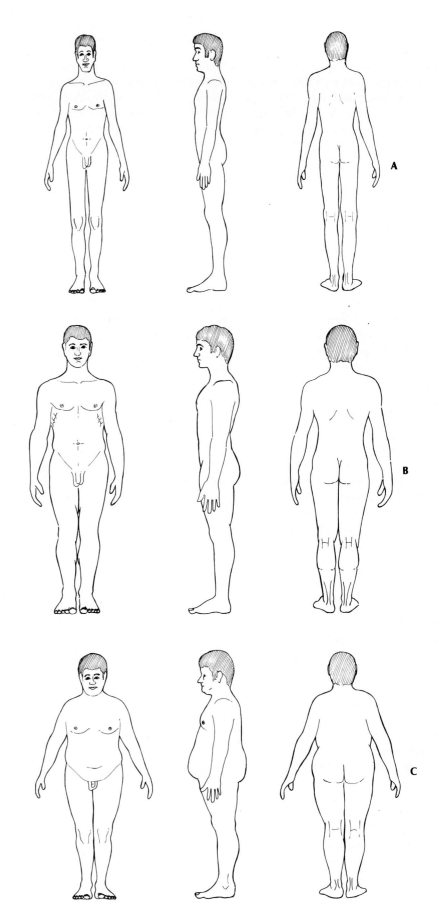

Fig. 3-3. A, Ectomorph. **B,** Mesomorph.
C, Endomorph.

dwarf or midget. The average height in the United States for men is 5 feet 9 inches with 90% between 5 feet 4 1/2 inches and 6 feet 4 1/2 inches. For women the average is 5 feet 3 1/2 inches, with 90% between 4 feet 11 1/2 inches and 5 feet 8 inches.[5] The term *stature* is broadened in general usage to include the relationship of arm and leg length to body length: the arm span of a healthy individual is usually approximately the same as the height, and the trunk is two thirds the length of the lower extremities. Major variations in the trunk-limb ratios suggest genetic diseases, such as Marfan's syndrome (Fig. 3-2), and birth defects such as were seen in the thalidomide-induced birth defects of the 1960s. There are many other syndromes and endocrine deficiencies that produce abnormal limb-trunk ratios. These become even more relevant to dentistry because many of these syndromes have oral manifestations.

Body type. The body build or type is determined by the relationship of the stature to skeletal size or frame and by the softness of tissues (muscles and adipose tissue). There are various classifications or ways of describing the body builds. One of the most simple is thin, well nourished, and obese. This is based primarily on the amount of adipose tissue and not on body build. One classification takes into consideration only the skeletal makeup or frame and classifies the frame as small, medium, or large.

Shelden[3] developed a system that he called somatotypes, which took into consideration all facets of the makeup of the body build. His somatotypes were ectomorph, mesomorph, and endomorph (Fig. 3-3). The ectomorph somatotype is characterized by a small frame, lightly muscled, with little adipose tissue. It is characterized as being derived from ectoderm. The mesomorph is a person with a medium body build, well muscled, with very little fat. The dominant structures are derived from the

mesoderm. The endomorph is characterized as a person with a soft, poorly muscled body with excess fatty tissue. The prominent developmental tissue is the endoderm. Each somatotype was described as having distinctive character traits.

Kampmeier and Blake[2] described the body types as sthenic, hyposthenic, and hypersthenic. These body types roughly correspond to the mesomorph, endomorph, and ectomorph of Shelden.

Height and weight tables give a guide for the evaluation of body builds. There are many tables available showing some variance in the ideal or recommended height-weight relationship. A frequently used table is published by the Metropolitan Life Insurance Company (Table 1). A recent survey by the National Center for Health Statistics shows that even though these are recommended weights, the American public averages well above these.[5]

Table 1. Recommended height-weight relationship

		Desirable weights Weight in pounds according to frame (in indoor clothing)			
	Height (with shoes on) 1-inch heels		**Small frame**	**Medium frame**	**Large frame**
	Feet	Inches			
Men	5	2	112-120	118-129	126-141
of ages 25	5	3	115-123	121-133	129-144
and over	5	4	118-126	124-136	132-148
	5	5	121-129	127-139	135-152
	5	6	124-133	130-143	138-156
	5	7	128-137	134-147	142-161
	5	8	132-141	138-152	147-166
	5	9	136-145	142-156	151-170
	5	10	140-150	146-160	155-174
	5	11	144-154	150-165	159-179
	6	0	148-158	154-170	164-184
	6	1	152-162	158-175	168-189
	6	2	156-167	162-180	173-194
	6	3	160-171	167-185	178-199
	6	4	164-175	172-190	182-204
	Height (with shoes on) 2-inch heels		**Small frame**	**Medium frame**	**Large frame**
	Feet	Inches			
Women	4	10	92- 98	96-107	104-119
of ages 25	4	11	94-101	98-110	106-122
and over	5	0	96-104	101-113	109-125
	5	1	99-107	104-116	112-128
	5	2	102-110	107-119	115-131
	5	3	105-113	110-122	118-134
	5	4	108-116	113-126	121-138
	5	5	111-119	116-130	125-142
	5	6	114-123	120-135	129-146
	5	7	118-127	124-139	133-150
	5	8	122-131	128-143	137-154
	5	9	126-135	132-147	141-158
	5	10	130-140	136-151	145-163
	5	11	134-144	140-155	149-168
	6	0	138-148	144-159	153-173

For girls between 18 and 25, subtract 1 pound for each year under 25.

From Metropolitan Life Insurance Company.

Evaluation of body build as to the relationship of frame and soft tissues may have direct importance for the dentist. The frame, musculature, and amount of fat should be in proportion. A small-framed person with large muscles has probably altered the expected somatotype with exercises to build up the muscles. The obese person, regardless of frame, probably will have some type of dietary problem and, as a general rule, will have a high carbohydrate intake, which is detrimental to dental health. Patients who have wasted musculature or who are very thin will appear to have either some type of chronic disease or a nutritional deficiency. The debilitated person will need evaluation of his or her health status. These patients may suffer from diseases such as chronic obstructive pulmonary disease, chronic coronary insufficiency, tuberculosis, malignancies, dietary deficiencies, or anorexia nervosa.

Posture. The patient's posture is observed. The healthy mature individual will stand straight with a slight kyphosis (posterior rounding of the thoracic spine), lordosis (anterior rounding of the lumbar spine), head up, and feet centered well under the body (Fig. 3-4). The healthy adult will sit with a basically straight back with the weight centered well over the buttocks and the feet either crossed or placed on the floor; the head will be erect and mobile. Children and the elderly will have variations of this posture: the young have a slightly exaggerated lordosis and the compensating head and leg position; the elderly tend to have an exaggerated kyphosis with the compensating head and leg position. Severe spinal deviations, such as scoliosis (lateral curvature of the spine, Fig. 3-5) or kyphosis (Fig. 3-6) and severe lordosis (Fig. 3-7), will produce abnormal postures and make movement difficult. Patients with degenerative arthritis or osteoporosis of the spine will become stooped and frequently humpbacked (kyphosis)

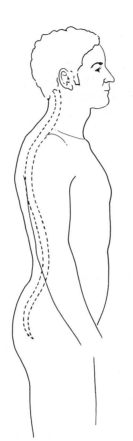

Fig. 3-4. Normal posture and curvature of spine.

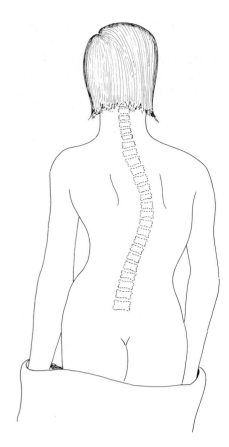

Fig. 3-5. Scoliosis (lateral deviation of spine).

with a very bent appearance. Patients with chronic obstructive pulmonary disease will have posture in which the shoulders will be up, producing a barrel chest to expand the lung capacity. Patients with pain will develop postures that are stooped or bent, designed to relieve some of the pain. The severely depressed person may have a drooping posture.

Gait. Observation of the patient's walk is done as the patient walks in the reception room and as the patient is moved from the reception room to the operatory or consultation room. Patients are observed for any abnormalities in the usual smooth movement in which they move one foot at a time in a smooth, rhythmic motion. Patients who have suffered cerebral vascular accidents will frequently have paralysis in which their gait

shows a leg that is dragged. Patients who have had a leg amputated either because of trauma or because of malignancy, diabetes, or blood clots will walk with a limp because of the artificial limbs they are wearing. A classic example of an abnormal gait is seen in tertiary syphilis in the form of tabes dorsalis. These patients' gait is very halty because they search for the ground with each step. The height to which the patient lifts the foot should be noted. Severely depressed patients frequently shuffle and drag their feet.

Mobility. Patients' mobility or ability to move all parts of their body is carefully observed. Healthy persons will be able to move all their limbs and their head and neck with smooth, easy movements. They will have a full range of movement of the arms so that they can make circular motions

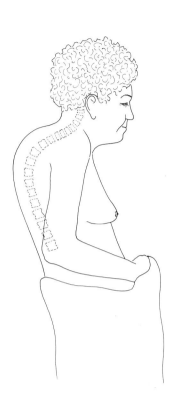

Fig. 3-6. Kyphosis (flexion of spine).

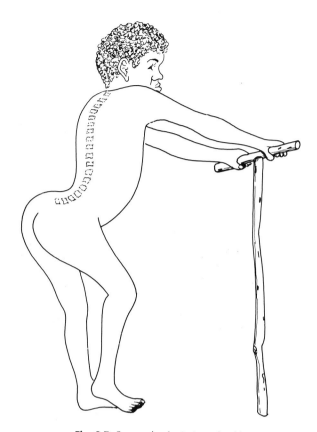

Fig. 3-7. Severe lordosis (swayback).

around the body both laterally and horizontally. The head will be able to be turned in approximately a 180° arc from shoulder to shoulder and moved down so that the chin will touch the chest and up so that the eyes are looking almost straight above the body. The legs and feet will be able to be moved in all directions but at a slightly decreased arc from that of the arms. Both the arms and legs can be straightened at the elbow and knee so that the arm and leg are straight. The fingers may likewise be straightened or extended so they are straight and closed to make a solid fist with fingertips in the palm of the hand. The patient who has rheumatoid or degenerative arthritis will have a greatly decreased mobility of arms, legs, and fingers. The patient who has neurologic disturbances or who has had a

cerebral vascular accident may have decreased mobility of the limbs. There are rare cases of hypomobility of joints. These patients are the so-called double-jointed and may not be able to grasp objects (including toothbrushes) well in their hands.

Symmetry. A person will normally be nearly bilaterally symmetrical; that is to say, the hands, arms, legs, feet, trunk, face, and head will be the same on each side of the body. Of course, there will be minor variations in the symmetry. Major variations would indicate diseases such as atrophies or hypertrophies that are due to neurologic or muscle disturbances. Tumors may be seen as asymmetrical growths; these may be benign or malignant.

Sex. Observation of the patient will generally give the observer enough information to determine the sex of the

patient. The observation of the dentist should be matched with the patient-completed form in which the patient has indicated what sex he or she is. Occasionally, patients will not dress and appear as the same sex that they are genetically.

Color. The pigmentation of the patient's skin needs to be observed carefully. Many diseases and physiologic processes produce alterations in skin pigmentation (Fig. 3-8).

Skin. The examination of the skin is discussed in detail in Chapter 10. The general observation of the patient includes observing the skin for any changes in color, texture, consistency, or symmetry.

Head, face, and neck. The head, face, and neck are part of the general observation. The details to be observed are explained in Chapter 8.

Hair. The hair is observed to determine the color, texture, brightness, and distribution. This includes the facial and body hair as well as the scalp hair. The hair color is described as brown, red, black, blonde, gray, or white and should be fairly uniform. Colors different from these should arouse suspicion that the hair is dyed by cosmetics or drugs. The texture of the hair is described as either fine or coarse. The degree of oiliness determines the brightness of the hair. Very dry hair will have a dull appearance, whereas clean, oily hair will have a sheen. The distribution of the hair is important. The male will have facial and body hair, whereas the female will have little or no hair in these areas. Excessive facial or body hair in the female suggest hormonal disturbances. Hormonal disturbances produce a lack of this hair in the male. Loss of hair may be either genetic, as the balding pattern in men, or pathologic, as a side effect of radiation or chemotherapy for malignancies. Certain fungus infections (as well as psychologic problems) will produce partial loss of hair (alopecia areata).

Hands. The patient's hands are observed to determine if all the fingers are present or if there are extra fingers. They are observed to determine if they are symmetrical. The palms of the hand can be observed to determine if there are deformities or skin diseases such as palmar keratosis, fungal infections of the hands, id reactions, or allergic reactions. The palms are also observed for callouses, which will give some idea as to the occupation of the patient. The person who does heavy work every day would be expected to have palms that are more heavily calloused than, say, the pianist, beautician, dentist, or surgeon who, because of necessity, maintains softer and less calloused hands.

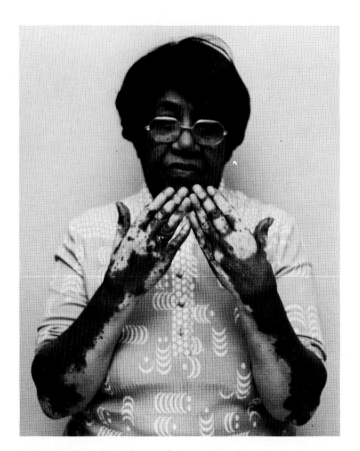

Fig. 3-8. Vitiligo (loss of normal pigmentation).

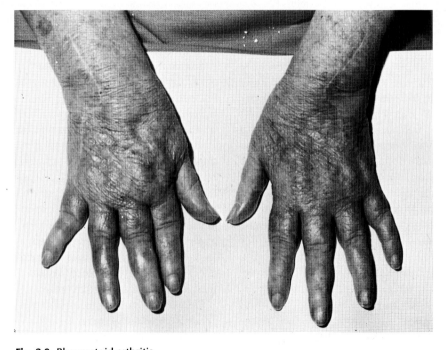

Fig. 3-9. Rheumatoid arthritis.

20

The ability to move the fingers is observed. Patients with rheumatoid arthritis (Fig. 3-9) have difficulty in bending their fingers, as do those with gout (Fig. 3-10). Old fractures or joint disturbances will inhibit the patient's mobility of the fingers. The patient who does not have full use of the hands will make it necessary to alter the standard of oral hygiene procedures. The patient who does not have good dexterity could not be expected to use dental floss effectively.

The fingers are observed for clubbing (Fig. 3-11). Clubbing, or pulmonary osteoarthropathy, is caused by a number of conditions. Clubbing can be congenital and of no significance from a disease standpoint. The most common cause of clubbing of the fingers is severe coronary or respiratory disease. Patients with severe ventricular septal defects or other congenital circulation problems fre-

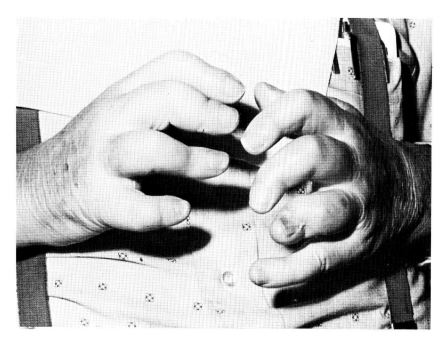

Fig. 3-10. Gouty arthritis.

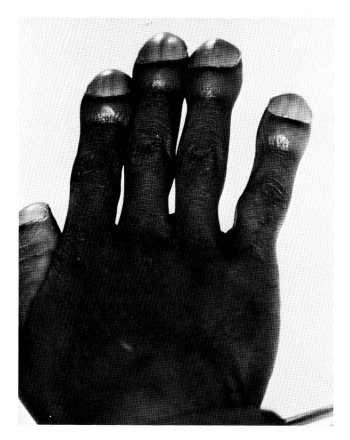

Fig. 3-11. Clubbing of fingers.

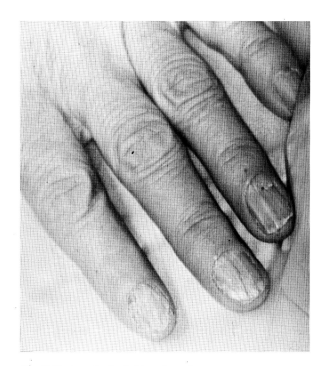

Fig. 3-12. Longitudinal ridges in nails.

quently have large clubbed fingers. Patients with chronic obstructive lung disease or any chronic heart disease that reduces the amount of blood circulated will frequently show large clubbing of the fingers.

The fingernails may indicate much about a patient's medical history. The classic splinter hemorrhage of endocarditis is caused by bacterial emboli in the fingernails, producing infarction and a hemorrhage that runs longitudinally in the fingernail (Fig. 3-12). Extended periods of severe illness produce horizontal lines in all the fingernails. These lines move as the fingernail grows. The fingernail grows from a bed and is constantly formed. A disturbance such as a myocardial infarct, a prolonged high fever, surgery, or other severe disease will disrupt the normal formation pattern of the fingernail and therefore produce the horizontal lines. Fingernails grow at the rate of 1.9 mm to 4.4 mm per month.[5] There is further discussion of nails in Chapter 10.

Responses and function. Observation together with the history taking and interview of patients should give the dentist a reasonable evaluation of hearing, vision, comprehension, and coordination. Details of examination of the eyes and ears are discussed in Chapter 9.

Dress and cleanliness. The patient's manner of dress and factors such as quality, fashionability, cleanliness, and coordination of clothing should be observed and may give some helpful insight regarding the patient's general health. These may also indicate the patient's mental attitudes and daily hygiene habits. Patients with self-respect are usually neat and clean, even though their clothing may be old or out of fashion.

Palpation

Palpation is the act of feeling by the sense of touch. It is usually accomplished through fingertip pressure applied lightly against the various body tissues. To become astute in the art of palpation usually requires much clinical experience and the development of a manual or digital sensitivity that can discern the many variations that exist between soft and hard or rough and smooth. Palpation carried out by an experienced clinician can allow perception of physical signs not detectable from inspection alone.

In order to realize the maximal benefit from palpation, the clinician must know normal gross anatomy, the location of tissues and organs, their extent, which plane they lie in, and their anatomic relationship to each other. In addition, knowledge of histology can be extremely helpful by allowing mental visualization of the tissues being palpated.

The palpation techniques or methods commonly used for the head, neck, and oral examination are illustrated in Figs. 3-13 through 3-15. The basic techniques of palpation can be described as bilateral, bimanual, and bidigital palpation. The particular method used depends on the area to be examined.

Bilateral and bimanual palpation techniques require the use of both hands. With the examiner standing behind the patient, the bilateral use of the fingertips (Fig. 3-13) with relatively light pressure, starting in the preauricular area and systematically palpating the head and neck, will allow evaluation of normal structures or detection of abnormal changes. A comparison of bilateral symmmetry and tissue consistency should readily distinguish between normal anatomic structures and pathologic changes. This technique should be performed in a systematic manner to include the head and neck down to the supraclavicular area.

The bimanual technique (Fig. 3-14) is an invaluable method when examining areas such as the floor of the mouth. With one hand supporting the submandibular area and serving as a base, the index finger of the other hand can carefully palpate the entire contents of each side of the mouth's floor. With light pressure from both hands, the submandibular gland and

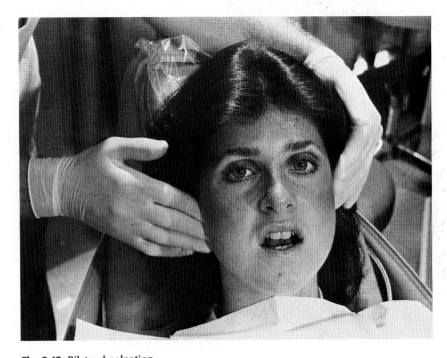

Fig. 3-13. Bilateral palpation.

22

other tissues can be rolled between the fingers.

Bidigital palpation (Fig. 3-15) can be used with the index finger and thumb of one or both hands pressing lightly and gently, rolling the tissues such as the lips or buccal mucosa between the two fingers. This will usually detect very early submucosal changes.

In general, structures that are palpable are bones, joints, muscles, tendon sheaths, ligaments, and organs. These structures can serve as a base on which to further palpate superficial arteries, thickened or thrombosed veins, superficial nerves, salivary glands and ducts, enlarged lymph nodes, and accumulation of body fluids, pus, or blood.

Some of the qualities that can be appreciated through palpation are consistency of tissues, textural change, presence of masses, tenderness, temperature, moisture, crepitus, and thrills or pulsatility from vascular structures. When masses are detected, features such as size, shape, consistency, mobility, and pulsatility may be evaluated.

Consistency of tissues refers to the degree of softness or hardness that is characteristic for each type of tissue. Consistency is often described as soft, cheesy, rubbery, firm, or bony hard. This scale reflects the relative compressibility of the tissues on palpation. Induration is another term used to indicate an abnormal firmness or hardness. It results from an infiltrating growth pattern of the disease process and is often associated with cancer.

Textural change denotes a variation from normal in the surface characteristics. Such changes as abnormal roughness, increased thickness, or crust formation indicate abnormal textural change for the skin or mucosa.

To detect the presence of masses requires thorough knowledge of normal structures and organs for the site being examined. When an abnormal mass is detected, the examiner must determine whether it is superficial or deep and whether it involves the skin, muscle, or any regional organs, such as glands.

Tenderness is the abnormal sensitiveness to touch or pressure, whereas pain is a sensation of discomfort resulting from the stimulation of specialized nerve endings; hence, pain may be spontaneous, but tenderness results from palpation or the application of pressure.

Temperature changes may indicate systemic change or regional surface change. The dorsum of the hands or fingers is best suited for evaluating

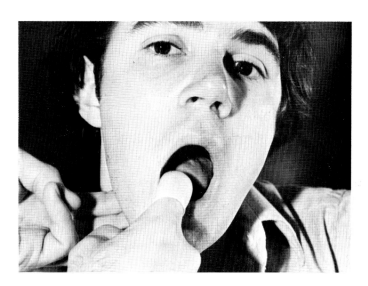

Fig. 3-14. Bimanual palpation.

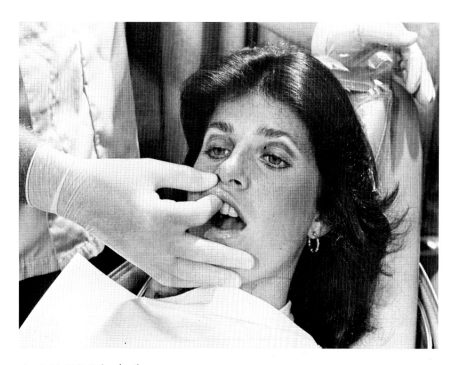

Fig. 3-15. Bidigital palpation.

temperature change, since the skin is much thinner in these areas. Increased systemic temperature is usually associated with fever resulting from infections, but regional surface increase in temperature may result from infection or from increased blood circulation in the area. Subnormal temperatures may result from a decreased circulation in the area.

The moistness of tissues is usually related to glandular secretions and results in degrees of dryness or oiliness, or sweating on the skin. The moistness of mucosal surfaces is usually related to mucous gland secretions, and in the oral cavity the moistness is affected by major and minor salivary gland secretions.

Crepitus is a crackling sensation that can be heard, palpated, or both. It is commonly associated with joint movement but can also be noted when air-filled tissues are palpated.

Thrills are palpable vibrations, usually caused by the flow of blood from one chamber to another through a narrowed orifice. The intensity of the thrill varies according to the velocity of the blood, the degree of narrowing of the orifice, and the difference in pressure between the two chambers. Rapid vibrations result in fine thrills, whereas slower vibrations produce coarser thrills.

Pulsatility refers to rhythmic pulsations associated with systolic and diastolic pressures resulting from heart contractions.

Fluctuant is another term commonly used to describe a palpable sensation. If the fingers sense a wave-like movement on compressing a fluid-filled mass, this is referred to as fluctuance.

For the dentist, routine palpation during the head, neck, and oral examination is the key in evaluating textural characteristics site by site. This may be the only means of detecting early submucosal changes, some of which may characteristically remain or persist as invisible submucosal le-

sions. Early carcinoma of the tongue may appear simply as a lesion with a firm change in consistency that can be detected only by palpation.

Some problems associated with palpation can be the limitations that swelling and pain may cause. Swelling tends to obscure definitive structures, and pain may inhibit the extent of palpation the patient can tolerate. Another problem unique to the head and neck is the distinction between enlarged lymph nodes and salivary glands. Lymph nodes are intimately associated with both the parotid and submandibular salivary glands and may enlarge within the substance or on the surface of the gland. Some hyperplastic, inflammatory nodes may persist indefinitely as palpable but inactive nodes.

Careful palpation is usually necessary to distinguish between glands and enlarged nodes (see Chapter 8). Normal lymph nodes may not be palpable, but following inflammation or other immune system stimulation, they may enlarge quite dramatically. Qualities of node palpation that may be significant in distinguishing inflammatory changes from neoplastic changes are consistency, size, tenderness, outline, and mobility. Neoplastic nodes tend to be firm to hard with a tendency to clump or mat together. Attachment to muscle or other structures tends to limit the degree of mobility. Inflammatory nodes usually have a rubbery consistency and are freely movable and tender.

Percussion

Percussion is the act of striking a portion of the body with the fingers or an instrument to evaluate the condition of the underlying structures by careful attention to the sound or echo produced. The response of the patient to the percussing may be as significant as the sounds produced.

The physician uses percussion to a much greater extent than the dentist does. Percussion of the chest wall

(see Chapter 12) can assist in identifying the demarcation and density of underlying organs such as the heart and lungs. Testing of neuromuscular reflex mechanisms is another routine use of percussion.

Sonorous percussion is the term applied to any percussion method that ascertains the density of the tissue by the sound emitted when struck. The percussion sounds or notes may be arranged in sequence according to the density that produces them, from least to most dense: tympany, hyperresonance, resonance, impaired resonance, dullness, and flatness. In general, the pitch or frequency of the sounds progresses through the series from lowest for tympany to highest for flatness.

The dentist primarily uses percussion in the dental portion of the oral examination. By striking the dentition lightly with the handle of the dental mirror, the examiner can evaluate changes in sounds from one tooth to another and may also elicit discomfort when inflammation is present. The quality of the sounds will vary according to the density of the underlying structures. Normal, healthy bone and periodontal membrane should give a rather sharp, crisp sound that has approximately the same character for similar teeth on each side of the arch. If there has been a loss of bony support or an alteration in the thickness and attachment of the periodontal membrane, the resulting sound will have a lower, dull quality. When discomfort is elicited, it then becomes the examiner's responsibility to determine the source of the inflammatory change, which is usually either periodontal or pulpal in origin.

Less frequently, percussion may be used in a more general manner (Fig. 3-16) by tapping the bony or muscular areas of the head and neck to detect possible sites of tenderness, hypertonicity of muscles, or marked change in density as a result of intrabony pathosis. Again, it is important to compare the sounds elicited from corresponding sites on each side of the body.

These specific examination techniques are referred to in more detail in the site-by-site examination chapters.

Auscultation

Auscultation is the act of listening to functional sounds of the body. The listening can be done with the unaided ear or with the stethoscope. The unaided ear can detect important signs related to breath sounds. The breathing sounds and patterns associated with such conditions as asthma, emphysema, and cardiac problems should all be of special interest to the dentist as well as to the physician. The detection of such abnormal sounds can provide a cross-check with the health history given by the patient. It is not unusual for dental patients to underestimate or fail to see the value or relation of such health problems to their dental treatment.

Other potentially significant sounds that may be readily heard are clicking and crepitus sounds associated with the temporomandibular joint. The astute listener may detect abnormal sounds, such as squeaks or premature contacts related to malocclusions. Similar clicking and abnormal occlusal sounds can be heard in denture wearers.

The stethoscope can provide enhancement to these and other sounds, which may be very significant in the clinical examination. Abnormal temporomandibular joint sounds inaudible to the unaided ear may be appreciated by simply listening through a stethoscope placed over the joint (Fig. 3-17). In addition to using the stethoscope for taking blood pressure, one can sometimes detect the bruit or vascular pulsation of developmental lesions, such as arteriovenous fistulas, which occur in the jaws and skull. Murmurs in the vessels of the neck, particularly the carotid, subclavican,

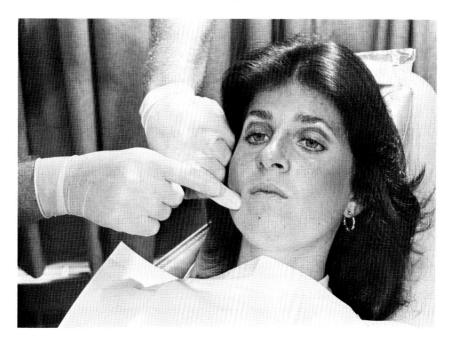

Fig. 3-16. Indirect percussion. Left index finger represents pleximeter and right index finger serves as plexor.

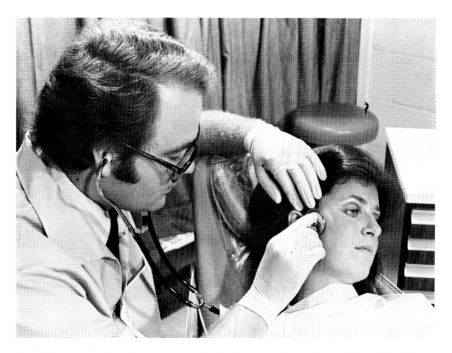

Fig. 3-17. Auscultation. Temporomandibular joint sounds can be greatly amplified by using stethoscope.

and thyroid arteries, and venous hums may also be detected by use of the stethoscope in the head and neck examination.

SUPPLEMENTAL DIAGNOSTIC AIDS

The basic techniques described above, when used intelligently, will provide a wealth of examination information. For many soft tissue diseases and developmental anomalies the diagnosis may be obvious at this point of the examination. However, since the dentist's primary concern must be the dentition and their supporting structures and contiguous osseous tissues, radiographic examination becomes an integral part of initial patient examinations. Radiographs alone seldom provide specific diagnoses, but when radiographic findings are combined with the clinical examination, they provide essential supplemental information. In subsequent examinations of the dental patient, radiographs become more of an elective supplemental diagnostic aid. Their use has to be based on sound clinical judgment as to the number and frequency of radiographs for each patient. Dental radiology is a comprehensive subject for which several textbooks are available.

Other supplemental diagnostic aids that the dentist may use according to the findings of the basic examination are transillumination and pulpal vitality tests in the dental portion of the examination. Biopsy, cytology, aspiration, and culture can serve as essential supplemental diagnostic aids in making specific diagnoses of various soft tissue and osseous tissue pathosis.

Laboratory tests are still another category of invaluable supplemental diagnostic aids that should be used to supplement the findings of the basic examination procedure. Certain laboratory tests have been suggested for routine use by the dentist for the purpose of screening. This subject is controversial, particularly as to the practicality of individual dentists using such an approach. All these diagnostic aids as well as others are discussed in more detail in the chapters dealing with site-by-site examination. Laboratory tests are the subject of Chapter 18.

REFERENCES

1. Judge, R.D., and Zuidema, G.D.: Methods of clinical examination, ed. 3, Little, Brown & Co.
2. Kampmeier, R.H., and Blake, T.M.: Physical examination in health and disease, ed. 4, Philadelphia, 1970, F.A. Davis Co.
3. Shelden, W.H., Stevens, S.S., and Tucker, A.B.: The varieties of human physique, New York, 1940, Harper & Row, Publishers, Inc.
4. Siginga, M.S.: Observations on growth of fingernails in health and disease, Pediatrics 24:225, 1959.
5. U.S. Department of Health, Education and Welfare: Height and weight of adults 18-74 years of age in the United States, Advanced data HE 20, 62-9/3:3, Nov. 19, 1976.

BIBLIOGRAPHY

Bates, B.: A guide to physical examinations, Philadelphia, 1974, J.B. Lippincott Co.

Clark, J.W.: Clinical dentistry, vol. 1, New York, 1976, Harper & Row, Publishers.

Halstead, C.L., and Weathers, D.R.: Differential diagnosis of oral soft tissue, pathosis, Disease Directory, P-3382, Washington, D.C., 1977, National Audiovisual Center.

Kerr, D.A., Ash, M.M., and Millard, H.D.: Oral diagnosis, ed. 5, St. Louis, 1978, The C.V. Mosby Co.

Merchant, H.W.: Clubbed fingers: indicators of serious illness, J. Am. Dent. Assoc. 96:96, 1978.

Strong, J.H.S.: The general examination and external features of disease. In Macleod, J. Clinical examination, ed. 4, Edinburgh, 1976, Churchill Livingstone.

Wood, N.K., and Goaz, P.W.: Differential diagnosis of oral lesions, ed. 2, St. Louis, 1975, The C.V. Mosby Co.

4 Health record

Information that is obtained while one is evaluating and managing a patient's health problems must be recorded in some way so that it is available for future reference. Because the amount of this information becomes voluminous at times, a system of indexing to facilitate its retrieval is necessary. The need for an organized record system becomes still more apparent when both the number of patients and the frequency with which they are seen by health care providers are considered. Unfortunately there is no unanimity as to a term for this repository of information, and many different terms are used to identify it. Some of the terms used include record, history, chart, and folder. These terms may be prefaced by words such as dental, medical, patient, clinic, or hospital. Invariably the terms that are used are dictated by local custom and the content of the record. Since a record frequently contains information pertinent to many aspects of the patient's health (medical, dental, and psychosocial), the term *health record* is used here.

FUNCTIONS OF A HEALTH RECORD

The principal reasons for maintaining a health record are the retrieval of information, communication, and education. The extent and importance of these general areas depend on the nature of the health care facility where the patient is being seen. The records in a private office would be used far less often for communication and education than those maintained in a large clinic or hospital. The following are more specific examples of the general functions of the health record that were cited.

Acts as the archives of health problems

The record contains information in regard to previous episodes of illness that may have some bearing on a patient's current problem or may influence how the patient is managed.

Facilitates the diagnostic process

The record aids in the acquisition, compilation, and storage of information obtained during the diagnostic process and serves as a source for the review of this information.

Helps ensure ongoing and quality care

The record helps ensure that a patient will receive uninterrupted and appropriate care by indicating: (1) the reason(s) for treatment (diagnosis), (2) the treatment considered most appropriate for the problem, (3) the sequence of treatment, (4) the treatment that has been provided up to the present time, and (5) the patient's response to the treatment. In situations where there are long intervals between patient-doctor contact or when multiple health care personnel are responsible for care, a central and current source of complete information is essential.

Serves as a legal record

The information in a record is useful for completing insurance forms, documenting injury claims, and providing evidence in malpractice litigation. The record should contain sufficient information to: (1) justify that care was required, (2) prove that care was rendered, and (3) document the results of the care provided.

Provides data for forensic odontology

Complete and accurate dental records are useful in identifying bodies and bite marks. The dentition is more resistant to destruction than other body tissues are and consequently is extremely useful in identifying bodies found in natural disasters, fires, and airplane crashes. Information from the analysis of bite marks found in food at the scene of a crime or on human bodies has been used to identify and convict individuals.

Serves as a source of teaching material

Information about the signs, symptoms, and laboratory results found in both common and rare diseases is listed in records and helps in developing a better understanding of these disease problems and their management. This information is used in teaching programs and in preparing publications.

ORGANIZATION AND CONTENT

The character of a health record can be quite variable, ranging from a few index cards with notes to an elaborate loose-leaf notebook with voluminous and assorted data that are indexed by dividers. Obviously the record system must suit the needs of the practitioner who may be treating patients either in a small private office or in a large medical center. Even though record systems are somewhat tailored to meet specific needs, they must be organized. Usually a health record contains a wide variety of information that, to be useful, must be categorized and indexed so that it is readily accessible for review. By tradition, various items of information have been categorized into specific divisions. Generally, health records are rather uniform in the divisions that are identified and the sequence in which they are listed, though there may be slight variations. The following is a listing of the major divisions usually found in a health record.

Identifying and biographic data
History and physical examination
Progress notes
Consultations
Laboratory reports

Divisions such as consultations and laboratory reports would probably be deleted by a general practitioner in dentistry, who would have infrequent occasion to use them. In contrast, a hospital record would require additional divisions for information obtained as a consequence of elaborate diagnostic studies and unique treatment procedures. This would require the addition of categories such as graphic charts, nurses' notes, reports of operations, and x-ray reports.

These various divisions are at times further subdivided into sections where specific bits of information are recorded. The following provides a brief discussion of the contents of the divisions and their subdivisions.

Identifying and biographic data

The information in this division should contain data that will identify the patient, provide a general background of the patient, and facilitate both oral and written contact with the patient or other appropriate individuals. The following is a common format.

Name: The family name (surname) and all given names should be recorded. The spouse's first name should also be recorded for married individuals. At times it may also be helpful to record a patient's maiden name.

Address: The residence number, street, city, state, and zip code should be listed. This is necessary for correspondence and may be useful for identification.

Telephone number: Both home and work numbers should be included.

Birth date: This is more desirable than just the patient's age, since it is more specific. The patient's age can be useful for identification purposes and may be significant in developing a diagnosis or determining treatment.

Sex: This also may be useful for identification purposes.

Race: This is useful because some diseases are limited to or occur more frequently in specific racial groups.

Marital status: A patient's marital status may be useful for identification, patient contact, and determining financial responsibility.

Occupation: This information may help provide an insight into the patient's temperament and may help identify environmental factors that could be responsible for disease.

Name, address, and telephone number of family physician: The telephone number of a patient's physician will facilitate contact for inquiries about health status or medications and is important for critical situations that may arise during treatment.

Name, address, and telephone number of person to contact in an emergency: Infrequent occasions occur when a family friend can provide assistance in emergency situations or support in postoperative periods. It is useful to be able to identify someone for this purpose.

History and physical examination

Of the entire health record, the history and physical examination have more subdivisions and may contain more information than the other divisions. Because of the nature of dental care and its prevention orientation, this division is usually less detailed and lengthy in records for dental patients than those for medical patients. The following is a rather typical outline of this segment of the record.

History
  Chief complaint (CC)
  Present illness (PI)
  Past history (PH)
  Review of systems (ROS)
  Family history (FH)
  Personal and social history (P/SH)
Physical examination
Diagnosis
Treatment plan

History. The history is the initial step in the diagnostic process and is the most important step in establishing the patient's problem. It should give a composite picture of the patient's problem, past and present health status, and an insight into the psychologic makeup. The history essentially consists of a summation of the information obtained from the patient interview, previous histories, and observations made by the examiner.

The *chief complaint* (CC) indicates the specific reason that the patient seeks health care. It should be expressed in a couple of words or as a short phrase, using the patient's own words (in quotation marks) when possible. The CC should not be expressed as a diagnosis unless the patient expresses it in those terms. If this happens, determine how the patient became aware of this diagnosis. At times there may be more than one complaint, all of which may or may not be interrelated. All the complaints (problems) that a patient identifies must be listed, with the major problem being listed first. In addition the duration of the complaint should be indicated. The following are examples: "toothache," 2 days' duration; "I have a sore in my mouth," 3 weeks' duration.

Because of the major emphasis on preventive care by the profession, many patients will be seeing their dentist for a routine examination or checkup. In these situations the CC would be listed as "checkup."

The *present illness* (PI) should record in a chronologic order a narrative account of the patient's problem from the onset to the present time, listing all symptoms, signs, diagnostic studies, and treatment. The preparation of this story is made easier by dividing it into specific segments dealing with the onset, the intervening period, and the current status of the problem. All the information that is pertinent should be recorded regardless of the time interval. Care must be exercised while obtaining the history so that the patient is not influenced by the examiner. The patient should be allowed to relate the story without leading questions. When a point is vague or requires further clarification, then questions are used to elicit the appropriate information. The dentist must listen carefully to sort the important facts from trivia. When appropriate, a typical attack or episode of disease should be characterized as well as possible. The information listed under PI should relate only to the problem that prompted the patient to see a dentist, that is, the CC.

When a checkup is listed as the CC, the PI will be rather brief. It should state the time interval since the last dental appointment and the nature of the dental care received at that time. There should also be a brief remark as to the patient's perception of his current oral health status.

With pain problems, the history becomes most critical, since it may be the only source of diagnostic information that is available. The following outline provides a format that is useful in characterizing a patient's symptoms. With slight modification it is also useful in developing a history for patients who have oral mucous membrane lesions.

Onset: When did the pain (lesion) first begin?

Duration: Is the pain (lesion) constant or intermittent? If intermittent, how long does it persist?

Frequency: How often does the pain (lesion) occur? Does the pain occur on a sporadic or regular basis, and does anything trigger it?

Location: Where is the pain located? Is it deep or superficial? Is it localized or diffuse? Does it radiate from one area to another? The location and distribution of lesions are important and can be of diagnostic significance.

Nature: The terms usually used to describe pain are dull ache, sharp or knifelike, throbbing, and sticking. The morphologic character (such as ulcer or papule) of lesions should be described.

Severity: The intensity of the symptoms is usually expressed in terms of mild, moderate, severe, and excruciating. In the case of lesions, the severity of the lesion seen at the time of examination should be noted.

Course of disease: Has the pain (lesion) changed since it began? Is it worse, better, or about the same?

Influencing factors: Is there anything that makes the pain worse or better, such as bending over or lying down? Do hot or cold liquids or foods aggravate or alleviate it?

Associated manifestations: Is there anything else that happens when the pain occurs (such as the nasal congestion, lacrimation, and flushing associated with cluster headache)?

As can be seen, the present illness represents a detailed story of the chief complaint.

The *past history* (PH) provides information about previous episodes of illness, its treatment, and the patient's response. The entries should list only previously established diagnoses, with dates of occurrence and details of severity or complications. This information may or may not be of significance in regard to the patient's CC (for example, the CC may represent recurrent disease, a complication of previous illness, or an entirely unrelated problem). The PH can provide important background and must always be reviewed. For our purposes, the PH should be divided into dental and medical.

The dental PH should include information about the patient's previous dental treatment. This will provide a basis for understanding the patient's current dental status and how the patient will respond to proposed treatment. Information about previous dental care, complications of previous care, and the patient's attitude toward dental care should also be obtained. In addition, information about chronic or recurrent diseases (such as lichen planus or herpes labialis) should be listed.

The medical PH essentially consists of a listing of previously known and established medical facts. The primary purpose for obtaining this information from a dental patient is to avoid complications during treatment. The importance of obtaining a medical PH cannot be overemphasized, since it serves to protect the patient. This history should identify any past or current medical problems (which fall in the PH category) that may require a change in the type of dental care provided or the manner in which it is provided. A few examples of such problems are drug allergies, previous irradiation for head and neck cancer, and bleeding dyscrasias.

The medical PH also has functions other than protecting the patient. It may serve to establish a relationship between oral disease and past or current systemic problems or medications. A patient's oral disease may represent an oral manifestation of systemic disease or a reaction to medication, and without appropriate information it may pose a diagnostic problem. The history also serves to alert the dentist and staff to infectious disease that the patient may have. Of these, the most notable is hepatitis B, a disease of serious consequence that can be passed from patient to dentist. Whenever a patient is identified as being hepatitis B_sAg positive, protective precautions must be taken. This, of course, should be true for a patient with any contagious disease.

Generally in a medical PH information pertaining to all major illnesses and injuries, especially those requiring medical attention or hospitalization, is obtained and recorded. The following are the general areas of inquiry.

Childhood diseases
Major illnesses
Previous hospital admissions
Operations
Pregnancies
Accidents and injuries
Allergies and immunizations
Current medications

For the dental patient an exhaustive inquiry into the medical PH is not essential, but the inquiry should be selective. The past and current systemic diseases that are of greatest concern to the dentist are those that place a patient at risk while receiving dental care. For most patients this involves cardiovascular problems, such as hypertension, angina pectoris, and rheumatic heart disease. There are numerous other diseases that are also of concern, but they are encountered less frequently.

A series of questions can be used to obtain information about previous episodes of illness. Specific questions are usually directed toward the more common and serious problems. Rather general and open-ended questions are used to identify less common problems. The following are types of questions that are used.

Have you had any serious illness or been hospitalized?

Have you had rheumatic fever or rheumatic heart disease?

Do you have or have you had a heart murmur (leaky valve)?

Have you been told that your blood pressure is too high?

Have you had hepatitis?

Have you been treated for a seizure disorder (convulsions or epilepsy)?

Have you had a tumor or disease that required x-ray, radium, or cobalt treatments?

Have you had excessive or prolonged bleeding following a cut, tooth extraction, or other injury?

Have you had an allergic or other unusual reaction to any drugs or medications (such as penicillin, codeine, or aspirin)?

Do you have any allergies?

Are you currently taking any drugs or medications (such as antibiotics, blood thinners, cortisone, or tranquilizers)?

Are you currently under the care of a physician (MD, DO)?

Approximately how long has it been since you were last seen by a physician?

Do you have any disease, condition, or problem not listed above?

A limited number of questions should be sufficient to obtain the necessary information. When there are serious problems, patients are usually prepared and willing to provide the necessary details. If some responses to questions are vague or equivocal, then a consultation with the patient's physician should be considered.

The *review of systems* (ROS) attempts to identify all current and pertinent past symptoms that may have been overlooked by the patient or dentist while obtaining the history. It has a twofold purpose. The review, through questions, is intended to detect other evidence of disease in the body that may be related to the CC. At the same time it also serves as a health-screening technique and is used to detect evidence of other unrelated but coincidental disease that the patient may have.

The ROS (or systems review) is conducted by asking the patient selected questions about symptoms of common problems. The pattern or sequence of questions is somewhat arbitrary, but usually follows an anatomic order.

The ROS for a medical history usually begins with some general questions and then covers the following areas and organ systems: skin, head, eyes, ears, nose, mouth, throat and neck, breasts, respiratory, cardiovascular, gastrointestinal, genitourinary, gynecologic-obstetric, musculoskeletal, neuropsychiatric, hematologic, and endocrine systems. A wide range of questions can be asked while reviewing each system, though usually the questions are limited to the more common symptoms. The following are a few examples of the types of information that are sought during a systems review.

General: Overall state of health, fatigue, unexplained weight changes, fevers, night sweats, frequent infections, exercise tolerance, and ability to carry out everyday activities.

Skin: Eruptions, pruritus (itching), ulcers, color changes, masses, and dryness.

Head: Headache, trauma, and syncope.

Throat and neck: Sore throat, hoarseness, hemoptysis (blood in sputum), dysphagia (difficulty in swallowing), swelling, neck mass, tenderness, and pain or stiffness of the neck.

Respiratory: Cough, hemoptysis, wheezing, shortness of breath at rest or with exertion, orthopnea (need to sit up for easier breathing), and date of last chest x-ray.

Cardiovascular: Chest pain, palpitations, heart murmur, hypertension, peripheral edema, and claudication (lameness or cramplike pains).

With the dental patient the review of systems would be used primarily as a health-screening technique. Generally, only a few inquiries that would identify overt disease are made. These would be questions such as: "Do you get pains in the heart or chest?" "Does climbing one flight of stairs make you tired and require you to stop and rest so that you can catch your breath?" Dentists who conduct a comprehensive evaluation of their patients usually incorporate a rather detailed ROS in the history.

The ROS can be adapted to evaluate the various areas of the stomatognathic system. The oral cavity can be arbitrarily divided for inquiry and examination purposes into the following systems: dental, periodontal, occlusion, soft tissue, and osseous. Inquiry into these areas is useful in identifying previous disease that was resolved without therapy or problems that are intermittent in nature and may not be present during the current examination. The following shows the types of information that might be requested.

Dental: Toothache, sensitivity of teeth to thermal change, and tenderness of teeth.

Periodontal: Bleeding gums, sore gums, shifting teeth, loose teeth, and grinding of teeth.

Occlusal: Sore teeth when chewing, tender or painful areas in the head and neck (muscles), tenderness or pain of temporomandibular joint (TMJ), clicking or crepitus in TMJ, and limitation of opening.

Mucous membranes: Any previous or current evidence of textural change, ulcerations, swelling, or other morphologic change, soreness, or color change.

Osseous: Swelling or soreness of the jaws or supporting areas of the teeth.

Some of the questions overlap and identify different diseases, but are still useful in alerting the dentist to potential problems that the patient may or may not be aware of.

The *family history* (FH) delves into diseases that are inherited or that follow a familial pattern. Moreover, it may also identify possible exposure to communicable diseases that may involve the patient. The following diseases are some examples: diabetes mellitus, hypertension, cancer, hemophilia, obesity, allergic disorders, coronary artery disease, tuberculosis, and mental illness. Information about the patient's mother, father, brothers, and sisters should be listed. Their ages and health status should be recorded, and if any are deceased, the age at death and cause of death should be listed.

Equally important is information in regard to the dental status of parents and siblings. The dentist should find out whether they have extensive caries, periodontal disease, or dentures. This information will provide an insight into the genetic makeup of the patient's dentition and supporting tissues.

The *personal and social history* (P/SH) contains information on the overall makeup of the patient. The dentist should attempt to gain some insight into the habits, occupation, and personality of the patient. According to the nature and extent of dental care required, this information may be important in determining the prognosis. The following are examples of the types of information that should be obtained.

Habits: Diet, regularity of eating, sleep, use of tobacco, alcohol, and other drugs, and frequency of toothbrushing.

Occupation: Nature of work, duration of current employment, and attitude toward work.

Personality: Easygoing, tense, or chronic worrier.

When there is suspicion that a patient has a problem related to psychophysiologic conditions, a careful assessment must be made of the patient's family life, work, financial status, and health status. Obtaining this type of information may be difficult and awkward, and cannot be approached in a casual fashion. It is facilitated by building patient rapport and confidence, which requires care and sensitivity by the clinician. This is essential to obtain meaningful information in these situations.

Physical examination. The physical examination of the patient involves a search for objective evidence of changes in form and function of the various body areas. The techniques of the physical examination and the significance of changes detected during this examination have been discussed in Chapter 3. More detailed information about changes in the various body areas is presented in subsequent chapters.

This section of the record usually consists of a listing of the areas that are routinely examined. It is important that a specific listing be established to ensure that all the areas are examined. Such a listing also helps establish a pattern for the examination, which makes it more consistent and efficient. A typical examination form would list, in addition to the vital signs and general observations, areas such as:

Extraoral: Head, skin, eyes, ears, nose, TMJ, salivary glands, and neck.

Intraoral: Lips, labial and buccal mucosa, palate, tonsils, oropharynx, tongue, floor of the mouth, gingiva, teeth, and occlusion.

These headings can be expanded by subdividing the areas or shortened by combining them. The listing, or headings that are used, will reflect in part the training and interest of the dentist.

While the physical examination is being conducted or shortly after it is completed, notations must be made about each area that was examined. If no abnormality or disease was detected, then an entry indicating that the area was normal or that findings were negative should be made. The dentist can use either the words or their abbreviations. The capital letter N is used for normal or a zero (0) for negative. If there is a positive finding, then a diagnosis should be listed if it is known. If the abnormality or lesion cannot be identified, then it should be described. Nothing is more frustrating than reviewing previous records to determine whether a lesion had been present previously, only to find a heading without an entry. Then the question arises as to whether the area was normal or not examined. Developing good habits can avoid these problems.

Diagnosis. The diagnosis essentially identifies or labels the problem (CC) that prompted a patient to seek care. It is a bringing together of all the pertinent information that was obtained and then recorded in the health record. The process that is involved in establishing a diagnosis has been discussed in Chapter 2.

If other diseases are found during the evaluation of the patient, the diagnoses of these should also be listed. The diagnosis relating to the CC should always be listed first, and then the others should be listed in order of their severity.

Treatment plan. *Management plan* and *disposition* are other terms used to identify this section. The type of information contained here varies according to how definitively the diagnosis is established. In those situations where a specific diagnosis cannot be established, this section lists the plan of study proposed to develop a final diagnosis. It indicates the various tests and observations that are planned to exclude or verify certain diseases. The less complex and more definitive studies are listed first so that unnecessary procedures can be avoided.

If a final diagnosis has been established, then the treatment plan indicates the nature and sequence of treatment that is considered most appropriate. If there is a question about the patient's response to treatment, an entry as to the prognosis should be made at this time.

A treatment plan must contain sufficiently detailed information so that any clinician who reads the health record can provide the patient with appropriate therapy. A sequence should be established so that the most urgent problems are treated at the onset and then the others in a logical and appropriate fashion.

In providing dental care, the treatment sequence can be extremely important. Inappropriate and inefficient treatment may be rendered unless the plan is carefully structured. The sequencing of care must be based on the desired final outcome and must logically progress from one aspect of treatment to another. The dentist must always keep in mind the various interrelationships that might exist. The sequencing of care should also consider the most effective use of both the patient's and the dentist's time. The following is a general list of a treatment sequence that is frequently used as a basis for developing a treatment plan.

Emergency care
Surgical procedures
Periodontal treatment
Endodontic treatment
Restorative dentistry
Orthodontic care
Fixed partial prosthesis
Partial or complete removable prosthesis

Before any dental treatment is undertaken, it is essential to determine whether a patient has any systemic disease (such as rheumatic heart disease) or is taking any medication (such as anticoagulants) that might modify the treatment plan or require specific precautions. Any special information that relates to treatment should be indicated in the treatment plan. When patients require prophylactic antibiotics or premedication for certain problems, this information must be clearly indicated in the treatment plan. It may be wise to have a method of flagging such records to prevent overlooking such information.

The treatment plan should be a dynamic program that is frequently reviewed for its appropriateness. If new information is obtained, the treatment plan must be reviewed to determine whether it should be modified in the light of this new information. The management of a patient's problem should never become static or perfunctory.

Progress notes

The progress notes essentially constitute a chronicle of the patient's treatment and health status during the course of treatment. If there is a diagnostic problem at the onset, the progress notes should detail the diagnostic procedures that were undertaken and contain the interpretation of their results.

During the treatment period, entries must be made in the progress notes recording the therapeutic measures and results for each visit. They should be brief but sufficiently detailed to document what happened. When some procedure is performed, the following types of information should be included.

Premedication, drug and dose
Anesthetic agent, type and quantity
Description of procedure performed
Complications, if any
Postoperative medication, drug and
   dose
Postoperative instructions
Date of next appointment

If an appointment relates to a follow-up visit to assess the progress of treatment, then entries should be made indicating both the subjective and objective changes. Any changes in treatment should also be noted.

While patient care is being provided, new information may become apparent that changes the diagnosis or the appropriateness of treatment. Also, new problems may occur in addition to those being treated. All this information is usually placed in the progress notes.

Each entry in the progress notes must be dated and signed. When treatment is completed, or if (for some reason) it is terminated before being completed, a discharge summary that indicates the patient's current status should be entered in the progress notes. This summary should list the treatment that was provided, the treatment that is still necessary, and the patient's response to treatment.

Consultation

Consulting with colleagues about patient problems and their management can be an important and at times an indispensable aspect of health care. These consultations may occur during a casual conversation or as a formal request for information. Whenever a consultation provides the basis for a diagnosis or treatment, this information should be included in the patient's record. Chapter 19 explains the reasons for requesting a consultation and describes the format that should be used.

Laboratory reports

Most record systems are structured so that there is a separate division for laboratory reports. When laboratory studies and diagnostic procedures are not a significant or major portion of patient management, this segment may be omitted or combined with another segment, such as the progress notes. Irrespective of the record structure, whenever any diagnostic studies are ordered, a note indicating this fact must be made in the patient's record. This note may be a part of the diagnostic plan or an entry in the progress notes.

In most instances the results of these studies are reported on a form that lists the study or procedure requested, the results, and (if appropriate) the normal values. These reports should be attached to the health record. In addition an entry must be made in the record, usually in the progress notes, indicating the results

of the laboratory study. If the report is an oral communication, then it is essential that the results be listed in the record as completely as possible. At times it may also be appropriate to comment on the significance of the results as it pertains to the diagnosis.

. Unless a careful inventory of the studies requested and their results are maintained, important information may be overlooked. This could also contribute to the ordering of additional, needless studies or the repetition of those already completed. Chapter 18 deals with the general concepts of laboratory studies and provides some details about the more routine studies.

METHODS OF OBTAINING INFORMATION

Information for the health record is obtained through interrogation of the patient. This may be accomplished in one of two ways: a patient interview or a questionnaire. Since each technique has its advantages and disadvantages, the best method is probably a combination of both.

The traditional technique has been the patient interview, in which the clinician obtains all the necessary information by a series of questions that follow a somewhat structured format. This allows a degree of freedom so that certain segments of the history can be expanded and others considered in less detail, according to their significance. Using the interview technique, the clinician usually develops a better rapport with the patient, which tends to lead to a more open discussion and a more complete exchange of information.

The use of a questionnaire has a more impersonal aspect and is somewhat limiting in the type of information that is acquired. It is a time-saving device in that large quantities of information can be obtained without requiring the clinician to be present while the patient considers the questions and lists the responses. The clinician can review the completed questionnaire and then confine the interview to the positive responses that require additional information. The validity of this technique is in large part contingent on the patient's ability to understand and interpret the questions correctly. If there is any doubt as to the patient's ability to respond to a questionnaire, the clinician or staff must assist the patient in completion of the form.

Though there are some disadvantages with the questionnaire technique, its application on a limited basis is useful in a dental office. Some studies in the techniques of history taking suggest that information obtained by questionnaires is more complete, more accurate, and recorded in a fashion that makes it more readily available for retrieval at a later date.[3,4] Much of the information that is of significance or interest in sections such as past history, review of systems, family history, and personal and social history is limited and can usually be obtained by the use of a questionnaire. The questionnaire is structured so that it delves only into the more pertinent areas and provides the type of information that is considered most critical. When there are positive responses in the pertinent areas, more detailed information is developed by patient interview.

The chief complaint and present illness sections contain a less stereotyped form of information that can be elicited only by a patient interview. Information relating to these sections covers a wide range of possibilities and is quite variable. It cannot be acquired by the use of questionnaires or standard forms because of their limitations. Pertinent and detailed information can be obtained only through the interview technique, which allows for a more explicit characterization of the information. The techniques used for information acquisition should be adapted to best suit the needs of the patient, clinician, and health care facility.

PROBLEM-ORIENTED RECORD

A modified system for organizing the health record, which is referred to as the problem-oriented record, has been proposed by Weed.[5] Though this system has essentially the same components as the traditional record system, it is structured in a fashion that facilitates the review of information. This system is purportedly responsible for improved patient care, better medical education, and an improved system for peer review. It is based on the concept that the patient's problems serve as an index for the record. Each problem is numbered, and then all plans and actions that are taken to resolve these problems are indexed by the same number that is assigned to the problem. Theoretically this system allows for a more rapid and complete review of all information pertaining to any one problem. The problem-oriented record has four major components: (1) the data base, (2) the problem list, (3) the plans, and (4) the progress notes.

The data base includes all the information that is currently available about the patient. This includes information such as the biographic data, chief complaint (problem) and other segments of the history, the physical examination, and the results from all laboratory studies and diagnostic procedures that have been conducted up to the present time. Though there are some general guidelines for the type of information that should be included in the data base, they have not been standardized. Generally it is assumed that the data base will be somewhat incomplete at the onset. As the clinician proceeds after the acquisition of the initial data base, new information will become available and be added to the data base. The data base should not be considered an isolated or static segment of the record, but one that is changing as more information becomes available.

The problem list serves as the basis of the record and is a listing of the concerns or reasons that prompted a patient to seek health care. These problems may be physical, psychologic, or social. The problem list may also include items that were not identified by the patient, but by the clinician. They would represent matters of concern to the clinician that were identified during the acquisition of the data base.

The clinician should be as specific as possible in identifying the problems and enter them in the record at the level of his or her understanding. The problem list usually includes signs and symptoms of disease and may include abnormal results of laboratory studies or diagnostic procedures. Occasionally some of the problems may be interrelated and in fact represent the signs and symptoms of one specific disease. When this becomes apparent, these interrelated problems are consolidated into one problem. There are also times when a diagnosis may be listed as a specific problem. The problem list essentially becomes an index or a table of contents and provides the basis for further action.

After a problem list is formulated, plans are developed for resolving the problems. Each problem has its own plan, which is indexed by the same number that refers to the problem. According to the nature of the problem, plans will fall into three general categories: diagnosis, therapy, and patient education. If the problem requires further study to develop a diagnosis, the plan lists the various diagnostic procedures that will be undertaken to establish a diagnosis. If a problem is listed as a diagnosis, then the plan details the therapeutic procedures or medications that will be used to manage the problem. The plan should also outline the action that will be taken to inform the patient about the disease and the way the patient will participate in the management of the disease. As can be seen, the plans provide an outline of the overall course of action that will be taken in managing the problems that have been identified at the onset.

The progress notes list the actions that are taken in implementing the plans. They include orders for diagnostic or therapeutic procedures, consultations, and additional information that might be obtained through subsequent histories and physical examinations. The accumulation of this new information leads to a new data base, which may modify the initial data base and require a reevaluation of the problem or its treatment.

The progress notes are dated, and each entry is identified with the problem title and number to facilitate its location and review. When appropriate, information should be entered in the progress notes using a SOAP format.

S: Subjective
O: Objective
A: Assessment
P: Plan

The S portion lists information that pertains to the patient's own perception of the problem and the progress that is being made in either diagnosis or therapy. It may include new symptoms that the patient has recently noted. The O portion lists the objective information that the clinician may identify during the examination. This may comprise new signs that become apparent or new laboratory data. The A portion lists the clinician's assessment of the patient's current situation according to the new information that has been obtained. This may pertain to diagnostic considerations or to the patient's response to therapy. The P portion of the progress notes lists any procedures that were performed at the appointment or indicates future plans, which may be either new plans or modifications of old ones. As problems are resolved, summary statements must be entered in the progress notes indicating the resolutions of the problems and the current status of the patient.

The problem-oriented record has stirred considerable controversy since its inception. Generally it is accepted as an improvement over the traditional form of record system. It is being used in many health care programs, but frequently modified from the form in which it was originally proposed. To a limited degree it has also been applied to the practice of dentistry, though with much less success and acceptance.[1,2] Since the practice of dentistry is confronted more with therapeutic than with diagnostic problems, the problem-oriented record has less practical application.

It is apparent that the health record is an important and integral part of providing health care. Without complete and accurate records, this care can be compromised and in fact be totally inappropriate. Good records reflect good habits and almost invariably represent an accurate measure of the type of health care that is provided by the clinician.

REFERENCES

1. Calhoun, N.R.: The problem-oriented health record system in dentistry, J. Oral Surg. **31:**756, 1973.
2. Ingber, J.S., and Rose, L.F.: The problem-oriented record: clinical application in a teaching hospital, J. Dent. Educ. **39:**472, 1975.
3. Gumpel, J.M., and Mason, A.M.S.: Self-administered clinical questionnaire for outpatients, Br. Med. J. **2:**209, 1974.
4. Simborg, D.W., Rikli, A.E., and Hall, P.: Experimentation in medical history-taking, J.A.M.A. **210:**1443, 1969.
5. Weed, L.L.: Medical records that guide and teach, N. Engl. J. Med. **278:**593, 652, 1968.

BIBLIOGRAPHY

Kerr, D.A., Ash, M.M., and Millard, H.D.: Oral diagnosis, ed. 5, St. Louis, 1978, The C.V. Mosby Co.
Malasanos, L., and others: Health assessment, St. Louis, 1977, The C.V. Mosby Co.
Sherman, J.L., Jr., and Fields, S.K.: Guide to patient evaluation, ed. 3, Flushing, N.Y., 1978, Medical Examination Publishing Co., Inc.

5 Patient interviewing and psychologic assessment

Patient interviewing and psychologic assessment are two subjects whose mastery enables the dentist to truly "know" the dental patient. Good interviewing skills enable the practitioner to efficiently gather all available information regarding the patient's problem. A good psychologic assessment aids in patient management, is central to the development of good communication and motivation strategies, and gives insight into any possible emotional components of the patient's problem. The purpose of this chapter is threefold: (1) to discuss patient interviewing techniques, (2) to provide an efficient method for the psychologic assessment of dental patients, and (3) to examine mental disorders that may affect diagnosis and treatment of dental patients.

PATIENT INTERVIEWING

Patient interviewing may be defined as an exchange of information between dentist and patient regarding a patient's health. This exchange of information enables the practitioner to acquire information necessary for diagnosis and treatment, to convey information to the patient concerning treatment, and to motivate the patient toward a philosophy of disease prevention. For purposes of discussion the interview will be divided into three parts: (1) preparation and initiation of the interview, (2) obtaining information, and (3) closing the interview.

Preparation and initiation of the interview

Before the interview is begun it is important to establish definite interview goals and to review any information available concerning the patient. These steps will help ensure a smooth and efficient interview. There are an abundance of goals appropriate for a patient interview. Generally, most goals will fall into one of two categories: goals relating to the acquisition of information and goals relating to the communication of information.

For example, if a patient appears with acute pain, interview goals would include obtaining a chief complaint, information regarding the present illness, and a past medical history (acquisition of information). On the other hand, if the patient came in for a checkup, goals would include all those listed above plus some assessment of the patient's attitude toward dentistry and oral health. In addition, the dentist may want to communicate his or her philosophies toward prevention and policies regarding fees and payments (communication of information). In either event, the interview will be more efficient if goals are planned in advance.

Before the interview it is also important to carefully review any information concerning the patient. If the patient is new, review the biographic data and medical history before entering the interview room. Was the patient referred? If so, by whom? For previous patients, make a mental note of when the patient was last seen and what treatment was provided. It is also wise to make a brief note on the patient's record about interests and hobbies. This information provides personalized material for discussion with the patient and will communicate respect for his or her individuality.

A dentist's private office or special interview room is the best place to conduct a routine interview. This room should be quiet and free of potentially anxiety-evoking dental stimuli, such as handpieces and casts. Both the patient and dentist should be seated in chairs of similar size, with the patient seated slightly to one side of the dentist at a distance of approximately $2\frac{1}{2}$ to 4 feet. Closer distances may make the patient uncomfortable, and greater distances may create an impersonal atmosphere. Seating the patient slightly to the side of the dentist prevents a potential face-to-face confrontation. If a desk is used, the patient should be seated at one end of it rather than directly opposite the dentist. This will prevent the desk from forming a barrier. In addition, communicating directly across a large desk may create an overly formal and authoritarian atmosphere.

Interruptions should be kept to a minimum, as they communicate nonverbally to the patient that his or her problem is relatively unimportant.

Routine interviews conducted in the operatory may save time; however, this environment may not be conducive to effective communication. This is because the operatory contains stimuli that may evoke anxiety in many patients (for example, syringe, handpiece, or dental chair). Furthermore, the operatory may also create an authoritarian atmosphere by having the dentist sitting and looking down on the patient.

Interviews with emergency patients, on the other hand, may be conducted in the operatory, for two reasons. First, an interview conducted in the operatory communicates to the patient nonverbally that something is being done as quickly as possible. Second, when emergency patients are being treated time is often limited, and conducting the interview in the operatory saves time. In short, in emergency situations the advantages outlined above may outweigh the disadvantages of creating anxiety and an authoritarian atmosphere.

A good beginning is vital to the success of an interview because it sets the mood for the balance of the dialogue. A good beginning may be achieved through a warm, friendly introduction or greeting and positive nonverbal communication. An interview with a new patient should begin with a cordial introduction, such as "Mr. Smith, I am Dr. Black." After the introduction, you may want to be a little less formal. This may be accomplished in the following manner : "May I call you Joe?" or "Do you care if I call you Mary?" Interviews with previous patients should begin with a cordial greeting, such as "Good morning, Mrs. Johnson; how was your vacation in Michigan?" Positive nonverbal communication may be accomplished by a friendly handshake and by looking directly at the patient.

Obtaining information

Information may be obtained in the patient interview through direct questioning and facilitation of patient dialogue.

Three types of questions are especially useful in patient interviewing. The first may be referred to as the open-ended question,[9] which solicits information of a broad, general nature and is useful in obtaining relatively large amounts of information. It is ordinarily not an efficient method for obtaining specific details. The following are several examples of open-ended questions:

Dentist: "What can we do for you today?"
Dentist: "Tell me about the pain in your tooth."
Dentist: "What is it about your front teeth that doesn't look good?"

These examples illustrate the potential of the open-ended question for gathering information. This fact makes the open-ended question a useful tool for initiating an interview or topic, since this type of question provides an ample base of information, which then may be pursued in detail.

The second type of question may be referred to as the "laundry-list" question.[9] This question supplies the patient with a list of potential answers. The laundry-list question is more specific than the open-ended question but still offers the patient some freedom in answering. For example:

Dentist: "Would you describe your pain as crushing, stabbing, drawing, or throbbing?"

When using the laundry-list question, the dentist must avoid suggesting the answer.[9] This may be accomplished by not placing the potential responses in any logical sequence and by making certain that the potential responses provide a range that exceeds what the patient might be expected to answer.[9] For instance:

Dentist: "Does the pain last for an hour, a day, a few seconds, or a minute?"

The laundry-list question is often beneficial in clarifying a response to an open-ended question:

Dentist: "How have you been getting along with that new crown?" (Open-ended question.)

Patient: "It hurts sometimes."

Dentist: "Does it hurt when you chew, when you eat something hot, when you eat something cold, or just for no reason at all?" (Laundry-list question.)

Patient: "It hurts for only a few seconds when I drink something cold."

The third type of question useful in patient interviewing is the direct question.[9] This question solicits a specific response, usually in a sentence or less. The following are examples of direct questions:

Dentist: "How often do these muscles feel sore?"

Dentist: "What type of toothbrush are you using?"

Dentist: "What does your blood pressure usually run?"

The direct question is usually most productive when it is preceded by an open-ended or laundry-list question:

Dentist: "Would you describe your pain as crushing, stabbing, drawing, or throbbing?" *(Laundry-list question.)*

Patient: "Kind of a dull throbbing."

Dentist: "Can you point to the tooth that hurts?" *(Direct question.)*

Patient: "I really can't tell, but it's one of these upper ones."

Dentist: "Do you have frequent sinus problems?" *(Direct question.)*

Patient: "Yes."

Direct questions that may be answered with "yes" or "no" should be used with care. Yes-or-no questions make it easy for the patient to answer in a manner just to please you or avoid further discussion.[9] Frequently, yes-or-no questions may be reworded to provide more information.[9] Consider the following examples:

Dentist: "Did you like that new toothbrush I gave you?"

Dentist: "Have you had trouble with your immediate denture?"

These questions would be more productive if stated in the following manner:

Dentist: "What about that new toothbrush I gave you?"

Dentist: "How have you been getting along with your immediate denture?'

Questions that anger, offend, insult, accuse, pass judgment, or ask the patient to justify his or her behavior should be avoided. Examples of this type of question include:

Dentist: "Why aren't you brushing the way I showed you?"

Dentist: "Did you take your penicillin as I instructed?"

Dentist: "Why did you wait so long to come in?"

Dentist: "You haven't been flossing, have you?"

Dentist: "Why did you let your teeth get in such bad shape?"

Questions such as these will certainly decrease the amount of dialogue and may compel a patient to give false information.

In summary, the open-ended question solicits a large amount of general information and is particularly useful in beginning an interview or topic. The laundry-list question offers the patient a list of potential answers and is beneficial in clarifying an open-ended question. A direct question focuses on small, specific pieces of information and functions primarily to clarify both open-ended and laundry-list questions.

In addition to direct questioning, information may be obtained through facilitation of the patient's dialogue—that is, by encouraging the patient to fully express his or her ideas, give thorough answers to your questions and not feel afraid to express himself or herself in an honest, open manner. There are five techniques that will facilitate patient dialogue: empathy, respect, reflection, interpretation, and silence.

The term *empathy* refers to the ability to accurately understand the patient's feelings and ideas. Empathy involves perceiving the patient's intellectual and emotional frame of reference—how do things look through

the patient's eyes?[3,5] Moreover, empathy involves being able to convincingly communicate this understanding.[3,5] Perhaps a few examples will help clarify this process.

Patient: "I'm sorry I'm late. I had to take Tim to the doctor today. He has been having a lot of trouble with his new contact lenses. Then the dog got sick and I had to make sure he didn't throw up on the new carpet. Well, anyway I'm sorry I'm late."

Dentist: "Everything is happening all at once today and you're in a real frenzy."

Patient: "I've been to at least three dentists and spent over $3500 in all these crowns and still my teeth keep rotting away and getting abscessed."

Dentist: "Saving your teeth seems like a futile effort."

Properly done, empathy will greatly increase rapport, encourage open expression, and facilitate trust.[3,5]

In order to make good empathic responses you must listen actively—that is, concentrate on what the patient is trying to say both verbally and nonverbally. Sometimes it is helpful to focus almost entirely on the nonverbal aspect of the patient's statement.[3,5]

Patient: (Cracking knuckles and talking fast.) "It sure is hot in here. Is this going to take long? Where is your assistant today?"

Dentist: "The thought of getting those sutures out makes you a little nervous, doesn't it?"

You also should keep your language at a level the patient can readily understand.[3,5] Furthermore, when you are trying to communicate empathically, it is helpful to make your responses with the same feeling as the patient's statement.[3,5] For example, if the patient is sad, then your response should be somewhat sad; if the patient is happy, your response should be happy.

Patient: (Talking softly and looking at the floor.) "You know, bad luck seems to come in groups of three.

First the car had to have new brakes. Then the water heater started to leak. That was a quick 200 bucks. Now this damn tooth breaks off.''

Dentist: (Responding in a relatively soft, slow manner.) ''Hardly seems fair, does it?''

Respect refers to a way of viewing the patient and is closely related to empathy.[3,5] Essentially, respect means that you regard each patient as a unique individual.[3,5] Respect is generally communicated not in words but by the way you work with the patient.[3,5]

Carkuff[3] and Egan[5] have offered several suggestions for communicating respect. First, demonstrate a willingness to work with the patient, and assume that the patient is willing to work with you. Second, regard each patient as a unique individual. Third, try to avoid critical judgments regarding the patient. This is especially important at the beginning of the interview. Fourth, and probably the best way to communicate respect, is empathy. Fifth, be sure to give the patient the opportunity to communicate information that will elicit praise from you. Finally, respect will be conveyed if you communicate in a genuine, spontaneous manner. Following are examples of responses that communicate respect.

Patient: ''I realize that fixed bridges would be better, doctor, but I just can't swing it now.''
Dentist: ''I can certainly understand where $4100 would be a great financial burden for you to manage at this time. Let's explore the alternatives.''
Patient: ''Well, how did I do with the injection this time?''
Dentist: ''Marvelous!''
Patient: ''I really am ashamed that I haven't taken better care of my teeth, but I'm ready to work now.''
Dentist: ''That's great. The important thing now is your willingness to work.''

Respect has essentially the same functions as empathy—facilitation of rapport, open expression, and trust.[3,5]

A *reflection* is a response that restates or repeats a segment of the patient's statement.[9] For example:

Patient: ''These dentures don't fit right.''
Dentist: ''Don't fit right?''
Patient: ''I'm not sure about that bridge.''
Dentist: ''Not sure?''

Reflection encourages the patient to continue communicating.[9] In reality, reflection is a subtle way of asking a question; however, it is generally less intimidating than asking a direct question.

An *interpretation* is an explanation of the patient's statement developed from your inferences.[9] The following is an example of how an interpretation might be used to facilitate patient dialogue:

Patient: ''Last week, when my mother-in-law was staying with us, the pain in my joints was really bad.''
Dentist: ''Sounds like your mother-in-law's visit was stressful and caused you to grind your teeth a lot.''

It should be noted that an interpretation may stimulate dialogue by compelling the patient to agree or disagree with your statement. An interpretation need not be correct in order to stimulate dialogue.

Patient: ''Doctor, this upper plate just isn't quite right.''
Dentist: ''You think those teeth might be just a little too yellow?''
Patient: ''No, it's the way this little tooth on the side overlaps this front one.''

Silence may often facilitate dialogue by stimulating the patient to break the silence with verbalization.[9] When silence is used to facilitate dialogue, it is important to communicate interest nonverbally.[9] This may be accomplished by nodding ''yes,'' shifting or moving toward the patient, and maintaining eye contact.[9] Looking away or moving back from the patient during a silent period might be inter-

preted as lack of interest.[9] Following are two examples illustrating the use of silence.

Patient: ''I really don't know what we are going to do with this partial.''
Dentist: (Silence, nodding ''yes'' and leaning forward.)
Patient: ''I mean about the color of these front teeth.''
Patient: ''I don't like this new filling you did.''
Dentist: (Silence, nodding ''yes'' and leaning forward.)
Patient: ''It looks too white.''

Closing the interview

There are two procedures that should take place during the close of an interview: a summarization and an explanation. A brief summary is an efficient way to make certain that you accurately understand what the patient has told you. At the end of the summary the patient should be given an opportunity to correct any misunderstandings or ask questions.

Dentist: ''Let me see if I understand this correctly. You first noticed this pain about 2 months ago. At that time it was triggered by cold foods and seldom lasted any longer than a few minutes. Then in the past week or so it began to ache spontaneously, and now it throbs constantly. Do I have an accurate picture?''

The closing should also contain an explanation of what will happen next; or, if the closing takes place at the end of an appointment, what the patient should expect between appointments and what will take place at the next appointment.

Dentist: ''As I said earlier, Mr. Jones, the pain in your jaws appears to be caused by muscle spasm. When you come back next Thursday I'll have your bite plane ready. In the meantime I want you to relax your jaw as much as possible, apply the moist heat like I showed you, and take the muscle relaxant that I prescribed. Do you have any questions?''

Summary

To summarize, there are several points to consider when conducting the patient interview. First, be well prepared for the interview by establishing definite goals and reviewing all available patient information. Second, a routine interview should take place in a private office or interview room, whereas emergency interviews are most efficiently completed in the operatory. Third, a good beginning is essential and may be achieved by a warm, friendly introduction and positive nonverbal communication. Fourth, information may be obtained through direct questioning or facilitation of patient dialogue. The three types of questions discussed were the open-ended question, which is useful for gathering relatively large quantities of general information; the direct question, which is advantageous in collecting small pieces of specific information; and the laundry-list question, which falls somewhere between the other two. Empathy, respect, reflection, interpretation, and silence are five methods helpful in facilitating patient dialogue. Finally, an explanation and a summarization should take place at the close of an interview.

PSYCHOLOGIC ASSESSMENT

Psychologic assessment is important to the dentist for at least three reasons. First, a good psychologic assessment provides insight into any possible emotional components of the patient's dental problem. This is especially important when assessing pain. Second, understanding the patient's psychologic state is useful in patient management. Finally, psychologic assessment is fundamental to developing good communication and motivation strategies.

The purposes of this section are to illustrate how the dentist may easily integrate an abbreviated psychologic assessment into the patient interview and dental-medical history and to discuss mental disorders that relate directly to dental care.

The American Psychiatric Association classifies mental disorders according to a "multi-axial" system.[1] This system consists of five axes or categories. Usually a patient will receive a diagnosis or assessment along each axis.[1] An outline of this system may be found in Table 2.

Interview and psychologic tests

The interview and psychologic tests are the two primary methods psychiatrists use to assess the psychologic state.[7] The interview may be divided into the psychiatric history and the mental status examination. The psychiatric history resembles the standard medical history in that it contains a chief complaint, present illness and past history.[7] However, a much greater emphasis is placed on the emotional, mental, and behavioral aspects of each of these entries.[7] For example, the personal history is considered in much greater detail and is usually divided into three parts: early childhood (birth to age 10), later childhood (puberty through adolescence), and adulthood.[7] In addition, entries such as medical history and current social situation may be included.[7]

The mental status examination serves as a record of the current findings and includes a description of the patient's appearance, mood, thought processes, intelligence, and other factors.[7]

Since a great many psychologic tests are standardized, they afford some degree of objectivity in diagnosis and evaluation of mental or personality disorders.[7] Objectivity is

Table 2. American Psychiatric Association classification system DSM-III

Axis I: Clinical syndromes
    Disorders usually first evident in infancy, childhood, or adolescence
    Organic mental disorders
    Substance use disorders
    Schizophrenic disorders
    Paranoid disorders
    Psychotic disorders not elsewhere classified
    Affective disorders
    Anxiety disorders
    Somatoform disorders
    Dissociative disorders
    Psychosexual disorders
    Factitious disorders
    Disorders of impulse control not elsewhere classified
    Adjustment disorder
    Psychological factors affecting physical condition
Axis II: Personality disorders
    Paranoid
    Schizoid
    Schizotypal
    Histrionic
    Narcissistic
    Antisocial
    Borderline
    Avoidant
    Dependent
    Compulsive
    Passive-aggressive
    Atypical, mixed, or other personality disorder
Axis III: Physical disorders and conditions
Axis IV: Severity of psychosocial stressors
Axis V: Highest level of adaptive functioning past year

From American Psychiatric Association: Diagnostic and statistical manual of mental disorders, ed. 3, Washington, D.C., 1980, The Association.

achieved by allowing the psychiatrist to compare the patient's behavior on a particular test with that of a large reference group.[7] The Minnesota Multiphasic Personality Inventory (MMPI) is an example of such a test. Psychologic tests may be classified according to the variable measured, such as intelligence or personality (Wechsler Adult Intelligence Scale and Rorschach, or ink-blot, test); according to the method of responding, such as the objective test in which the questions have obvious meanings (MMPI); or according to the projective test in which the questions are not obvious and the patient must project his or her own needs into the answer (Thematic Apperception Test).

It is not the intention of this section to suggest that every dentist conduct an elaborate psychologic assessment on every patient. This would obviously be impractical and beyond the abilities of most dentists. However, with a little extra effort it is possible to effectively integrate an abbreviated version of the psychiatric history and mental status examination into the patient interview and dental-medical history.

It would obviously be awkward for a dentist to pursue in any great detail the emotional, mental, or behavioral aspects of the patient's history. Nevertheless, with little modification, the dental-medical history may often reveal a great deal about the patient's psychologic state.

To begin, the dental-medical history should ask specifically if the patient has suffered any psychologic, psychiatric, or mental difficulties. A history of mental difficulties may not appear in response to an inquiry regarding major illnesses or hospitalization for two reasons. First, the patient may assume you are asking about, or are only interested in, physical disease. Second, many people believe there is a stigma associated with psychologic or psychiatric problems and do not wish to acknowledge a positive history. At times they may use such

terms as "nervous breakdown." If a positive history is encountered, record the date of occurrence, duration, diagnosis, and any medication the patient is taking.

The dental-medical history should also be designed to reveal any history of diseases that are a result of psychologic factors (psychophysiologic or psychosomatic diseases). Examples of such diseases include peptic ulcer, asthma, muscle-tension headaches, migraine headaches, ulcerative colitis, essential hypertension, and rheumatoid arthritis.[1] Inquiries regarding diseases that are the result of psychologic factors may be asked as a single question ("Have you ever had a peptic ulcer?") or each disease may be placed in its appropriate area of the history (for example, peptic ulcer under gastorintestinal system and asthma under respiratory system). A positive history of psychophysiologic disease indicates that emotional factors may play a significant role in the patient's disease processes.

Finally, the section of the dental-medical history containing a list of the patient's current medications may indicate the presence of a mental disorder. Mental disorders are treated with several categories of medications: major tranquilizers (antipsychotic drugs), antidepressant drugs, minor tranquilizers, antianxiety agents, sedatives, and hypnotics. Examples of these medications are listed in Table 3.

Generally, major tranquilizers are used to treat psychotic symptoms, whereas minor tranquilizers are used to reduce anxiety in patients with affective disorders (variations in mood), anxiety disorders, somatoform disorders (the presence of physical symptoms without organic cause) and dissociative disorders (confusion or loss of memory). Antidepressant drugs are, of course, used to treat depression. If a patient is taking one of these medications, an entry should be made regarding the reason and the length of time.

As stated previously, the mental status examination serves as a record of current psychologic findings. During the patient interview it is often possible for the practitioner to conduct an abbreviated mental status examination. In fact, most dentists do this without realizing it.

Several factors are usually evaluated in the medical status examination. Each factor and some suggestions for evaluation are listed below.[6,7]

1. Appearance: What are the patient's facial expression, mannerisms, eye contact, posture, type of clothing, and grooming?
2. Speech: Does the patient exhibit a fast or slow rate of speech? What about the flow of speech? Are there frequent interruptions? Is the volume loud or soft? Does he or she have difficulty finding the correct word?

Table 3. Examples of psychoactive medications

Major tranquilizers (antipsychotic drugs)	Antidepressants	Minor tranquilizers, antianxiety agents, sedatives, and hypnotics
Chlorpromazine (Thorazine)	*Tricyclic*	Meprobamate (Miltown)
Triflupromazine hydrochloride (Vesprin)	Imipramine (Tofranil)	Chlordiazepoxide (Librium)
Promazine hydrochloride (Sparine)	Desipramine (Norpramin)	Diazepam (Valium)
	Amitriptyline (Elavil)	Hydroxyzine (Vistaril)
Prochlorperazine (Compazine)	Nortriptyline (Aventyl)	
Trifluoperazine (Stelazine)	Doxepin (Sinequan)	
Thioridazine (Mellaril)	*Monoamine oxidase inhibitors*	
Haloperidol (Haldol)	Isocarboxazid (Marplan)	
	Phenelzine (Nardil)	
	Tranylcypromine (Parnate)	

3. Motor activity: Does the patient appear agitated, usually still, or switch back and forth? Are there tics or an unusual gait present?
4. Mood: This is sometimes called the patient's affective state. Assess whether the patient feels happy or sad. Does his or her mood vacillate? Is it appropriate for the circumstances?
5. Thought: Is the patient's thinking accelerated or retarded? Are his or her interests realistic, or do they have no basis in reality? Does the patient show evidence of delusions (false beliefs or ideas retained even in the face of contradictory evidence), obsessions (persistent, unwanted thoughts), or phobias (persistent, intense, irrational fears)?
6. Perception: Perceptual variation may occur with regard to the patient himself or herself or to the environment. Illusions (perceptual distortions) and hallucinations (perceiving something that is not there) may occur in any of the senses.
7. Orientation and memory: Can the patient properly orient himself or herself in time and space? Does the patient have difficulty remembering recent and past facts and experiences?
8. Attention and concentration: Does the patient have difficulty concentrating and maintaining attention?
9. Intelligence: A cursory assessment may be made from the patient's ability to reason and from his or her accomplishments, education, and occupation.

Information acquired from the mental status examination is useful in screening for mental disorders of interest to the dentist.

Mental disorders

Mental disorders that may profoundly affect the diagnosis and treatment of dental patients include anxiety disorders, affective disorders, so-matoform disorders, and paranoid disorders.

Anxiety disorders. The most common anxiety disorder encountered in a dental office is the simple phobia. A simple phobia is a persistent, irrational fear of and desire to avoid a particular situation or object.[1] Generally, the patient recognizes that his or her fear is irrational and excessive. One study[8] has estimated that approximately 5% to 9% of the general population avoid dental treatment because of anxiety, and the rate may be as high as 16% among school-age children.[16]

The signs of anxiety are generally easy to recognize and may be grouped into three categories—verbal, behavioral, and physiologic. Verbal signs of anxiety include rapid and voluminous speech, a large number of questions, argumentative words and phrases, frequent use of words that connote compulsion (such as "I had to!" or "You must!") and inappropriately loud or soft speech. Examples of the behavioral signs of anxiety are difficulty in sitting still, trembling or clenched hands, cancelled or broken appointments, and consistent lateness. Physiologic signs of anxiety are the result of sympathetic nervous system stimulation and include rapid respiration and heart rate, perspiration, dry mouth, and dilated pupils.

Affective disorders. A disturbance in mood is the primary characteristic of the affective disorders. This disturbance in mood may take the form of depression, elation, or a combination of the two. Depression is the most important of the affective disorders with respect to dentistry.

Depression has been called the "common cold of psychopathology" and may be defined as an emotional state characterized by feelings of guilt, grief, worthlessness, dejection, and despair. Depression may range from mild disturbances in mood, which are common among normal persons, to neurotic depression that may involve serious symptoms, to psychotic depression with serious distortions of reality and a potential of suicide. The National Institute of Mental Health has estimated that approximately 15% of all adults in this country have symptoms of at least a mild depression in any given year.[2]

It is important that the dentist be able to recognize depression because it has been associated with the following oral-facial pain syndromes: (1) atypical facial pain, (2) myofascial pain-dysfunction syndrome (MPD), and (3) glossopyrosis (burning tongue).[2]

Atypical facial pain is a poorly defined syndrome referring to a heterogeneous cluster of discomforts that localize in the lower half of the head.[13] This syndrome is characterized by a deep, drawing, burning, or boring pain that generally does not reach excruciating proportions or have trigger areas.[12,13] Atypical facial pain usually occurs unilaterally in the area supplied by cranial nerves II, III, V, or IX, but does not always follow the peripheral distribution of these nerves.[12,13] This syndrome is seen more frequently in women.[13]

Though many patients with atypical facial pain are depressed,[12-14] it remains unclear whether atypical facial pain is a cause or a sequela of depression. Evidence supporting depression as a cause of atypical facial pain is based on the observations that patients with atypical facial pain do not have apparent organic cause for their pain, generally have the symptoms of depression, and often obtain relief with antidepression therapy.[12,14] However, it should be emphasized that chronic pain such as that of atypical facial pain could be a precipitating factor of depression.[4]

MPD (Chapter 15) has been defined as a functional disorder of the masticatory system.[4] Symptoms of MPD include chronic, generally unilateral pain of the temporomandibular joint and masseter and temporal muscles; temporomandibular joint noises; and limitation of mandibular movement.[4] MPD, like atypical facial pain, has been implicated as both a sequela and a cause of depression.[4,11] In either case, depression appears to be an important component of the MPD syndrome and may need to be treated specifically in order to eliminate MPD symptoms.[10]

Glossopyrosis is a third oral-facial pain syndrome that has been associated with depression.[15,17] This syndrome, characterized by painful or burning tongue, has been reported as a symptom of depression.[15] It has also been suggested that glossopyrosis may be precipitated by a dental procedure.[15]

In addition to the pain syndromes, depression may create potential difficulties and frustrations in the provision of dental care.[2] For example, a depressed patient is generally less likely to accept elaborate or expensive dental treatment or comply with suggested measures of oral hygiene.[2] Finally, depression may directly or indirectly reduce the rate of salivation.[2]

Many of the signs and symptoms of depression center on self-reports of the patient's emotional state.[2] With mild depressions these may include feelings of disappointment in oneself, lack of self-confidence, and a sense of inadequacy. There may be lowered enthusiasm for life, a distaste for ordinary activities, and sometimes an increased desire to be left alone. The mildly depressed patient will frequently display speech retardation and have difficulty with the elaboration of ideas. In addition, there may be mild distortions of body image as a result of excessive concern with physical appearance. This may become evident with excessive complaints of ''unattractive'' features, such as facial wrinkles and dark teeth. Indecisiveness is also present in mild depressions.

Patients suffering from severe depression may blame all misfortune on their own ineptness and have considerable difficulty making even the simplest of decisions. Furthermore, they may often harbor feelings of self-hate, apathy, and worthlessness. Increased distortions of body image may make the patient feel ugly and repulsive. The severely depressed patient may express suicidal wishes along with feelings of despondency and helplessness.

Even though depression is an affective disorder, physical manifestations may be apparent.[2] These include poor appetite, weight loss, sleep disturbances, and decreased or absent sex drive.

Somatoform disorders. Somatoform disorders are distinguished by the presence of physical symptoms without evidence of organic changes or apparent pathophysiologic mechanisms.[1] These symptoms are not under voluntary control and are believed to be linked to psychologic factors or conflicts.[1] Two somatoform disorders that are discussed briefly here are psychogenic pain disorder and hypochondriasis.

The central feature of the psychogenic pain disorder is severe, prolonged pain for which no organic pathologic or pathophysiologic mechanism may be demonstrated.[1] In addition, it is believed that psychologic factors are involved in the etiology.[1] For example, pain may provide the patient with some type of environmental support or reinforcement (such as special favors from friends and time off work) that otherwise might not be obtainable or permit the patient to avoid some disliked or threatening activity (such as taking an examination). This pain generally arises abruptly, and then increases in severity after a period of several days to weeks.[1] Psychogenic pain may diminish with treatment or elimination of the precipitating psychologic event.[1] However, if the patient receives reinforcement for his or her pain, it may persist for months to years.[1]

Hypochondriasis is an obsessive concern with one's health or body functions when there is no detectable cause for worry. Hypochondriasis is characterized by an increased sensitivity or heightened awareness to irregularities in physical or emotional functioning and a fear or a belief of having a serious disease. Typically, patients suffering from hypochondriasis will appear with a lengthy, detailed medical history and will have visited numerous physicians and dentists.[1] Frequently these patients feel that they are not receiving good medical or dental care.[1]

The hypochondriac dental patient may create several problems. First, since professional reassurance does little to relieve the patient's unrealistic fear of disease,[1] managing hypochondriac patients may become a source of frustration. Second, after numerous ''false alarms,'' the dentist may become complacent and overlook true disease. Last, the dentist might be tempted to perform unnecessary diagnostic procedures or treatment in a misguided effort to help the patient.

Paranoid disorders. Paranoid disorders are characterized by delusions.[1] These delusions may be of persecution, grandeur, or jealousy and are generally well organized and developed in a logical progression.[1] With the exception of the delusional system, the paranoid patient appears normal.[1] There are no hallucinations, emotional responses are appropriate, and social behavior is usually well maintained.

Since the paranoid patient has difficulty trusting people, especially those in an authoritarian role, he or she may feel the dentist is trying to cause harm. Consequently, complications or a poor therapeutic response may be interpreted as an attack, with the end result being a lawsuit. In short, if you suspect that the patient has paranoid tendencies, be certain that there is sound evidence of organic pathosis before initiating treatment.

Summary

In summary, the psychologic assessment is important because it gives insight into any possible emotional components of the patient's problem, is useful in patient management, and is fundamental to developing good communication and motivational strategies. An abbreviated psychologic assessment may be easily done through careful design of the dental-medical history and thoughtful execution of the patient interview. Anxiety disorders, affective disorders, somatoform disorders, and paranoid disorders may all affect the diagnosis and treatment of dental patients. It is important to remember that pain may rise from psychologic factors alone. Consequently, be certain that there is evidence of organic disease before treating patients in pain with irreversible procedures, such as endodontic therapy or extractions.

REFERENCES

1. American Psychiatric Association: Diagnostic and statistical manual of mental disorders, ed. 3, Washington, D.C., 1980, The Association.
2. Beck, F.M., Kaul, T.J., and Weaver, J.M.: Recognition and management of the depressed dental patient, J. Am. Dent. Assoc. **99**:967, 1979.
3. Carkhuff, R.A.: Helping and human relations: a primer for lay and professional helpers, Vol. I, New York, 1969, Holt, Rinehart & Winston, Inc.
4. Dworkin, S.F., Ference, T.P., and Giddon, D.B.: Behavioral science and dental practice, St. Louis, 1978, The C.V. Mosby Co.
5. Egan, G.: The skilled helper: a model for systematic helping and interpersonal relating, Monterey, Calif., 1975, Brooks/Cole Publishing Co.
6. Enelow, A.J., and Swisher, S.N.: Interviewing and patient care, ed. 2, New York, 1979, Oxford University Press, Inc.
7. Freedman, A.M., Kaplan, H.I., and Sadock, B.J.: Modern synopsis of comprehensive textbook of psychiatry/II, ed. 2, Baltimore, 1976, The Williams & Wilkins Co.
8. Friedson, E., and Feldman, J.J.: The public looks at dental care, J. Am. Dent. Assoc. **57**:325, 1958.
9. Froelich, R.E., Bishop, F.M., and Dworkin, S.F.: Communication in the dental office: a programmed manual for the dental professional, St. Louis, 1976, The C.V. Mosby Co.
10. Gessel, A.H.: Electromyographic biofeedback and tricyclic antidepressants in myofascial pain-dysfunction syndrome: psychological predictors of outcome, J. Am. Dent. Assoc. **91**: 1048, 1975.
11. Gregg, J.M.: Functional anatomy of facial pain. In Alling, C.C., and Mahan, P.E., editors: Facial pain, Philadelphia, 1977, Lea & Febiger.
12. Lascelles, R.G.: Atypical facial pain and depression, Br. J. Psychiatry **112**:651, 1966.
13. Paulson, G.W.: Atypical facial pain, Oral Surg. **43**:338, 1977.
14. Poswillo, D.E.: Headache as a symptom of maxillofacial disorders. In Alling, C.C., and Mahan, P.E., editors: Facial pain, Philadelphia, 1977, Lea & Febiger.
15. Schoenberg, B.B.: The burning mouth. In Zegarelli, E.V., Kutscher, A.H., and Hyman, G.A., editors: Diagnosis of diseases of the mouth and jaws, ed. 2, Philadelphia, 1978, Lea & Febiger.
16. Stricker, G., and Howitt, J.W.: Physiological recording during simulated dental appointments, N.Y. State Dent. J. **31**:204, 1965.
17. Zucker, A.H.: A psychiatric appraisal of tongue symptoms, J. Am. Dent. Assoc. **85**:649, 1972.

6 Characteristics of skin and mucosal lesions

When the examiner has a thorough knowledge of the normal anatomy and physiology of the head and neck, oral mucosa, and skin, careful inspection and palpation will reveal various abnormal changes. Abnormal changes may be functional (physiologic) or structural (anatomic). Abnormal structural changes are commonly referred to as lesions.

Lesions of the skin and mucosa are basically very similar. The difference in degree of keratinization of the upper strata of the epithelium and the presence of various skin appendages, such as hair, sebaceous glands, and sweat glands, can account for a few lesions unique to the skin that are not found on the oral mucosa. These are discussed in Chapter 10, which deals with the skin.

A computerized analysis of approximately 200 oral soft tissue lesions[1] has established the importance of accurate descriptions of the site, the morphologic characteristics, and the color of these lesions as the most significant three factors in making differential diagnoses of oral lesions.

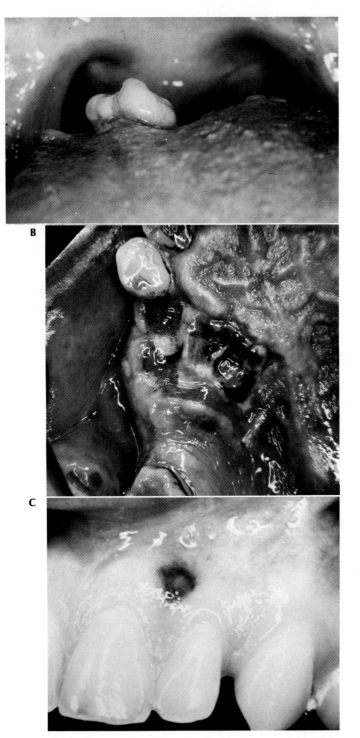

Fig. 6-1. Three basic morphologic categories. **A,** Elevated (very firm pedunculated nodule). Diagnosis: Soft tissue chondroma. **B,** Depressed (large traumatic ulcer). **C,** Flat (pigmented macule). Diagnosis: Tattoo.

TYPES OF LESIONS

Most lesions of the skin and oral mucosa can be placed in one of three broad morphologic categories: (1) elevated, (2) depressed, or (3) flat (Fig. 6-1).

Another broad classification for lesions is primary versus secondary. Primary lesions are the initial manifestations of a disease, whereas the secondary lesions result from modification or changes that occur after a period of time following the onset of the primary lesion. For example, elevated lesions in the mouth that contain fluid will usually rupture from normal masticatory function and result in a depressed lesion. Determining the characteristics of the initial lesion may be significant in making a diagnosis.

Unfortunately a standard, precise nomenclature or classification of oral mucosa lesions has never been established. The classification that follows is a suggested one that was developed in the computer analysis project referred to previously.[1]

Fig. 6-2. Various morphologic categories of elevated lesions.

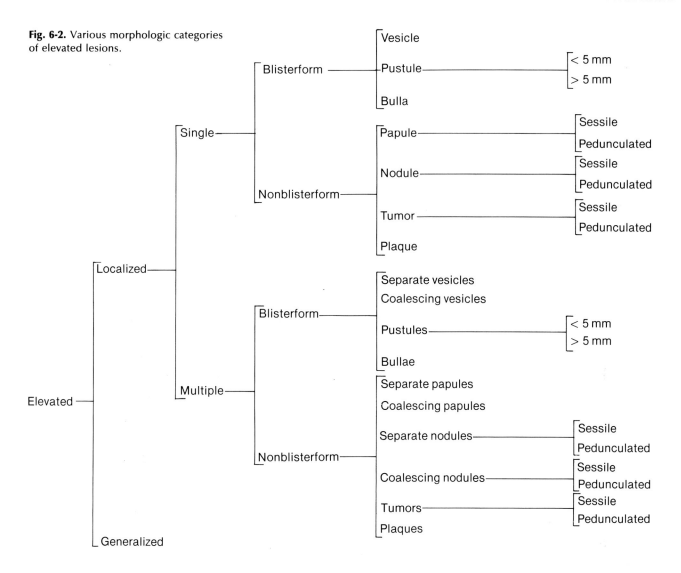

Morphology of lesions

Elevated lesions. An elevated lesion is one in which the surface is above the normal plane of the mucosa. Elevated lesions may be categorized according to a number of different characteristics, as shown in Fig. 6-2. Elevated lesions may be localized or generalized. A localized elevated lesion is limited to a small focal area. A generalized elevated lesion involves most or all of an area or site. Some generalized lesions may involve more than one site. It is usually easier to determine the limits of involvement of localized lesions than of generalized lesions. Localized lesions may be single or multiple. The number of lesions is often characteristic for a particular disease. A single lesion is one lesion of a particular morphologic type. Where more than one lesion of a particular morphologic type is present, they are considered multiple lesions.

Elevated lesions may be further divided into blisterform or nonblisterform lesions. Blisterform lesions are those that contain a body fluid. They are usually identified by their characteristic translucent appearance. Tactile examination of a blisterform lesion will reveal a soft rebounding sensation. In contrast nonblisterform lesions are solid and contain no fluid. They are recognized by their opaque appearance. When they are palpated, they feel firm and solid.

The size of a lesion is often a clue to its diagnosis. It is not necessary to exactly measure the size of a lesion. Only a reasonably accurate estimate of the lesion's size is expected. Size of lesions is best estimated by comparing the lesion with familiar landmarks of known size immediately adjacent to it. These landmarks include teeth, parotid papillae, lingual papillae, and incisive papilla. For example, lower incisors are approximately 5 mm in their greatest width, and up-

47

per central incisors are 8 to 9 mm in their greatest width. Molars are approximately 10 mm, or 1 cm, in their mesiodistal aspect. The lingual filiform and fungiform papillae are less than 1 mm in diameter.

By common usage, blisterform lesions are given descriptive names, depending on their size and the material contained within the blister. A blisterform lesion is either a vesicle, pustule, or bulla (Fig. 6-3). A vesicle is a blisterform lesion that is less than 5 mm in its greatest diameter and contains serum or mucin. The serum of mucin gives the vesicle a clear or translucent, slightly white appearance. A pustule is a blisterform lesion that contains pus that imparts a yellowish color. It may be greater or less than 5 mm. A bulla is a blisterform lesion larger than 5 mm in its greatest diameter that may contain serum or mucin. It may occasionally contain extravasated blood. The color may appear pink, red, or blue, according to the fluid content.

Nonblisterform lesions are also given descriptive names according to their size and pattern. A nonblisterform lesion is either a papule, nodule, tumor, or plaque (Fig. 6-4). The term *tumor* is used here in a general sense meaning a nonspecific tumescence. It is recognized that popular usage of this term has implied a neoplasm, either benign or malignant. A papule is a lesion that consists of tissue and is less than 5 mm in its greatest diameter. A nodule is similar to a papule in that it consists of tissue, but it is greater than 5 mm and less than 2 cm in its greatest diameter. A tumor is similar to a nodule in that it consists of tissue, but it is greater than 2 cm

in its greatest diameter. A plaque is a slightly raised nonblisterform lesion that has a broad flat top like a plateau. It has a "pasted on" or "stuck on" appearance and is usually greater than 5 mm in diameter.

A papule, nodule, or tumor may be classified as sessile or pedunculated according to its base or attachment to the mucosa. A sessile lesion is a

papule, nodule, or tumor whose base or attachment to the normal mucosa is the greatest diameter of the lesion. A pedunculated lesion is a papule, nodule, or tumor that has an attachment of the normal oral mucosa that is smaller than the greatest diameter of the lesion itself. In other words, the lesion is attached by a stalk or pedicle.

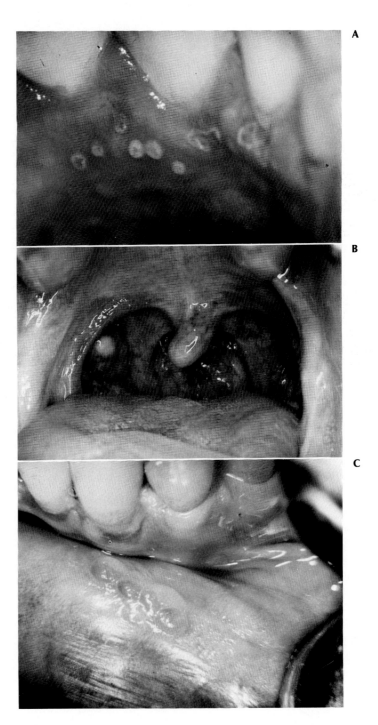

Fig. 6-3. A, Typical cluster of vesicles in varying stages of degeneration, which usually results in small, punctate ulcers in 24 to 48 hours. Diagnosis: Recurrent herpes simplex. **B,** Pustule resulting from abscess formation of pharyngeal tonsil. **C,** Bulla that developed from eliciting Nikolsky's sign during oral examination. Diagnosis: Pemphigus vulgaris.

Multiple lesions with any of the morphologic characteristics so far described can be separate or coalescing. However, in the oral cavity, small lesions coalesce more frequently than large ones do. Separate lesions are usually few in number and relatively widely spaced. They will remain individual, distinct lesions, even if they tend to enlarge after their initial appearance. Conversely, coalescing lesions are numerous and in proximity to one another. Their margins may merge and leave a single lesion, even if they enlarge only slightly after their initial appearance. With multiple lesions that vary in size, the morphologic type of peripheral lesions becomes important in deciding whether the lesions should be considered as separate or coalescing.

Fig. 6-4. A, Single, slightly pedunculated papule. Diagnosis: Mucous retention phenomenon (fibrosed). **B,** Multiple, small, coalescing papules forming linear and reticular patterns. Diagnosis: Lichen planus. **C,** Pedunculated nodule. Diagnosis: Irritation fibroma. **D,** Pedunculated tumor. Diagnosis: Peripheral ossifying fibroma. **E,** Single plaque. Diagnosis: Hyperkeratosis without atypia.

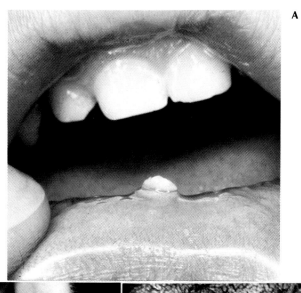

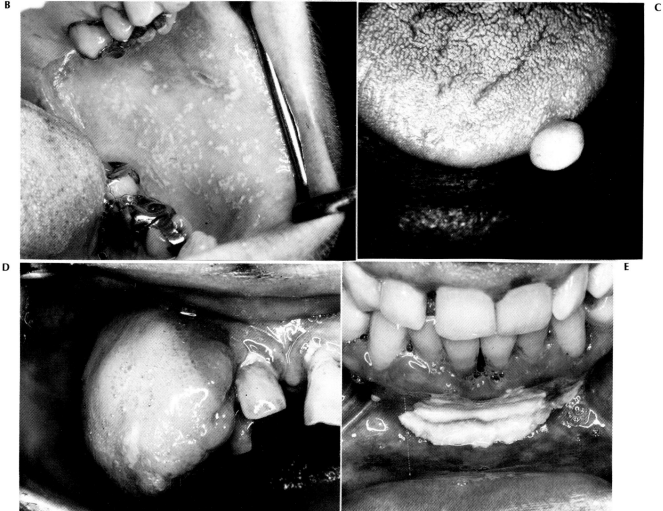

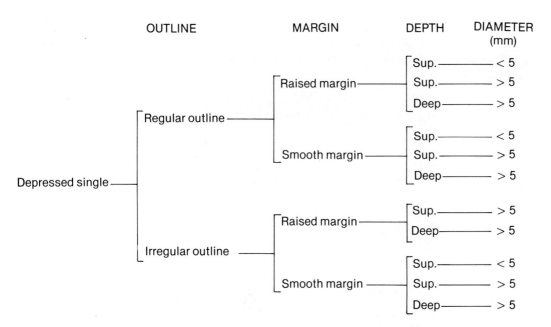

Fig. 6-5. Various morphologic categories of single depressed lesions, most commonly ulcers. Emphasis is placed on outline, margin, depth, and diameter characteristics.

Fig. 6-6. Similar classification for multiple depressed lesions.

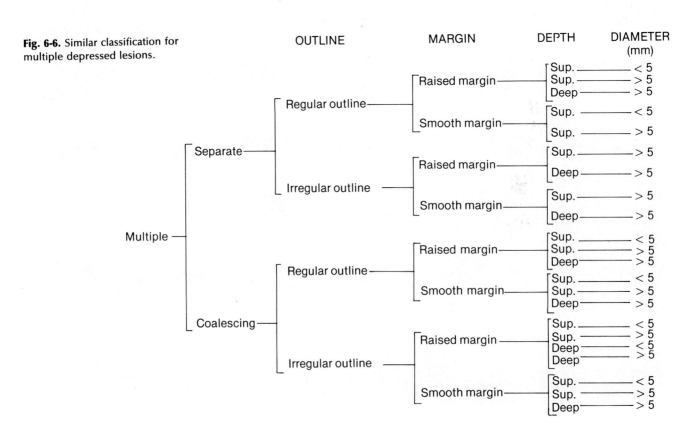

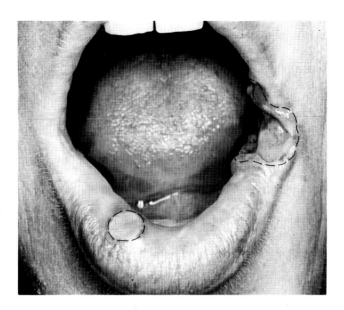

Fig. 6-7. Two large ulcers demonstrating regular and irregular outline. Diagnosis: Periadenitis mucosa necrotica recurrens (major aphthae).

Depressed lesions. A depressed lesion is one in which the surface is below the normal plane of the mucosa. Most depressed lesions are ulcers. An ulcer is a loss in continuity of the oral epithelium. Clinically, the center of the ulcer is often yellow to gray with a red periphery. Occasionally, a red center may be observed. Ulcers often result from the rupture of elevated lesions, such as vesicles, bullae, and pustules. Some ulcers may result from ischemia, which is the loss or reduction of blood supply to an area. This leads to necrosis and sloughing of the epithelium, which then becomes an ulcer. Some depressed lesions are the result of atrophy or scarring and have an intact epithelial surface. Other depressed lesions may be pits or blind ''pouches'' caused by a failure of complete fusion during embryologic development.

Depressed lesions may be single or multiple. The charts illustrated in Figs. 6-5 and 6-6 classify the possible characteristics that may be found when depressed lesions are seen clinically. Employment of the terminology used in Figs. 6-2, 6-5, and 6-6 will assist the dentist in describing lesions more accurately and in formulating a reasonable differential diagnosis.

Single depressed lesions may be divided, according to their outline, into regular and irregular. A depressed lesion is said to have a regular outline if the border is a continuous linear outline and resembles a circle or an oval (Fig. 6-7). A lesion is irregular in outline if the border has numerous deviations from a circular or oval pattern (Fig. 6-7). The determination of whether the outline is regular or irregular should be made at the normal viewing distance of about 30 to 40 cm, since most lesions, if inspected more closely, would show irregularities in their outlines.

Regardless of the outline, the margin of a single depressed lesion may be raised or smooth. When the margin is above the plane of the normal mucosa, the margin is raised. If the margin of a depressed lesion is on the same plane as the normal mucosa, the margin is said to be smooth (Fig. 6-8).

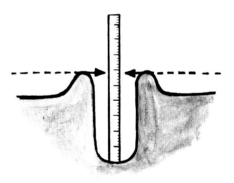

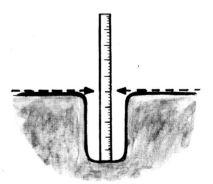

Fig. 6-8. Raised and smooth margins. Same lesions as in Fig. 6-7 show regular outlined ulcer to have smooth margins and irregular lesion to have raised margins.

51

A depressed lesion may vary in its depth, being described as superficial or deep. Depth is defined as the distance from the base of the depression to the plane of the margin of the depression. This depth can be estimated by comparing this distance with the known sizes of landmarks. It has been arbitrarily suggested that a superficial lesion is one that is less than 3 mm in depth. A deep lesion is one that is greater than 3 mm in depth (Fig. 6-9).

Depressed lesions vary in diameter. They have been arbitrarily divided into those that are less than 5 mm and those that are greater than 5 mm in their greatest diameter. The diameter of depressed lesions can be estimated by comparing the greatest diameter of the lesion with structures of known

size. Theoretically, all lesions of the morphologic types discussed can be less or greater than 5 mm. In practice, however, some lesions are almost always of a particular diameter. For example, most deep depressed lesions are greater than 5 mm in diameter.

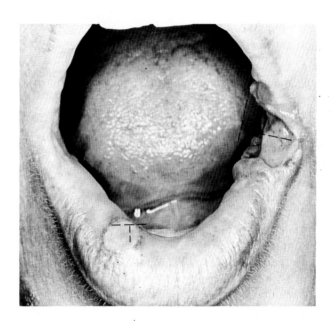

Fig. 6-9. Same lesions as in Fig. 6-7 also illustrate superficial versus deep ulcer.

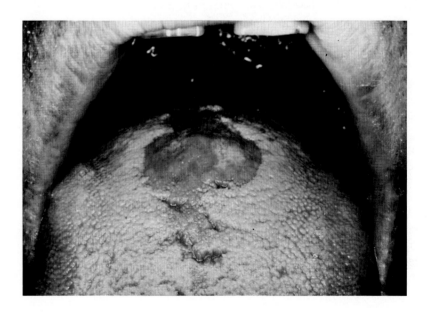

Fig. 6-10. Flat lesion of tongue resulting from loss of normal papillae. Diagnosis: Median rhomboid glossitis.

Multiple lesions may have the same morphologic descriptions as discussed for single lesions: outline, margin, depth, and diameter. In addition, multiple lesions may be either separate or coalescing. Separate lesions are few in number or widely spaced and are not likely to merge or blend into one another, even if they enlarge. They remain distinct. Coalescing lesions are usually numerous and in proximity. After minor enlargement, they may merge or blend into one another. When this occurs, a single lesion is formed. The orginal outline of the initial lesions may or may not still be detectable.

Each of the morphologic types of depressed multiple lesions theoretically can be divided into those less than 5 mm in their greatest diameter and those greater than 5 mm in their greatest diameter. In practice, however, some combinations are so rare as to be unimportant. For example, since depressed multiple separate lesions that have a regular outline and raised margins and are deep are almost always greater than 5 mm, the less than 5 mm category has been omitted from the chart in Fig. 6-6.

Flat lesions. A flat lesion is one in which the surface is on the same plane as the normal oral mucosa. Because of this, any lesion of normal mucosal coloring would be undetectable (except on the dorsum of the tongue). Therefore, the only way most flat lesions can be detected is through a change in color. A flat lesion with an abnormal color is called a macule (see Fig. 6-1, *C*).

Since the tongue is anatomically unique, special consideration must be given to flat lesions occurring on the dorsal and lateral borders of the tongue (Fig. 6-10). Loss of papillae results in an apparent depressed lesion, but since the mucosal surface is not involved, it is in fact a flat lesion. Since it does not involve an abnormality of color, it is not a macule.

Lesions resulting from a loss of papillae may be single or multiple. Single and multiple lesions may be regular or irregular in outline. Multiple lesions are almost always irregular.

COLOR OF LESIONS

Most oral soft tissue lesions demonstrate some color change. The following predominant colors are seen in oral soft tissue lesions: red, pink, white, red and white, blue, gray, yellow, purple, black, and brown. The graph in Fig. 6-11 shows the relative frequency of the various colors as they occur in the oral soft tissue lesions. As you can see, red, pink, and white are the most common colors, whereas blue, gray, yellow, purple, black, and brown are relatively rare.

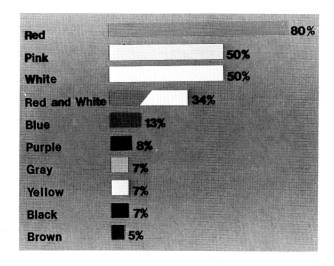

Fig. 6-11. Possible colors that approximately 200 diseases of oral mucosa may manifest. Obviously, many diseases may have different predominant color patterns.

Color that is perceived by the human eye represents light that is reflected from an object (Fig. 6-12). The human skin and oral mucosa are translucent, which allows the light to penetrate the covering epithelium to the various underlying layers of tissue (lamina propria and submucosa). As the incident light strikes each layer of tissue, a portion is transmitted, absorbed, scattered, and reflected (Fig. 6-13). We perceive the normal oral mucosa as pink because of the reflection of light after it strikes the capillary bed.

Pigments are present in all layers and influence the resultant tissue color. Normal tissue contains four primary endogenous pigments or biochromes: oxyhemoglobin, reduced hemoglobin, melanin, and carotene (Fig. 6-14). *Hemoglobin,* which is present in red blood cells, is of two types, *oxyhemoglobin* and *reduced hemoglobin,* according to the oxygen concentration. Oxyhemoglobin has more oxygen and imparts a bright red color. Reduced hemoglobin is less oxygenated and imparts a bluish color. *Melanin* is a brown pigment formed in specialized cells known as melanocytes. The pigment particles are transferred to malpighian cells of the epithelium. Since melanin is a significant diagnostic indicator, it is discussed in detail with brown and black lesions. *Carotene* is a yellow pigment of the submucosal fat that is also found in the cornified superficial layer of the epithelium, sebaceous glands, and blood plasma.

The blood contributes more to normal and abnormal tissue colors in the oral mucosa than any other single factor does. The color imparted by blood is due primarily to hemoglobin. The redness or blueness of tissue reflects the relative proportion of oxyhemoglobin and reduced hemoglobin in the underlying vessels. The arterioles contain approximately 95% oxyhemoglobin and 5% reduced hemoglobin. The capillaries contain approximately 70% oxyhemoglobin and 30% reduced hemoglobin. The subpapillary venous plexus contains approximately 50% of each.

Fig. 6-12. Passage of light through different levels of tissue and reflection of light resulting in pink color.

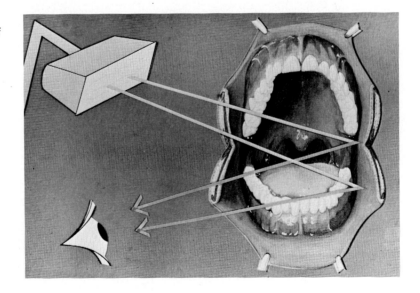

Fig. 6-13. Portions of light. **A,** Transmitted.
B, Absorbed. **C,** Scattered.
D, Reflected.

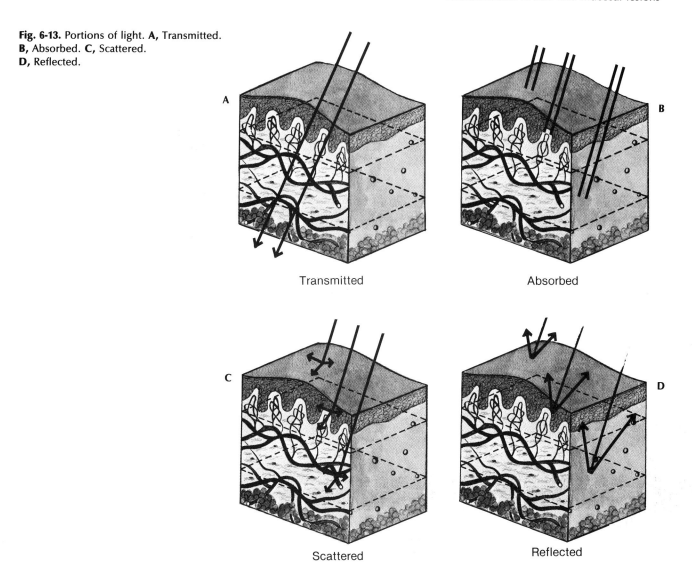

Transmitted

Absorbed

Scattered

Reflected

Fig. 6-14. Primary sources of four endogenous biochromes.

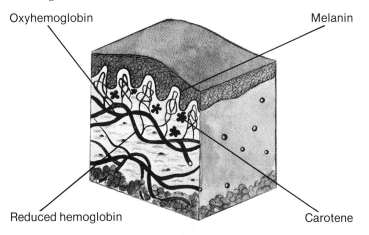

Oxyhemoglobin

Melanin

Reduced hemoglobin

Carotene

The other factors related to the effect of blood on tissue color are: (1) the number of blood vessels concentrated in an area, (2) the degree of dilatation or constriction of the vessels, and (3) the thickness of the overlying connective tissue and epithelium or the proximity of vessels to the surface (Fig. 6-15).

Because of the complex interaction of the tissue biochromes and other secondary factors affecting tissue colors that this unit discusses, it should be noted that single colors, as we normally interpret or see them, are rarely seen when soft tissue lesions are dealt with. When the color of soft tissue lesions is determined, the predominant color, which is the color involving the greatest surface area, should be noted first. Other lesser color changes involving smaller areas of the lesions may or may not be helpful in making a diagnosis. This complex interaction of color changes is discussed as it may relate to each predominant color.

The normal color of the oral mucosa is predominantly pink. Some areas, such as the vermilion zones, alveolar mucosae, soft palate, and pharynx will show more variation in color, usually more red, because of the prominent vascularity and nonkeratinization of the epithelium (Fig. 6-16). The other normal variations from the pink color of the oral tissues are related to localized concentrations of melanin pigment. This pigment is normally more prominent in black and other dark-skinned races. Normal melanin pigment concentrations are most common in the buccal mucosa, attached gingiva, and hard palate

Fig. 6-15. Effect of blood on mucosa color. **A,** Varying number of capillaries in lamina propria papillae and various stages of dilatation and constriction of these capillaries. **B,** Varying thickness of epithelium and collagen, which alters light effects, resulting in different shades of pink and red color.

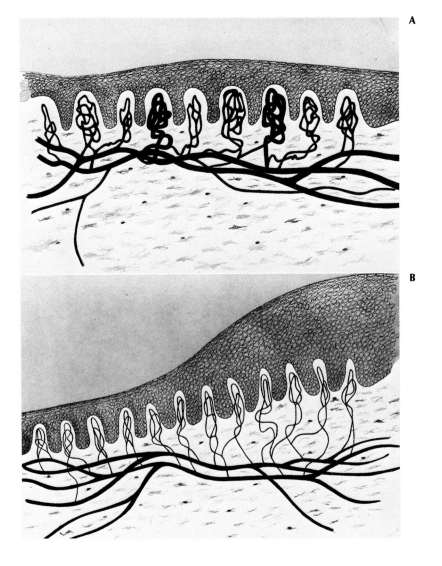

A

B

(Fig. 6-17). Normal melanin pigment may be patchy or diffuse in distribution. This may cause the color of the mucosa to be brown to bluish black, according to the amount of melanin present.

As indicated in the graph in Fig. 6-11, pink is a relatively common color for oral soft tissue lesions. Most lesions with a pink color are elevated lesions, and this indicates that the pathosis is submucosal in origin, the surfacing mucosa has not been altered significantly, and the pink color is intact. The elevated morphologic character of most pink lesions may be due to several forms of underlying pathosis. The lesions most commonly indicate (1) hyperplasia, (2) neoplasia, (3) fluid accumulation, and (4) cyst formation.

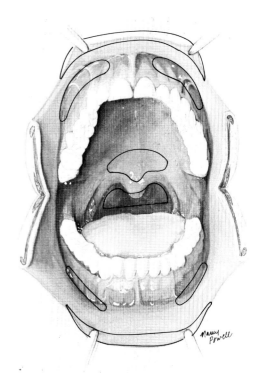

Fig. 6-16. Oral cavity with outlines indicating areas appearing more red than pink.

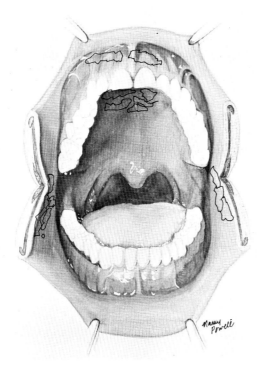

Fig. 6-17. Same drawing of oral cavity, indicating areas more likely to have physiologic melanin pigment, which alters normal pink color.

1. *Hyperplasia* results from an increased quantity of normal tissue. In the oral cavity, pink elevated lesions resulting from hyperplasia most commonly indicate hyperplasia of connective tissue or bone (Fig. 6-18).
2. *Neoplasia* is an abnormal new growth of tissue or cellular infiltrate that may indicate various benign or malignant proliferations (Fig. 6-19).
3. *Fluid accumulation* resulting in elevated pink lesions may be generalized or localized. Fluid accumulation as edema may be generalized or localized. Fluid accumulation in the form of mucin usually appears as a localized lesion (Fig. 6-20). The depth of the fluid accumulation beneath the surface will affect the color. If the lesion is deep, the surface often has a pink color. If the fluid accumulation is very superficial, the lesion will be more translucent, and the color will vary according to the color of the underlying structures.
4. *Cysts* are generally well-localized lesions that indicate a fluid-filled, epithelial-lined cavity (Fig. 6-21).

Fig. 6-18. Photograph, **A,** and drawing, **B,** illustrating clinical and histologic changes seen in one example of hyperplasia. Diagnosis: Fibroma.

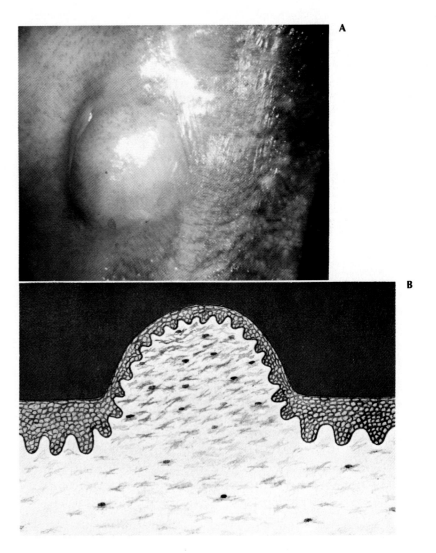

A

B

Elevated lesions with a pink color most commonly appear clinically as nonblisterform lesions, either as generalized lesions, tumors, nodules, or papules. Less frequently, blisterform lesions, such as bullae and vesicles, may have a pink color. Depressed lesions having a normal pink color are rare. However, such unusual lesions as developmental pits, clefts, or perforations will often have a pink color.

Atrophic scars may also have a pink color. Some flat lesions of the tongue may also be pink. These are unique lesions that result simply from the loss of normal lingual papillae. Some tongue lesions that result from loss of papillae may appear as dark pink or red as the result of contrast with the surrounding papillae, which are heavily keratinized.

A
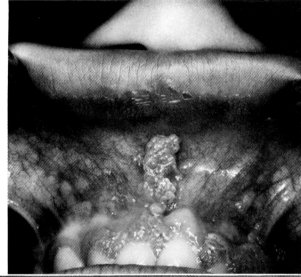

B
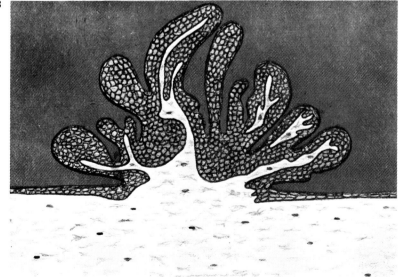

Fig. 6-19. Photograph, **A,** and drawing, **B,** of clinical and histologic changes seen in benign form of neoplasia. Diagnosis: Papilloma.

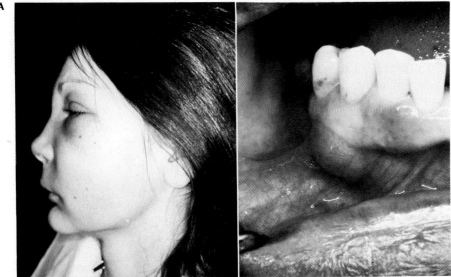

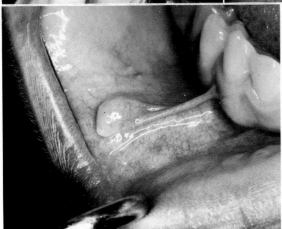

Fig. 6-20. A, Fluid accumulation as generalized swelling. Diagnosis: Cellulitis from periapical abscess. **B,** Localized fluid accumulation. Diagnosis: Periodontal abscess. **C,** Localized accumulation of mucin. Diagnosis: Mucous retention phenomenon (mucocele).

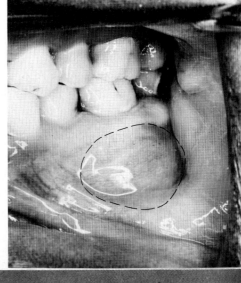

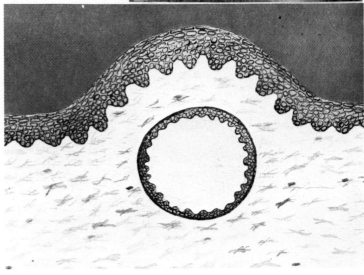

Fig. 6-21. Photograph, **A,** and drawing, **B,** showing clinical and histologic features of cyst. Diagnosis: Dentigerous cyst.

Red lesions

As was discussed earlier, blood is the most significant factor influencing red color change. An increased quantity of blood to an area will result in an increased redness, or erythema. Erythema may be localized or widespread, ranging from minute macules to involvement of large areas of skin or mucosa. These erythematous changes may occur without alteration in the morphologic character of the site. Red may be the predominant color in lesions of any morphologic type

An increased quantity of blood may be due to intravascular or extravascular changes (Fig. 6-22). Intravascular changes are the result of dilatation of blood vessels or proliferation of new vessels. The increased quantity of blood resulting from the dilatation is called *hyperemia*. Proliferation of new vessels may be associated with developmental anomalies or with benign or malignant neoplasms. Intravascular lesions resulting from either dilatation or proliferation of new vessels may often be diagnosed by pressing a clear microscopic glass slide on the lesion. This technique is called *diascopy* or *diascopic examination* (Fig. 6-23). If momentary blanching is observed, the lesion is intravascular in origin. If blanching does not occur, the lesion is usually extravascular or is due to other causes.

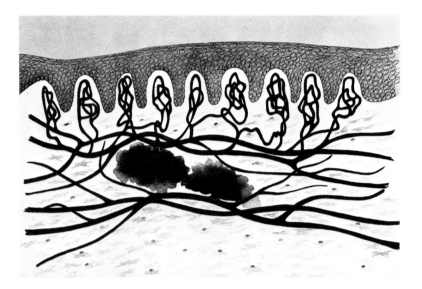

Fig. 6-22. Extravascular change or extravasation of red blood cells from altered blood vessels.

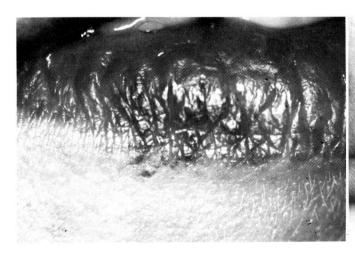 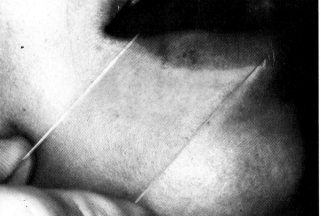

Fig. 6-23. Diascopy technique. Diagnosis: Capillary hemangioma.

Extravascular changes are due to the escape of erythrocytes into the surrounding tissue. This is called *extravasation*. When extravasation of blood occurs, the general term *purpura* is used to denote the discoloration of the skin or mucous membranes. There are three basic types of purpuric lesions: petechiae, ecchymoses, and hematomas (Fig. 6-24). *Petechiae* are small red macules 1 to 5 mm in diameter, sharply outlined, and may be slightly elevated but not elevated enough to be considered vesicles or papules. Purpuric lesions that are larger and slightly deeper in origin than petechiae are called *ecchymoses*. Ecchymoses appear as macules. When a large area of skin or mucosa is involved by extravasation, which causes an elevated tumescence, the lesion is referred to as a *hematoma*. As the blood is resorbed, the lesions flatten and undergo multiple color changes. Both ecchymoses and hematomas are characterized by multiple color changes following the initial red phase. The red color changes discussed thus far are due to increased quantities of hemoglobin pigment from intact red cells. Following hemoglobin breakdown, its products result in multiple color changes. Hemoglobin is transformed into biliverdin, bilirubin, and eventually hemosiderin. With these changes the ecchymoses or hematomas turn from bluish red to bluish green to yellow green to somewhat brownish.

The most common condition resulting in abnormal redness is inflammation. Inflammation can occur in the oral cavity as a result of trauma or infection. Although inflammation is characterized by intravascular and extravascular changes, dilatation is the predominant underlying factor caus-

ing the red color change. Many lesions that initially appear as pink in color can become partially or predominantly red lesions as a result of secondary inflammation.

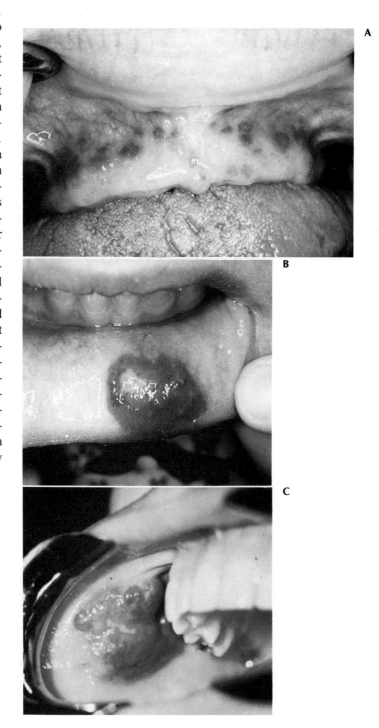

Fig. 6-24. A, Petechiae. Diagnosis: Contact allergy. **B,** Ecchymosis from trauma. **C,** Hematoma from trauma.

White lesions

White lesions of the oral mucosa may be due to alterations in the epithelium or in the connective tissue. In some instances the changes may be a combination of epithelial and underlying connective tissue changes. The most common causes of white lesions in the oral mucosa relate to changes in the epithelium. These are (1) hyperkeratinization, (2) acanthosis, (3) necrosis, and (4) fluid accumulation (Fig. 6-25).

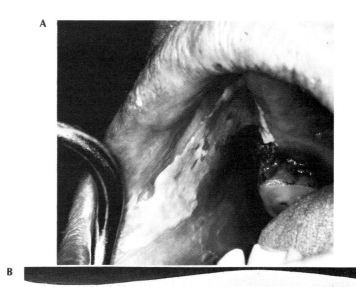

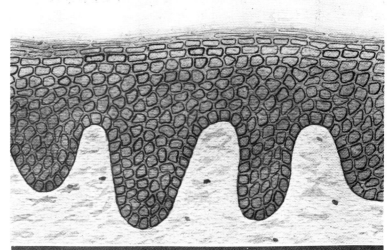

Fig. 6-25. A., Hyperkeratinization. **B,** Orthokeratin (absence of nuclei); parakeratin has residual nuclei. Diagnosis: Keratosis without atypia. **C** and **D,** Acanthosis; this is strictly microscopic change; no characteristic clinical changes are associated with it.

Continued.

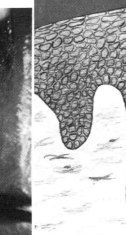

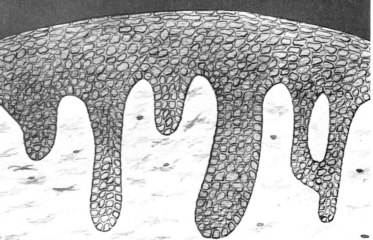

C

D

Hyperkeratinization is a thickening of the outer surface of the epithelium, similar to a callus on the skin. This excessive buildup and retention of surface cells alters the translucency of the epithelium. Chronic irritations and various other etiologic factors can cause an alteration in epithelial cell maturation, which results in hyperkeratinization.

E

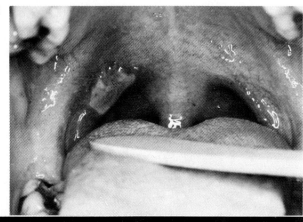

F

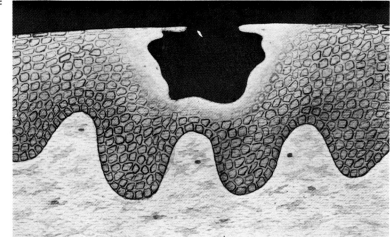

Fig. 6-25, cont'd. E and **F,** Necrosis. Diagnosis: Aphthous ulcer.
G and **H,** Intracellular fluid accumulation. Diagnosis: White sponge nevus.

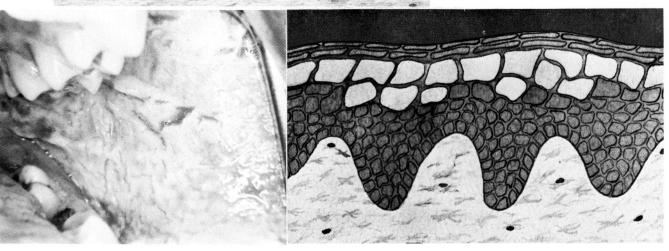

G

H

Acanthosis is another common epithelial change. Acanthosis is an increased thickening caused by hyperplasia of the prickle cell layer. When the epithelium becomes thickened by acanthosis, it becomes less translucent and more whitish because of decreased reflection of light from the normal capillary bed.

Necrosis of the epithelium is still another common cause of white color change. Necrosis is the death of cells in a localized area, which can result in a slough when extensive areas of the epithelium become necrotic. Necrosis frequently follows moderate or severe inflammation, but it may also be the result of physical or chemical trauma.

An increased *fluid accumulation* may be seen within the cells of the epithelium or beneath it. Intracellular edema can cause a pale white appearance of extensive areas of the oral mucosa. This is often associated with conditions involving the labial and buccal mucosa. Extracellular accumulation of fluid beneath the epithelium can also alter light reflection, resulting in a white color change. This may be true of cysts or of the accumulation of other fluids, such as edema or mucin.

Fig. 6-25, cont'd. I and **J,** Subepithelial fluid accumulation. Diagnosis: Mucous membrane pemphigoid.

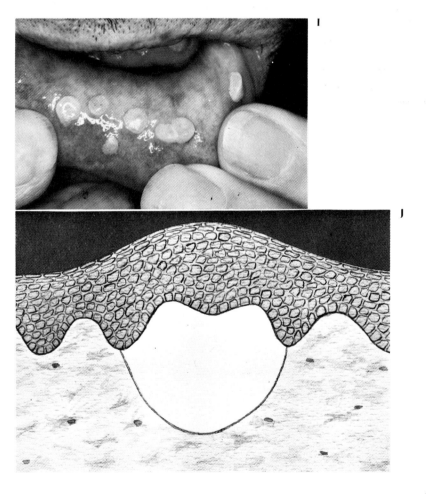

I

J

In addition to changes in the epithelium, other white lesions may result from changes in the connective tissue. These changes are primarily due to (1) an increased quantity of collagen or (2) an alteration in the maturity of collagen (Fig. 6-26).

An increase in the quantity of collagen above the capillary bed can decrease the reflection of red color to the surface. Examples of this change can be seen in fibromas and scars.

An alteration in the maturity of collagen usually results in decreased vascularity. Since there is less vascularity from which light can be reflected, the color perceived is more white. Some white lesions may be due to both epithelial and connective tissue changes (Fig. 6-27).

The morphologic characteristics that are most likely to be associated with white lesions are plaques and papules, because these are primarily due to epithelial alteration. Nodules and tumors are usually due to changes in the connective tissue. If allowed to persist, they will frequently show a white color change because of secondary hyperkeratinization. This hyperkeratinization is the result of mechanical friction from opposing structures during normal masticatory function.

A unique condition involving white color change is pallor. Pallor is a minimal white change of the skin or mucosa most commonly seen in nonkeratinized and melanin-free sites, such as the vermilion zones, fingernail beds, and conjunctival mucosa of the eyes. Pallor may be due to a decreased flow of blood, decreased hemoglobin content, or an actual loss of hemoglobin.

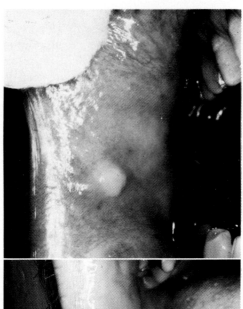
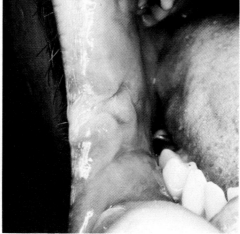

Fig. 6-26. A, Hyperplasia of collagen. Diagnosis: Fibroma. **B,** Scar formation. Diagnosis: Major aphthous ulcer.

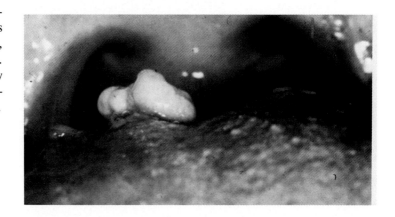

Fig. 6-27. Lesion having cartilage and hyperplasia of epithelium. Diagnosis: Soft tissue chondroma.

Red and white lesions

Red and white lesions commonly indicate inflammation. An inflamed lesion that was originally red may exhibit some white coloration as a result of necrosis and sloughing. Conversely, lesions originally white in color may undergo some red changes as a result of inflammation. For example, lesions such as superficial burns or fungal infections are white lesions initially, but rubbing them results in the partial loss of the necrotic white surface. This leaves a denuded red area due to exposure of the capillary bed. Some large elevated lesions having a white hyperkeratotic surface undergo trauma, which causes thinning and loss of the epithelial surface, resulting in a red and white lesion. The most common morphologic characteristics associated with red and white lesions are large ulcers and depressed lesions.

Gray lesions

The color gray is not due to biologic pigment but usually to deposition of foreign material in the connective tissues. The gray color may be localized or diffuse. Localized gray pigmentation usually results from implantation or deposition of foreign materials into lacerations or abrasions of the mucosa. The most common foreign particles encountered in the oral mucosa are amalgam particles. Diffuse gray pigmentations may result from heavy metal ingestion with subsequent systemic deposition of the material. This is seen in silver, lead, bismuth, or mercury poisoning. The color may vary from gray to dark brown to black. Occasionally, natural brown pigments, such as melanin and hemosiderin, may appear as gray clinically. Since some of the reflected light from the material is absorbed as it passes through the thickness of the mucous membrane, it appears gray rather than brown. This gray color change may be localized or diffuse. The natural grayness of some of the oral mucosa in blacks is an example of a brown pigment, melanin, appearing as a gray color clinically. Heavy concentrations of a pigment in the lamina propria may make the gray color very dark, appearing almost black. The color gray is most often associated with macules, since usually the amount of pigmented material is not sufficient to raise or otherwise alter the normal contour of the mucosa.

Blue lesions

There are no biologic pigments that are blue. However, the color blue is usually associated with two types of lesions. Some cystic lesions containing clear fluid appear blue, and some vascular lesions may be blue. Cysts, within soft tissue, that contain clear fluid, such as mucin, appear pale blue clinically. This blue appearance is related to the absorption and reflection of light passing through the overlying soft tissue and the contents of the cyst itself. Vascular lesions may appear blue when the blood within the lesion contains a large amount of reduced hemoglobin. This blue color can be seen through the translucent mucosa. The shade of this blue color may be altered by the thickness of the overlying mucosa. A darker blue is seen with a more superficial lesion. A lighter blue is seen with a deeper lesion. Since cystic and vascular lesions are relatively large blisterform lesions, the morphologic characteristic most often associated with a blue color is a bulla. Tattoos from foreign bodies may appear as blue macules.

Purple lesions

Factors that are most often associated with purple lesions include vascular lesions and deposition and interaction of pigments. Although some vascular lesions appear blue, others may appear purple. The purple color may be due in part to the basic bluish color's being modified by the normal pink or reddish mucosa; it may also be due to the combination of both oxygenated and reduced hemoglobin in the blood. Deposition and interaction of pigments from breakdown products of extravasated blood may cause a purple discoloration. Purple vascular lesions are usually bullae. Purple lesions resulting from deposition and interaction of pigments are usually nodules or tumors. Occasionally, bleeding into blisterform lesions and hematomas may cause a purple discoloration.

Brown lesions

Brown coloration may be caused by melanin or hemosiderin (Fig. 6-28). Melanin is a substance produced within melanocytes by structures called *melanosomes* (Fig. 6-29). Melanocytes are normally found near the basal layer of cells within the epithelium. Since not all melanocytes are functionally active at any particular time, even oral mucosa that is not pigmented clinically does contain melanocytes. An increase in brown pigmentation may be brought about by an increased number of melanocytes, increased melanin synthesis of available melanocytes, or an increased size of melanosomes. Increased numbers of melanocytes may form various benign and malignant neoplasms. Increased melanin synthesis may be stimulated by radiant energy, such as ultraviolet light, roentgen rays, and heat. Increased melanin synthesis may also result from unknown factors. Diffuse melanin synthesis may occur in some systemic diseases in which there is increased production of pituitary adrenocorticotropic hormone (ACTH). Brown pigmentation because of melanin usually appears as a macule but may also appear as a nodule or tumor. In addition to melanin, hemosiderin may also be a cause of brown coloration. Brown color resulting from hemosiderin is most frequently associated with crusting and drying of ulcerated lesions on the vermilion zones and skin.

Fig. 6-28. A, Melanin accumulation. Diagnosis: Ephelis. **B,** Hemosiderin accumulation. Diagnosis: Well-differentiated carcinoma.

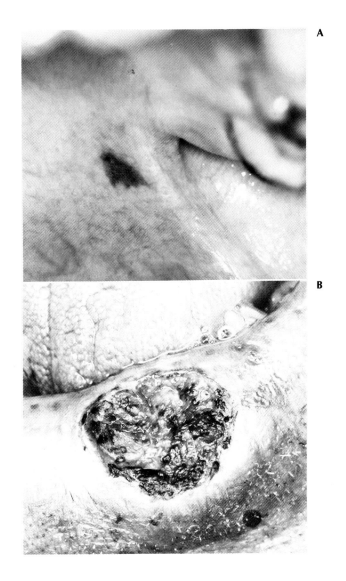

Fig. 6-29. Melanin formation in epithelial cells.

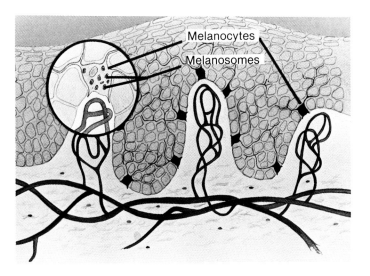

Black lesions

The most common cause for black color in the mouth is foreign body deposition. Less frequently, a black color may result from altered blood pigments, necrosis and gangrene of tissue, and dense accumulations of melanin pigment (Fig. 6-30). Any darkly colored foreign materials beneath the oral mucosa may appear as black. Amalgam particles beneath the oral mucosa, although usually gray, sometimes appear as black. Loss of epithelium in ulcerative lesions may allow the escape of blood onto the surface of the mucosa. If an alteration in blood pigments occurs, such as with oxidation and drying, a black color may appear in the crust. Extravasated blood that is undergoing degradation may appear as a black lesion. Death of tissue, or necrosis with invasion of saprophytic organisms, is termed *gangrene*. This process results in a black color. Heavy concentrations of foreign or biologic pigments may also result in a black appearance. For example, melanin, which is brown, in very heavy concentrations may appear black. Black lesions caused by foreign body deposition or breakdown of blood pigments are usually macules. When necrosis and gangrene of tissue result in a black color, the lesion usually undergoes a macular change. As the dead tissue sloughs, a depressed lesion with a black periphery is formed. Dense concentrations of melanin pigment causing a black lesion usually appear as a macule but may also appear as a nodule or tumor.

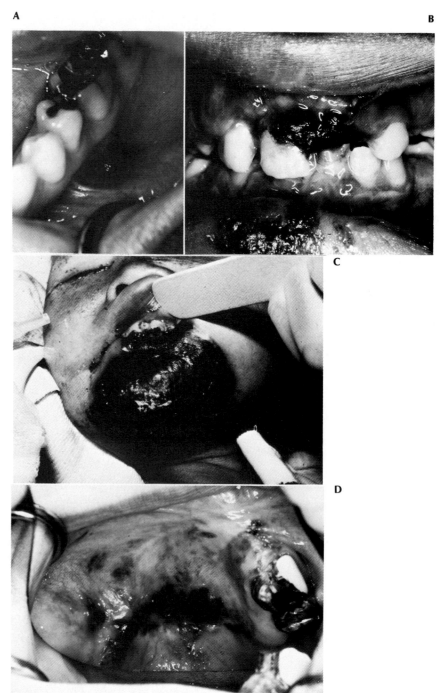

Fig. 6-30. A, Foreign body. Diagnosis: Amalgam tattoo. **B,** Altered blood pigments in coagulated blood. Diagnosis: Erythema multiforme. **C,** Necrosis and gangrene. Diagnosis: Noma. **D,** Accumulation of melanin. Diagnosis: Melanoma.

Yellow lesions

Yellow color may be caused by carotene. It may also result from other causes, such as (1) accumulation of pus, (2) aggregation of lymphoid tissue, (3) exudation of serum, (4) degeneration of blood pigments, (5) lipid-containing structures and neoplasms, and (6) extrinsic stains (Fig. 6-31).

Accumulation of pus resulting from degenerating leukocytes usually takes on a yellowish tinge. This is seen in an acute inflammatory process. Therefore, a yellow color may be seen in association with ulcers or pustules.

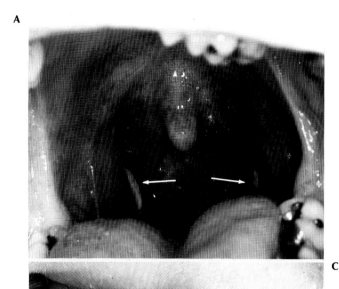

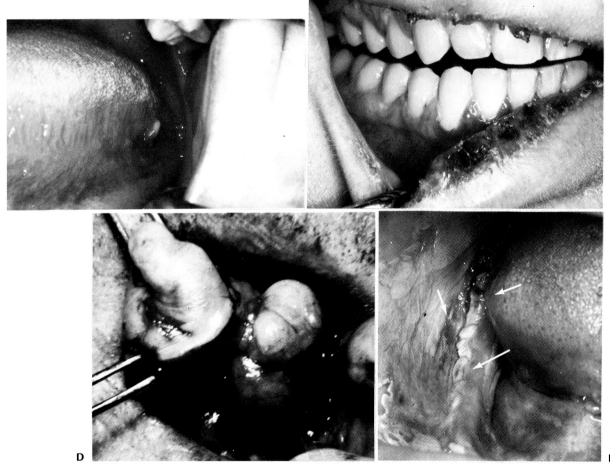

Fig. 6-31. A, Accumulation of pus. Diagnosis: Tonsillar abscesses. **B,** Aggregate of lymphoid tissue. Diagnosis: Lingual lymphoid tissue. **C,** Exudation of serum. Diagnosis: Erythema multiforme. **D,** Lipid-containing structures and neoplasms. Diagnosis: Lipoma. **E,** Extrinsic stains. Diagnosis: Nicotine stain on keratosis without atypia.

Lymphoid tissue that is located superficially beneath the oral mucosa may appear as yellow papules or nodules. This is a common finding on the posterior tongue or pharynx.

Serum is normally a yellow or straw-colored fluid. Exudation of serum in an inflammatory reaction may reach the surface if loss of epithelium has occurred. If drying occurs, as on the lips, a crust may form. This crust may take the form of a rough yellowish plaque or may be seen at the periphery of an ulcer.

Degeneration of blood pigments, particularly in the formation of bilirubin, may cause a yellow color that may be either localized or diffuse. A diffuse yellow color may occur if there is excess bilirubin in the tissues because of breakdown of bile pigments, such as occurs in liver disease, blockage of the bile ducts, or excess bilirubin formation in hemolytic disease. This condition is *jaundice* and is a diffuse macular change.

Lipid, or fat, is yellow in color. Accumulation of fat near the surface, such as occurs in obesity and neoplasms and as a result of abnormalities of lipid metabolism may cause a yellow color. Normal lipid-containing structures, such as Fordyce's granules, usually appear as yellow papules. A localized accumulation of fat, such as a fat-producing neoplasm (lipoma or liposarcoma), produces a yellow lesion with the morphologic characteristics of a nodule or tumor. A localized deposition of fatty substances may occur in systemic abnormalities of lipid metabolism. These appear as papules, nodules, or plaques.

Extrinsic stains of tissues, especially of white lesions, may cause a yellowish color. For example, the use of tobacco may cause a white lesion to assume a yellowish color. Extrinsic stains usually involve hyperkeratotic areas, such as plaques or nodules. Yellow may appear in any morphologic type, with the possible exception of a bulla.

Translucent lesions

Many blisterform lesions can be distinguished from nonblisterform lesions by their translucent quality. Lesions that appear translucent are blisterform lesions. The translucency and the associated color of oral lesions can be significant factors in differential diagnosis. Both the translucency and associated color change of a lesion are accurate indicators as to the nature of the fluid content and its proximity to the surface. Translucent pink lesions usually indicate an accumulation of a relatively clear fluid, such as serum, mucin, or lymph. The covering mucosa has a relatively normal thickness. Blue translucent lesions may indicate clear fluid or blood accumulation. The blue color from clear fluid accumulation indicates a superficial lesion covered by a thin mucosa that causes absorption of most of the visible wavelengths of light, except blue, which is reflected. Red or purple translucent lesions usually indicate blood accumulation, which may be either intravascular or extravascular. Most lesions that demonstrate a translucent quality are bullae or vesicles.

Summary

The nine colors associated with oral soft tissue lesions have been reviewed. Pink, red, white, and combinations of red and white are the most common colors encountered, whereas blue, yellow, purple, gray, brown, and black are uncommon colors for oral lesions. It should be evident after this review that pure colors are extremely rare when dealing with soft tissue pathosis. The primary and secondary factors causing and influencing tissue colors are varied and complex. It should be noted that blue and gray lesions may be extremely difficult to distinguish. In general, the more common colors such as pink, red, white, and red and white are less significant in leading to a differential diagnosis; however, colors such as blue, gray, yellow, purple, black, and brown may be highly significant in making diagnoses.

TEXTURE OF LESIONS

One other characteristic of lesions that may yield significant diagnostic information is surface textural change. These changes often indicate secondary changes to previous existing lesions and may be related to local irritation, secondary inflammatory changes, or habits. For example, the rough white surface associated with mechanical friction is commonly referred to as frictional keratosis. This change indicates an excessive accumulation of keratin and is somewhat analogous to the scale characteristics of numerous skin lesions.

A corrugated white textural change is often associated with long-term tobacco use, particularly snuff use.

Irregular, shaggy, sloughing, or desquamating epithelial remnants may indicate secondary change as a result of ruptured or collapsed bullae. This textural change can also occur with chewing, biting or other nervous habits, or chemical burns; it may also be characteristic of such diseases as candidiasis and of contact allergy reactions.

Crust formation represents an additional texture change, and it was explained under Yellow Lesions.

Careful analysis and consideration of all these lesion characteristics must be an integral part of the diagnostic process.

OTHER MISCELLANEOUS TERMS

contusion (bruise) A superficial injury, usually painful or tender, produced by impact without laceration, which may or may not have color change because of hemorrhage.

erosion A depressed lesion that results from the incomplete loss of the epithelial surface.

eschar A slough produced by burning or a corrosive application.

fissure A linear cleavage that may or may not extend through the epithelial surface.

pseudomembrane A membranous layer of exudate containing organisms, precipitated fibrin, necrotic cells, and inflammatory cells that is produced by an inflammatory reaction on the surface of a tissue.

slough A mass of dead tissue.

telangiectasia Permanently dilated, superficial small vessels.

annular Shaped like a ring.

punctate Resembling or marked with points or dots.

reticular Resembling a net.

stellate Shaped like a star.

verrucal Resembles or is shaped like a wart.

In addition to accurate descriptions of the size, morphologic type, color, and textural characteristics, there is often other pertinent information that should accompany the above data. The duration of the lesions, the presence of other lesions, change in character of the lesions, and associated systemic disease are factors that may greatly assist the clinician in making a more specific diagnosis.

REFERENCE

1. Halstead, C.L., and Weathers, D.R.: Differential diagnosis of oral soft tissue pathosis, morphology and color units, S-3380 and S-3381, Washington, D.C., 1977, National Audiovisual Center (NAC).

7 Vital signs

The vital signs include blood pressure, pulse rate, respiration rate, and temperature. These important indicators of health (vital: pertaining to life) are normally measured as part of the physical evaluation procedure and are traditionally recorded at regular intervals on all hospitalized patients. These intervals may vary from once-a-day recordings for the relatively healthy patient to frequent recordings (perhaps continual recordings) for the critically ill patient.

Measurements of weight and height are sometimes categorized as "vital signs," although these are not true indicators of life. It is seldom necessary for the general dentist to be concerned with a patient's height and weight, although orthodontists and pedodontists interested in skeletal growth patterns may find these values to be very important. Considerable variations from the normal height-weight ratios may indicate disease. For some conditions weight registrations may be necessary one or more times a day. Extreme weight gain, such as that which occurs in abnormalities of fluid retention or hypothyroidism, or the rapid weight loss seen in uncontrolled diabetes or in certain widespread malignant diseases may require that careful weight recordings be made at relatively short intervals.

This chapter deals with the techniques of detecting and recording blood pressure, pulse, respiration, and temperature and briefly reviews the more common variations that the dentist may encounter.

BLOOD PRESSURE

Several factors influence blood pressure. Cardiac output clearly plays an important role, as does the blood volume and the viscosity of the blood. The vessels, particularly the arterioles, are very important. They can dilate or constrict, thereby tending to lower or raise the blood pressure. The composition of the vessel walls will significantly affect the pressure within their lumina. Between each contraction of the heart the pressure within the arterial system varies between a maximal (systolic) pressure and a minimal (diastolic) pressure. The difference between these two levels, the pulse pressure, is determined by the condition of the arterial walls. For example, if the normally elastic walls lose their elasticity and become more rigid, they may be unable to "absorb" the pulse wave generated by each contraction of the ventricle. Consequently, the systolic pressure would rise, leading to an increase in the pulse pressure.

One of the earliest attempts to measure blood pressure was made at the end of the eighteenth century by Hales, who placed a glass tube in the femoral artery of a mare. The blood rose over 8 feet in the tube! It was noted that alterations in the blood pressure occurred with each heartbeat and respiration. This technique of measuring blood pressure has little use these days. Nowadays blood pressure is usually determined indirectly by the sphygmomanometer method (sphygmos: pulse). Direct methods of measuring blood pressure will naturally be more accurate than the indirect sphygmomanometric method. Sometimes, when it is most necessary for the physician to determine blood pressure very accurately, intraarterial recording devices are used. However, for most purposes, the indirect sphygmomanometric method is considered accurate enough.

Riva-Rocci (an Italian physician) developed the indirect method at the end of the nineteenth century. The sphygmomanometer consists of an inflatable bag covered by a cuff, an inflating bulb that permits the intrabag pressure to be increased, an exhaust valve by which the pressure in the bag can be lowered and the lowering carefully controlled, and a manometer that registers the pressure within the bag (Fig. 7-1). The two most common sphygmomanometers in current use are the mercury gravity and the aneroid. The special advantages and disadvantages of each are discussed later.

The unyielding cuff is applied to a limb, usually the arm, and then inflated so that increasing pressure is applied to the limb, compressing the underlying tissues. The blood vessels are compressed, and if there is sufficient pressure, their lumina are occluded. The pressure within the cuff is indicated at all times by the manometer.

An assessment of the arterial pressure can be made in several ways. The occlusion of a major limb vessel by the inflated cuff will result in the absence of a pulse distal to the cuff. If the pressure within the cuff is gradually reduced, a point will be reached at which the systolic pressure within the vessel can overcome the extraluminal pressure and permit a pulse wave to travel beyond the cuff. Pulsation in the arteries distal to the cuff may be detected with the fingers. It is

believed that the pressure registered in the cuff at this time will normally be some 10 to 15 mm Hg below the true systolic blood pressure. An alternative method of assessing the blood pressure is recording the pulsations of the air in the cuff by an oscillometer, the first appearance of oscillations indicating the systolic blood pressure, and the point of maximal oscillation the diastolic blood pressure. Although these two techniques may be of some value occasionally, it is much more usual for blood pressure to be measured indirectly by the auscultatory method. This technique involves hearing the sounds that the blood makes in a major artery immediately distal to an occluding pressure cuff in which the pressure is gradually reduced.

These sounds were first described by Korotkoff in the early part of the twentieth century. Their significant

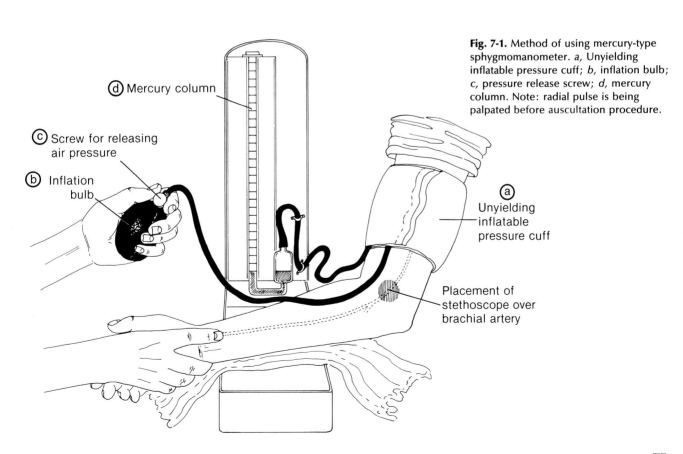

Fig. 7-1. Method of using mercury-type sphygmomanometer. *a,* Unyielding inflatable pressure cuff; *b,* inflation bulb; *c,* pressure release screw; *d,* mercury column. Note: radial pulse is being palpated before auscultation procedure.

ⓓ Mercury column

ⓒ Screw for releasing air pressure

ⓑ Inflation bulb

ⓐ Unyielding inflatable pressure cuff

Placement of stethoscope over brachial artery

features are as follows: as the pressure in the occluding cuff falls, the first spurt of blood that passes through the almost completely constricted artery beneath the cuff distends the wall of the artery, producing the first sound. This clear, tapping sound is coincident with each systolic beat. As the pressure falls, the sound increases in intensity and then changes, and a murmur becomes apparent. This murmur then disappears, and the intermittent tapping sounds become crisper and louder. This phase is then followed by an abrupt loss of the sound, or a change to a soft blowing sound. It should be understood by anyone beginning to learn blood pressure recording techniques that the various Korotkoff sounds may not always be heard easily. The systolic pressure is normally that point at which the initial tapping sound can be heard for at least two consecutive beats. It has been shown that the systolic pressure recorded in this way is normally only a few millimeters lower than that which would be obtained by direct measurement within the artery. The diastolic pressure is usually recorded as that point at which the heart sounds suddenly disappear or change quality. Further reference is made to this later in the section Technique of Recording Blood Pressure.

In view of the widespread practice of determining and recording patients' blood pressure in dental practice, the subject is covered in considerable detail. The following is based on the American Heart Association's recommendations for human blood pressure determination using sphygmomanometers.

Selection of cuff

It is important that the bag and cuff be appropriate for the patient. Since arm sizes vary, the inflatable bag must be the correct size. If it is too narrow, the blood pressure reading will be too high, and if the bag is too wide, then the reading will be too low. It is recommended that the bag be 20% wider than the diameter of the arm. The average adult patient requires a bag of about 12 to 14 cm wide. Smaller cuffs for children or wider ones for obese adults (or for blood pressure measurements that have to be made on the thigh) are available. The main factor in selecting the right cuff is the size of the arm itself, not the age of the patient.

The inflatable bag must be placed over the artery to be compressed. The cuff should be unyielding so that even pressure can be exerted throughout the cuff. It should be wrapped around the arm and secured in place. Fastening may be done by tucking the tail of the cuff into itself, by metal fasteners, of by simply pressing mating surfaces of an interlocking fabric together. It is important that this be securely done, because a slipping cuff will tend to give a higher false value.

Manometers

There are several points to remember concerning the use of either a mercury gravity or an aneroid manometer.

Mercury gravity manometer. Care must be taken not to lose mercury from the instrument and to ensure that the mercury "at rest" is always at zero. The mercury column should be vertical when it is read. The tubes containing the mercury must be cleaned regularly, and the air vent at the top of the mercury manometer column must be open, as clogging will affect the mercury column's rise and fall.

Aneroid manometer. Modern aneroid manometers, if well cared for (cleaned and checked periodically), can be as accurate as mercury gravity instruments. In these instruments a metal bellows elongates with pressure, and this elongation is transferred to a needle and scale. The aneroid manometer should be calibrated regularly over a wide range of values. Calibration is easily done by connecting an aneroid manometer by a Y connector to a mercury manometer and then comparing values.

Inflating bulbs and valves. Bulbs and valves should be checked to see that there are no leaks and that the valves, both inlet and exhaust, are functioning satisfactorily.

Stethoscope. A wide variety of styles of stethoscopes are available, and any one of several standard types (in good repair) is adequate. A brief discussion about the various types of stethoscopes is given in Chapter 12.

Technique of recording blood pressure

The person recording the blood pressure should be sitting or standing comfortably and should be able to see the manometer easily. If a mercury manometer is used, the observer's eye should be level with the mercury column meniscus. In view of the lability of blood pressure in some people, it is important that the pressure be taken on several occasions.

The patient should be seated comfortably with the arm fixed and the forearm supported on a flat surface at the level of the heart (Fig. 7-1). Readings taken in the standing or lying positions should be recorded and specified as having been determined in those positions, for example, RA (right arm), L (lying), or St (standing).

In some people, pressures may vary considerably among the sitting, standing, and lying positions. If possible, all factors that might conceivably affect blood pressure levels should be noted and recorded along with the blood pressure; examples of such factors include cold weather and patient pain, distress, or anxiety. The clothing on the upper arm should neither interfere with the placing of the cuff nor constrict the arm.

A full cardiovascular examination normally requires that the blood pressure be determined in both arms. In dental practice, however, unless there is some definite indication, it is more usual to record the pressure in one arm only. The deflated cuff should be applied to the arm about 2.5 cm above the antecubital space with the rubber bag applied over the inner aspect of the arm. An evaluation of systolic pressure should be made first by palpation, that is, by obliterating the brachial or radial arterial pulse by inflating the bag, then gradually deflating it and determining the level at which the brachial or radial pulse can first be felt returning. The bag should next be completely deflated and then reinflated, this time with the stethoscope placed over the brachial artery. The previous palpation of the brachial artery will permit the observer to determine exactly where the stethoscope should be placed. The stethoscope should be firmly applied against the skin, but not pressed, as heavy pressure can distort the artery and affect the sounds heard. The stethoscope should be free, not touching any clothing or the pressure cuff. The bag should be inflated to about 30 mm Hg above the point at which the pulse disappears and then released at a rate of about 2 to 3 mm Hg per heartbeat. Faster or slower deflation may cause errors.

As soon as the cuff pressure falls to just below systolic pressure, blood slips through the artery during the peak of systolic pressure, and the observer hears tapping sounds coincident with each heartbeat. This level, the onset of tapping sounds, should be recorded as the systolic pressure. As the pressure in the cuff is lowered further, the sounds continue their tapping quality until the pressure falls to equal diastolic pressure. Below this pressure the artery is no longer compressed during systole, which means that the basic factor causing the sound is no longer present.

The tapping quality of the sound changes to a muffled quality, or the sounds may disappear entirely. The diastolic pressure will normally be recorded when the sound quality changes from a tapping to a muffled sound or becomes inaudible. The neophyte should not be too concerned if at first there is difficulty in identifying

each of the various Korotkoff sounds. In some patients there may be an audible sound down to 0 mm Hg. In such cases the diastolic point is considered to be that level at which the regular tapping sounds suddenly change their quality, becoming muffled and less intense with more thumping than tapping.

Some hypertensive patients demonstrate an auscultatory gap. For example, a person with a systolic pressure of, say, 190 mm Hg may demonstrate the usual sharp tapping sounds as the sphygmomanometer cuff pressure is reduced down from 190 mm Hg. These sounds may then become inaudible, return again at around 140 mm Hg, and then finally change, indicating diastolic pressure. Clearly, if the blood pressure cuff were pumped up only to 160 mm Hg at the beginning of the blood pressure determination, then an erroneous systolic pressure might be recorded. It is always wise to gain a rough estimate of the blood pressure by palpating the pulse before auscultation.

BLOOD PRESSURE DETERMINATION STEP BY STEP

1. Seat patient comfortably.
2. Place and support forearm level with heart with palm up.
3. Move clothing to expose upper arm. Apply proper cuff snugly and fasten.
4. Identify brachial or radial artery and inflate bag to obliterate arterial pulse. Deflate bag and estimate systolic pressure when pulse returns.
5. Place stethoscope over brachial artery.
6. Inflate bag to about 30 mm Hg above estimated systolic pressure.
7. Deflate bag slowly, say, 2 to 3 mm Hg per heartbeat.
8. Record systolic pressure at onset of tapping sounds.
9. Record diastolic pressure when sounds become muffled or inaudible.

10. Wait until bag completely deflates (at least 20 to 30 seconds) before taking blood pressure.

PULSE

Palpation of the pulse is an ancient practice in medicine. The pulse is produced by the force imparted to the arterial blood each time the left ventricle contracts and expels blood into the aorta. The pulse wave travels through the various arteries, arriving at the wrist about 0.1 to 0.2 second after the contraction. The blood itself takes much longer to make the journey from the aorta to the wrist.

The pulse wave depends on the stroke volume (the quantity of blood expelled at each ventricular contraction), the "force" of expulsion, and the rigidity of the blood vessels. The pulse is most usually examined at the wrist by palpating the radial artery. Other convenient sites to examine the pulse are the neck (carotid), temporal region (temporal), groin (femoral), knee (popliteal), the posterior tibial artery at the ankle, and the dorsalis pedis vessel on the foot.

When the radial pulse is examined, the patient's hand should be held palm upward with the examiner's middle three fingers gently placed over the artery, the index finger being the nearest the heart (Fig. 7-2). This technique facilitates evaluating the characteristics of the pulse and gaining information about the vessel wall. The following characteristics should be noted and recorded:

1. Rate.
2. Rhythm.
3. Character.
4. Volume.
5. Condition of the vessel wall.

Rate

The average pulse rate in adults is 60 to 80 per minute. In children the pulse rate is usually higher, 90 to 140. The heart rate is normally regular but shows slight variations with respiratory movements. During inspi-

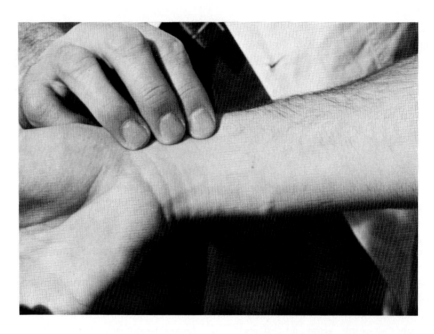

Fig. 7-2. Radial pulse is palpated by examiner with index finger closest to heart. Pressure on index finger and palpation of pulse by other fingers help determine thickness of vessel wall.

ration there is a slight acceleration of the pulse and during expiration a slight deceleration (sinus arrhythmia). A high pulse rate (tachycardia) is quite normal after eating, during and after exercise, and during emotional excitement. The pulse rate may be quite rapid during the physical examination and then return to normal levels when the patient relaxes. Tachycardia is seen in most febrile diseases, and there is a relationship between the elevated pulse rate and the temperature rise. Increased pulse rates occur frequently in anemia, after a severe hemorrhage, in thyrotoxicosis, and persistently in certain forms of heart disease. The dentist should be aware of the condition of paroxysmal atrial tachycardia (PAT). This condition is characterized by episodes of very fast heart rates. They may last for a few minutes or as long as weeks. These attacks do not necessarily signify underlying heart disease, but the extreme tachycardias may produce symptoms in the chest and head, and patients may become quite disturbed by the attacks.

Bradycardia, or slowing of the pulse, may be found in well-trained athletes and in patients with some disease states, such as myxedema and certain infections. Disturbances of the heart's conduction system may produce degrees of heart block to the degree that the ventricle contracts less frequently or so inefficiently that the aortic valve is not opened and no pulse is sent to the peripheral vascular system. Such circumstances may lead to a "pulse deficit"; that is, the pulse rate at the wrist will be less than the number of beats felt over the chest. Severe degrees of heart block may lead to Adams-Stokes attacks, in which patients develop very slow pulse rates and may suffer from cerebral arterial insufficiency and lose consciousness.

Rhythm

Apart from the slight variations in rate that occur during respiration (sinus arrhythmia), the normal pulse has a regular rhythm. Abnormalities of rhythm can be considered in two main groups: (1) regular irregularities and (2) irregular irregularities.

Regular irregularities may appear in several forms, and some specific terms have been applied to such pulses: *pulsus paradoxus* (the pulse becomes weaker or disappears at the end of inspiration) occurs in pericardial effusions; *pulsus alternans* (alternate strong and weak beats) occurs in severe myocardial damage. Generally, such variations are better appreciated by examining the electrocardiogram.

Irregular irregularities may appear when the atrium is fibrillating; that is, when there is a totally uncoordinated, irregular contraction of the atrial muscle, the pulse is totally irregular. Impulses from the atrial muscle arrive at the atrial ventricular (AV) node at different times. Some arrive when the AV node is refractory, and others arrive when it can respond to and transmit them to the ventricle. The net effect is that the ventricle beats irregularly, and because for some beats the ventricle is stimulated to contract before it has time to fill completely, there is a variable volume of blood expelled each time. The volume of the pulse therefore also varies. Atrial fibrillation may develop in several conditions, such as thyrotoxicosis or heart disease, and may exist for many years. It should not necessarily be considered an indicator of serious disease, and an irregular pulse should not always be considered a portent of imminent catastrophe. Premature ventricular contractions (sometimes called extrasystoles or PVCs) are very common but do not necessarily indicate serious heart disease. The heart "skips a beat." The ventricle contracts prematurely, and then there is a pause until the heart regains its normal rhythm. When a series of ectopic beats occurs for every second beat, the pulsus bigeminus results (coupled rhythm). A normal beat is followed quickly by a second slightly weaker beat (the ventricle did not have time to fill completely), followed by a prolonged pause, and then the process starts again. Extrasystoles are usually reduced or abolished by exercise.

Character

The character or form of an individual pulse wave may be of diagnostic value, particularly when there is cardiac valvular disease. Although pulse waves are better evaluated from a tracing than from palpation, the skilled examiner may learn much by concentrating on the form of a pulse.

One example of a pulse that can be readily detected on palpation is the so-called collapsing pulse. This is found in aortic incompetence. At the end of systole, because the aortic valves are incompetent, blood falls back from the aorta into the relaxing ventricle, and the aortic pressure falls dramatically. The body compensates for this "loss" of blood during each beat by increasing the systolic pressure and stroke volume. This increase of systolic pressure and the much lower diastolic pressure result in a large pulse pressure (the difference between systolic and diastolic pressures). A large pulse pressure results in a sudden rise and then a sudden fall in the pulse—the pulse is full but of short duration. Such a collapsing pulse has been described frequently as a "water hammer pulse."* The pulse in aortic stenosis is the opposite of that seen in aortic insufficiency. The pulse is small and rises and falls slowly.

---

*A water hammer was a nineteenth century toy consisting of a glass tube about 10 inches long, which was about one third filled with water. The air was evacuated from the tube before filling, and consequently, when the tube was inverted, the water fell through the vacuum as a solid body and produced a short, hard tap as it hit the bottom of the tube.

Volume

The pulse volume is the movement of the arterial wall during the passage of the pulse wave. It can be readily evaluated by gently pressing the index finger against the vessel. Generally, if there is no other vascular obstruction, the pulse volume is related to the left ventricular stroke volume. A *full* pulse is found during and after exercise, in fevers, and in certain emotional states. A *weak* pulse occurs after severe hemorrhage and in other types of shock. It is often referred to in these circumstances as "thready." In older people, thickening or calcification of vessel walls may reduce the pulse volume. In certain arrhythmias there is a variation in the volume of each pulse. Reference has already been made to the fact that, if the ventricle beats before it has been adequately filled, then the output for that stroke will be reduced.

Condition of the vessel wall

Some information concerning the vessel wall may be obtained while the pulse is being examined. If the examination is conducted in the way shown in Fig. 7-2, sufficient pressure should be exerted by the index finger to empty the blood vessel. This vessel should then be rolled against the bone by the distal two fingers. In young people the empty artery should not be palpable, but in older people the vessel wall may be thickened or even calcified and feel tortuous or like a "pipe stem."

RESPIRATION

The examination of the respiratory system, including the chest, is discussed in more detail in Chapter 12. In the present section the main features of the respiratory movements that should be noted and evaluated in a routine "vital signs" examination are discussed. These factors include:

1. Rate.
2. Rhythm.
3. Type.

Rate

In the normal healthy adult the frequency of respiration at rest is about 14 to 18 per minute. As respiration is normally an involuntary movement, it is a good practice to note the respiratory rate without drawing the patient's attention to the fact that the respiratory movements are being counted. This can be conveniently done by noting the respirations while palpating the pulse. The ratio of pulse rate to respiration rate is usually 4 or 5 to 1. The rate may vary if the patient is aware of the examiner's measurement of the respirations. An increase in the respiration rate (tachypnea) may occur under different conditions. Tachypnea occurs in febrile diseases, during and after exercise, and during emotional excitement. The purpose of this increase is adaptation to a need for increased gas exchange as the result of increased metabolism. Some patients with conditions that interfere with gas exchange or that restrict the full expansion of the lungs, for example, pulmonary fibrosis, may breathe rapidly and shallowly. Hyperventilation may occur if the patient is very anxious or is suffering from severe brain damage, such as from a cerebral vascular accident. Hyperventilation may lead to a disturbance in consciousness, a result of the respiratory alkalosis that develops following excessive exhalation of carbon dioxide.

Rhythm

The control of respiration is a complex process involving not only the nervous system, but also the gaseous tensions of oxygen and carbon dioxide in the blood, and also the pH. In certain conditions the normal neurologic mechanisms go awry, and strange patterns of breathing develop. One of the most well recognized of these is Cheyne-Stokes breathing, a condition described by Hippocrates. It is believed that there is a decreased sensitivity of the respiratory center to carbon dioxide. The depth of breathing varies cyclically. The cycle, which may take 1 to 3 minutes, is characterized by a phase of no breathing (apnea), followed by the onset of shallow breaths that gradually become more and more intense and then cease, only to be followed by another period of apnea, starting a new cycle. Cheyne-Stokes respiration may occur with cardiac or renal disease, brain tumors, and meningitis.

Kussmaul respiration (heavy labored breathing) is seen in uncontrolled diabetic patients who have severe acidosis. Because the body attempts to exhale the excess acid, the patient breathes frequently and deeply. This ''air hunger'' may also be seen in renal acidosis or after certain drug intoxications.

Type

Most people inspire by using their intercostal muscles and diaphragm. Expiration is a more passive process, resulting from the elasticity of the lungs. Women generally use the intercostal muscles more than the diaphragm, and for men the opposite is true. Clearly, any pain arising in the chest wall, say from pleuritis, will inhibit chest movement, and the breathing will more likely be diaphragmatic. Such patients often ''catch their breath'' when the chest and lungs expand, causing the painful rub. Abdominal pain from a distended bowel or some other condition worsened by the descent of the diaphragm tends to encourage thoracic movements. Severe difficulty in breathing (dyspnea) may result from many different conditions; among them is obstruction of any part of the respiratory tree. Pulmonary edema, pulmonary embolism, or food or other foreign body impaction in the trachea may produce disturbances in the respiratory pattern (see Chapter 12). In asthma there is intense constriction of the bronchioles. This necessitates that the patient forcibly expire, a phase of respiration that is normally passive. One of the

characteristics of the asthmatic attack is the wheezing, which is more pronounced during the expiratory phase. If adequate ventilation cannot be obtained by the normal respiratory movements, additional movements are used. The accessory muscles of respiration, the cervical muscles, attempt to lift the thoracic cage to assist in the expansion of the thoracic cavity. Tension in these neck muscles and possibly distension of the alae of the nose usually indicate some respiratory difficulty. During this phase, particularly if there is some obstruction of the respiratory tract, there may be marked sucking in of the supraclavicular and suprasternal areas.

In severe cases of emphysema, in which the elasticity of the lung is insufficient to expel the air during the expiratory phase, the patient has to force the air out. This forced expiration can be accomplished by contracting the abdominal muscles, thereby increasing intraabdominal pressure and forcing the diaphragm up to increase the thoracic pressure. The muscles of the back, the latissimus dorsi, may also be used to pull the ribs together. Patients often sit upright, holding a chair firmly, as this ''firms'' the shoulders so that the latissimus dorsi muscles can be used exclusively for their effect on the chest wall.

TEMPERATURE

Galileo is credited with having invented the thermometer, and Santorio (1561-1636), Professor of Medicine at Padua, was the first physician to use a clinical thermometer. Systematic temperature records of patients were first begun in the middle of the nineteenth century, and now routine temperature recordings of hospital patients are commonplace. The range of body temperature does not normally exceed 98.6° F (37° C) by mouth or 99.6° F (37.5° C) by rectum. There is a normal diurnal variation, the temperature being lower in the morning and higher in the evening. It is occa-

sionally necessary for an axillary temperature reading to be made, and this is usually approximately 97.6° F (36.5° C). A variety of clinical thermometers are available, and the method of taking an oral temperature is so well known that a lengthy description is unnecessary, although one or two points are worthy of mention. Clinical thermometers may be classified as $^1/_2$-minute, 1-minute, and 2-minute instruments. These times indicate how long a particular thermometer should be left in place. They should be regarded as minimal times, as it is usually advisable to leave the thermometer in place for at least twice the recommended time. Recently, disposable temperature-sensitive individualized tapes have become available. When these are held in the patient's mouth for about 30 seconds, the temperature is shown in figures on the heat-sensitive tape.

It should be noted that the temperature of the skin does not necessarily relate to the body temperature. A hot drink just before an oral reading may give a falsely elevated temperature, a trick that has been used on occasions by malingerers feigning illnesses! The mercury thermometer, whether oral, anal, or axillary, should be well cared for, and, when it is appropriate, should be ''shaken down'' before using. Thermometers for oral temperatures and anal temperatures should be kept separate, and care taken that they are not mixed inadvertently. From the dentist's point of view, the oral temperature is nearly always satisfactory, and it is seldom necessary to seek anal or axillary readings. On occasion, when the dentist is dealing with a fractious or uncooperative child who refuses to permit the thermometer to be placed in the mouth, it may be necessary to take an axillary temperature. There are several ''dental'' conditions in which the temperature is elevated, including severe dental abscesses, cellulitides, and acute herpetic stomatitis.

SUMMARY

The vital signs are baseline indicators of disease. More detailed assessment of a patient may require definitive evaluation of the cardiovascular and respiratory systems. In Chapters 11 and 12 the basic examination of the heart and lungs is discussed.

BIBLIOGRAPHY

Guyton, A.C.: Textbook of medical physiology, ed. 6, Philadelphia, 1981, W.B. Saunders Co.

8   Head, face, and neck

Many important and complex structures are located in the relatively small region of the head, face, and neck. Within this small region there is a wide range of problems that can involve these structures either as primary disease or as local expression of systemic disease. Although significant or serious disease is detected infrequently in the routine dental patient, a careful examination of the head, face, and neck is important and can lead to the early detection of disease.

A sound knowledge of the normal structures in this area and of the techniques used in their examinations is essential in conducting a meaningful evaluation of the patient. When these examinations are performed in a thorough and diligent fashion, they can result in early diagnosis and treatment that significantly reduce mortality and morbidity.

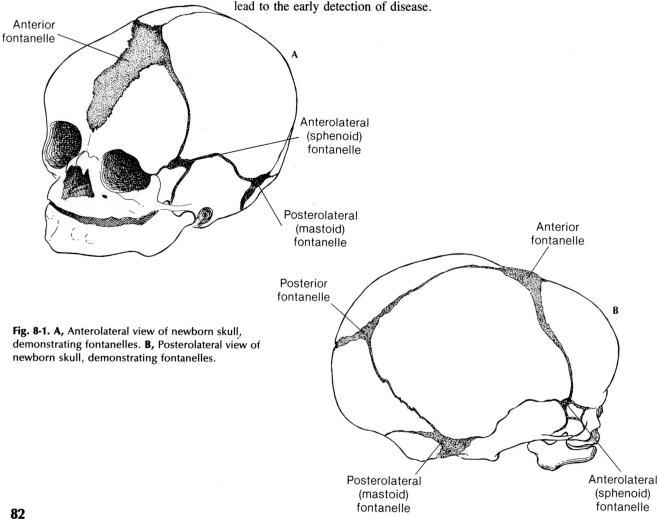

Fig. 8-1. A, Anterolateral view of newborn skull, demonstrating fontanelles. **B,** Posterolateral view of newborn skull, demonstrating fontanelles.

HEAD
Anatomy

At birth, the bones that compose the cranium are not fused and are separated by six membrane-filled gaps called fontanelles (Fig. 8-1). Usually these fontanelles are completely closed by ossification within 2 years after birth. The fibrous union between the cranial bones are referred to as sutures and fuse at maturity (Fig. 8-2). They appear as uneven and irregular lines on the skull. Secondary centers of ossification may appear in the suture lines and form small bones that are referred to as wormian bones.

The frontal bone develops as two bones with the frontal (metopic) suture between them. This suture usually disappears, but does persist in approximately 10% of the population. The point of intersection between the coronal and sagittal sutures is called the *bregma*. A similar intersection between the sagittal suture and lambdoidal suture is named the *lambda*. The highest point of the skull as seen from a lateral view is referred to as the *vertex*. Names for areas of the skull are usually derived from the names of the underlying bones (frontal, parietal, temporal, and occipital).

The skin covering the calvarium is referred to as the *scalp*. It is dense, uniformly thick, and tightly adherent to the bone. Hair normally covers the scalp.

Examination

A general observation is made of the head with special attention taken to note any abnormalities in size, shape, or symmetry. The character, condition, and distribution of the hair are observed. When involved by disease, it may become fine, coarse, or oily. Areas of hair loss or color change are noted. The scalp is inspected for changes in surface texture and lesions. Gentle palpation should be used to locate small nodules or areas of tenderness and to characterize any swelling.

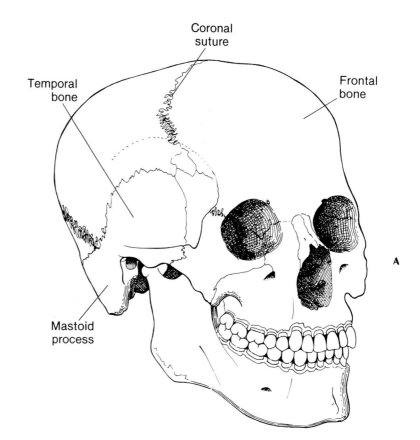

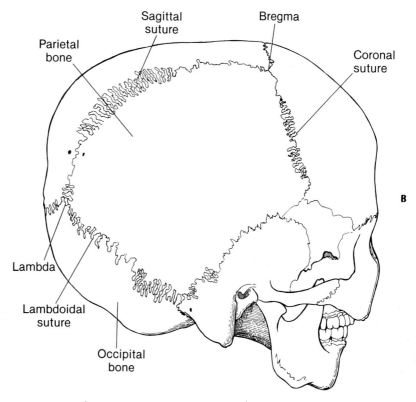

Fig. 8-2. A, Anterolateral view of adult skull, demonstrating sutures and bones. **B,** Posterolateral view of adult skull, demonstrating sutures and bones.

Abnormalities

Extreme variation in skull size is an easily noted and dramatic example of disease that usually has occurred during the first few years of life. As the brain enlarges during growth, the skull also enlarges so that it can accommodate the brain. If there is a lack of brain growth or a destructive lesion of the brain early in life, a small head (microcephaly) will result. Enlargement of the head (macrocephaly) occurs with abnormal enlargement of the brain (megalencephaly) or with an abnormal accumulation of fluid in the cranial cavity (hydrocephalus).

Normal skull shape depends on the proper sequential closing of sutures. The premature closure of cranial sutures (craniosynostosis) produces an unusual or deformed shape of the skull (craniostenosis). If a suture closes prematurely, compensatory growth occurs in other directions, and an abnormal head shape results. The head will become long and narrow (scaphocephaly or dolichocephaly) if the sagittal suture fuses too early. Premature fusion of the coronal suture causes the head to be wider than it is long (brachycephaly), producing a rounded head. Early closure of the coronal and another suture produces a pointed or tower skull (oxycephaly or turricephaly).

Fontanelles may not close but persist as "soft spots" in the skull. The anterior fontanelle is the largest of the six and usually is the most apparent. This lack of closure is found in a variety of syndromes, such as cleidocranial dysostosis and progeria.

Enlargement of the head in adults is usually the result of acquired diseases, such as acromegaly (Fig. 8-3) or Paget's disease. In patients with acromegaly there is an increase in the size of the head, hands, and feet. Rather coarse facial features result because of enlargement of the nose, lips, and mandible. The jaw may be quite prominent, and as a result of the enlargement there may be spacing between the teeth. Macroglossia

has also been noted. In Paget's disease a slow, asymptomatic enlargement of the calvarium occurs that produces an acorn-shaped head. Some patients complain of facial pain or headache. Classically, the patient becomes aware of the enlargement of the skull because of increasing hat size. The jaws may show marked enlargement if involved.

Endocrine disorders, chemical agents, genetic factors, nutritional factors, and severe chronic illness are a few of the reasons for the premature partial or complete loss of hair (alopecia). The most dramatic changes are seen in patients undergoing chemotherapy for cancer. Depending on the chemotherapeutic agents, some

patients may lose all their hair during therapy. Alopecia areata produces a patchy loss of hair that is usually asymptomatic and noticed by someone other than the patient. The patch is often rounded or oval, clearly defined, and increasing in size. Reportedly, patients with this problem are frequently under emotional stress. A patchy alopecia that has a "moth-eaten" appearance may be seen occasionally in patients with secondary syphilis.

Depigmentation that produces a few strands or a patch of white hair (poliosis) is found in patients with hereditary or acquired abnormalities. Among the hereditary defects are Waardenburg's syndrome and tuber-

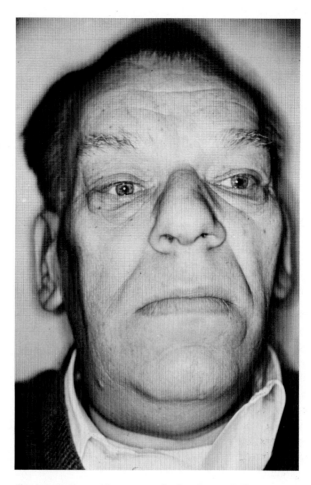

Fig. 8-3. Patient with acromegaly showing typical coarse facial features.

84

ous sclerosis. Permanent loss of hair pigment may occur after localized inflammatory disease or radiation injury to the scalp.

Endocrine disorders can produce changes in hair character, distribution, and growth. In hypothyroidism the hair becomes coarse, dry, and brittle. In hyperthyroidism the hair tends to be fine and soft, and there may be thinning.

Lesions of psoriasis, lichen planus, and lupus erythematosus are found on the scalp. These diseases usually involve other regions of the body concurrently and are more apparent in those locations. These skin lesions are discussed in Chapter 10. Seborrheic keratosis, a circumscribed, greasy, pigmented plague, is common in older patients and may be found not only on the scalp but also on the face and upper trunk. Cysts and tumors occur in the scalp, but infrequently. The most common lesion is a sebaceous cyst that appears as a well-defined mobile nodule with a doughy consistency. In elderly patients the sudden appearance of solitary or multiple nodules should arouse a suspicion of metastatic carcinoma.

FACE
Anatomy

The face develops through a rather complex system of union and fusion of "processes" and is a composite of a number of anatomic structures. It is difficult to characterize the end result, the normal adult face, other than to note that it shows relative symmetry and harmony. The symmetry is not absolute in that slight deviations are seen with critical observation. A "sense" of the appearance of the normal face is developed through general observations in everyday situations and frequent contacts with patients.

Developmental and acquired abnormalities usually produce a defect or asymmetry that is apparent to the careful examiner. The normal dentition is important in providing support for the facial tissues. This becomes most apparent as individuals become edentulous. Their facial tissues lose tone and collapse.

Landmarks such as the nasolabial groove, philtrum, and labiomental groove are useful in identifying disease or specifying the location of abnormalities (Fig. 8-4). These landmarks or surface anatomy may be altered by facial paralysis, space-occupying lesions, or other similar problems. Discussion of the surface anatomy of the eyes, ears, and nose is presented in Chapter 9.

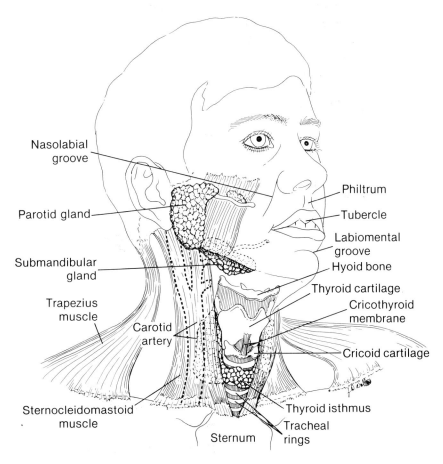

Fig. 8-4. Surface anatomy and major structures of head and neck.

Examination

When the face is inspected, the size and location of landmarks on each side are compared. The general symmetry of structures and movement are noted. Isolated large areas of swelling are usually apparent, but diffuse swellings may be subtle, requiring more than a casual glance to detect.

Facial expressions can show evidence of organic disease, particularly neurologic disease, but may also provide a great deal of information about the emotional status of the patient. The face can express a range of emotions, such as happiness, sadness, surprise, anger, disgust, and fear. The appearance or movement of facial areas such as the forehead-brows, eyes-lids, and mouth-chin-jaw can convey useful and important information. For this reason the face deserves constant study during the initial examination and at subsequent visits.

Palpation is primarily used to detect small tissue masses and to identify the character of larger swellings (see Chapter 3). When the lips and cheeks are palpated, a bidigital (thumb and index finger) technique should be used so that the tissue is supported. In areas supported by bone, the tissue should be palpated by direct pressure with the fingertips. Since a significant number of tumors occur in the parotid region, this area should be examined carefully to facilitate early detection of lesions.

Abnormalities

Patients with Parkinson's disease have a mask-like, expressionless face. They remain immobile for prolonged periods, have diminished eye blinking, and tend to drool. Some patients with hyperthyroidism may have a startled and anxious appearance characterized by protruding eyes (exophthalmos, Fig. 8-5). In Down's syndrome (monogolism) the eyes slant upward and outward and have a medial epicanthal fold. The nose appears broad and flat, and the ears are set low.

In myxedema (hypothyroidism) the face appears puffy and swollen. The nose is broad and the eyelids are edematous. The eyebrows and lashes may be sparse. Patients with Cushing's syndrome have a rounded face referred to as "moon facies." Preauricular fullness and bulging cheeks occur because of fat deposition and produce this rounded appearance. In females, acne and hirsutism are also frequently seen. The hair appears as a fine downy coat on the forehead and face. Patients who are receiving prolonged or large doses of steroids will show changes similar to those seen in Cushing's syndrome. Although wide separation of the eyes (ocular hypertelorism) is an infrequent finding, its presence usually suggests that the patient has other birth defects.

Facial paralysis ranging from a mild facial weakness to a disfiguring palsy occurs with a lesion of the seventh cranial (facial) nerve (see Chapter 14). On the affected side of the face these patients cannot close their eyelids, smile, or show their teeth. The corner of the mouth droops, and the nasolabial fold disappears. If the lesion involving the nerve is peripheral, they also cannot wrinkle their foreheads. The forehead can be wrinkled when the lesion occurs in the brain. The most common reason for facial paralysis is Bell's palsy (see Chapter 14). It may also be seen in the Ramsay Hunt syndrome, the Melkersson-Rosenthal syndrome, uveoparotid fever (Heerfordt's disease), malignant parotid tumors and vascular lesions or tumors of the brain. Unilateral and bilateral drooping (ptosis) of the eyelids caused by weakness of the ocular muscle may be the first sign of myasthenia gravis. Subsequent weakness of the facial muscles results in a smooth and relatively immobile facies. Patients complain of easy fatique with mastication and speech. The speech becomes feeble and develops a nasal quality.

Fig. 8-5. Marked exophthalmos in patient with hyperthyroidism.

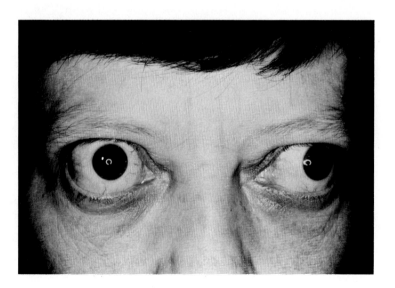

The facial profile reflects the relationship of the patient's jaws. A retruded mandible (Angle's Class II) is characterized by a small jaw that may be the result of the patient's genetic makeup or may represent the sequela of injury to the growth centers before development is complete. When there is a prognathic relationship (Angle's Class III) the mandible is proportionally too large. Again, this may reflect the patient's genetic makeup, which is usually the case, or represent changes in a disease such as acromegaly.

Mandibular asymmetry accounts for most individuals who have developmental facial asymmetry (Fig. 8-6). There is continued growth in either the condyle or body of the mandible, which produces a unilaterally enlarged mandible, a shift in the midline, and varying degrees of malocclusion. These changes range from subtle to severe. More dramatic changes are seen in patients who have hemifacial hypertrophy. The soft tissues and bone of both the facial and

oral structures are enlarged in these individuals. This enlargement is almost always apparent at birth and at times may involve half the body. Conversely, a striking loss of soft tissue is seen in hemifacial atrophy (Romberg's syndrome). This atrophy is unilateral and progresses to produce a distinct facial deformity. In advanced stages, both the muscle and bone become atrophied.

Facial clefts may follow a variety of patterns and be quite variable in their expression. The defect produced may be extremely severe or appear only as a cutaneous scar or depression. A lateral facial cleft will produce a macrostomia. A cleft of the upper lip, which is the most common, occurs in about 1 per 1000 white births, and may involve the nostril. Clefts are usually unilateral, though they may be bilateral, and are found most frequently on the left side (70%). Oblique facial clefts, median cleft upper lip, and median cleft lower lip do occur, but they are rare.

Small nodules or masses may be found in the cheek. These swellings may indicate enlarged buccal lymph nodes or epidermal cysts. Distinguishing one from the other may be difficult. The epidermal cysts are well circumscribed and mobile, and they usually appear tethered to the surface. Buccal lymph nodes tend to be deeper in the tissue and may be tender. Infrequent adnexal tumors may simulate these lesions. Mandibular lymph nodes that are located on the lateral surface of the posterior mandible may become enlarged when the site of an oral lesion is drained. Unless the examiner is familiar with their location and character, a tumor may be erroneously suspected.

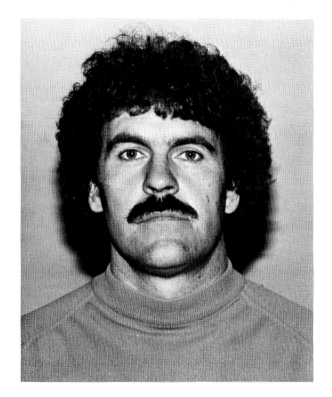

Fig. 8-6. Patient with mild facial asymmetry as a result of right mandibular hypertrophy.

Localized or diffuse parotid enlargement may occur for a variety of reasons. The swelling itself is usually relatively nonspecific, but additional information provided by a history and specific characteristics of the swelling (consistency, tenderness, and extent) frequently helps categorize the nature of the problem. Isolated parotid lymph nodes may become enlarged and simulate tumors. The reason for lymphadenopathy is frequently not apparent on examination, and as a result an enlarged node may be managed as a possible tumor. Benign parotid tumors usually are painless and nontender (Fig. 8-7). They are slow-growing and feel relatively firm. Malignant tumors tend to occur in an older age group and enlarge relatively rapidly (Fig. 8-8). They are firm to hard and usually fixed to the surrounding tissue. These lesions may invade nerves to produce pain or paralysis. At times the surface ulcerates.

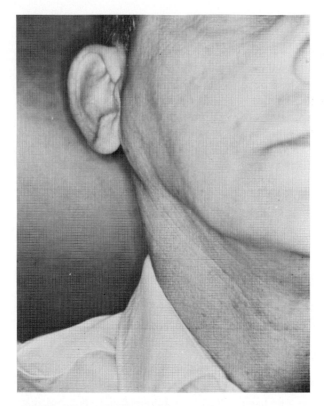

Fig. 8-7. Patient with pleomorphic adenoma in right parotid gland that has produced a diffuse swelling anterior to ear.

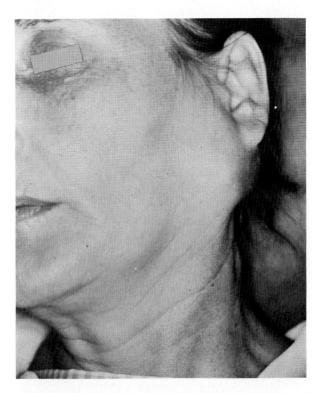

Fig. 8-8. Rapidly growing adenocarcinoma of parotid gland that is about to perforate skin.

Diffuse unilateral or bilateral enlargement may be related to nutritional deficiencies, drug idiosyncrasies, or involvement by systemic disease. Salivary gland enlargement is seen in alcoholics (Fig. 8-9). The exact mechanism is not know but is probably related to nutritional deficiencies. Enlargement has also been associated with diabetes, though its relationship is not clear. Diseases such as sarcoidosis, leukemia, and lymphoma can involve the parotid and produce localized or diffuse swelling. This involvement of the parotid gland by a systemic disease has been referred to as *Mikulicz's syndrome*.

A diffuse, firm, and usually painless parotid enlargement occurs in approximately one third of patients who have an autoimmune disease of the salivary glands, Sjögren's syndrome. The syndrome is characterized by dryness of the eyes, mouth, and other mucous membranes. Frequently these patients have an associated connective tissue disease, the most common being rheumatoid arthritis. When this autoimmune disease is localized in the salivary and lacrimal glands, the terms *benign lymphoepithelial lesion* and *Mikulicz's disease* have been used.

The parotid gland may be involved by obstructive disease, but far less frequently than the submandibular salivary gland. Classically these patients have swelling and tenderness of the obstructed gland that occurs during meals and persists for hours afterwards. Acute suppurative parotitis appears as a sudden and tender swelling. The gland may feel rather doughy or tense. A purulent discharge can almost always be expressed from the orifice of the gland. This type of parotitis is seen most frequently in debilitated and dehydrated individuals. Mumps (epidemic parotitis) appears as a diffuse and tender, unilateral or bilateral (75%) swelling of the parotid glands. The papilla of Stensen's duct may be red and swollen. The patient, usually a young child, may have flu-like symptoms.

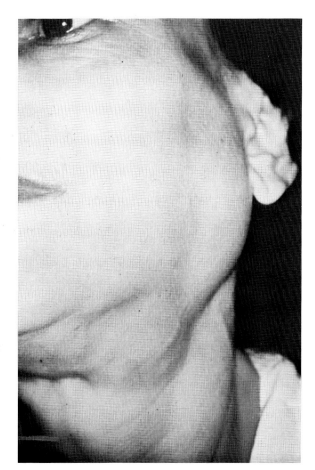

Fig. 8-9. Patient with long history of alcoholism who has marked enlargement of parotid and submandibular salivary glands.

NECK
Anatomy

A clear conception and understanding of the structures in the neck are essential for a good examination. Traditionally the neck is divided into two triangles by the major neck muscles, the sternocleidomastoid and trapezius. The anterior triangle is bounded superiorly by the mandible, laterally by the sternocleidomastoid muscle, and medially by the midline. The posterior triangle is bordered by the sternocleidomastoid muscle anteriorly, the trapezius muscle posteriorly, and the clavical inferiorly. During an examination the sternocleidomastoid muscle can be made more apparent and identifiable by turning the patient's head to the side opposite the side being examined.

The major structures of interest are found in the anterior triangles (Fig. 8-4). These are the hyoid bone, thyroid cartilage, cricoid cartilage, tracheal rings, and thyroid gland. The hyoid bone lies immediately below the mandible and can be best identified by palpating the area with the thumb and index finger. At times the greater horn of the hyoid is mistaken for a neck mass or lymph node. The thyroid cartilage is shaped somewhat like a shield and has a notch in its superior edge. The upper anterior area of the thyroid cartilage is more prominent than other areas and produces a projection on the neck termed the *laryngeal prominence* (Adam's apple), which is larger in males than in females. The superior edge is at the level where the common carotid artery bifurcates. Immediately below the thyroid cartilage, the cricoid cartilage can be identified. A small, distinct depression can usually be palpated between the thyroid and cricoid cartilages. This represents the cricothyroid space, which is covered by the cricothyroid membrane. If an emergency tracheostomy (cricothyreotomy) is inidcated, this space is used to establish an airway. The tracheal rings begin below the cricoid cartilage and are smaller and less rigid than the cricoid. They are palpable down to the jugular notch, which is located at the upper border of the sternum between the sternal heads of the sternocleidomastoid muscles.

The thyroid gland has two lateral lobes and an isthmus that connects the lobes at the lower third, resulting in a shape that somewhat resembles a butterfly. The isthmus is located immediately below the cricoid cartilage and extends laterally to the lobes. Curving posteriorly, the thyroid covers the lateral portion of the trachea and is itself covered by the sternocleidomastoid muscle.

The major vessels of the neck, the carotid artery and internal jugular vein, are located deep and medial to the sternocleidomastoid muscle. Careful and gentle palpation will readily identify the pulse of the carotid. The external jugular vein crosses the sternocleidomastoid muscle diagonally, running from near the angle of the mandible to the midclavicular region.

In the upper neck the transverse process of the atlas can be palpated below the ear and between the ramus and the sternocleidomastoid muscle. In thin and less muscular individuals the process is rather apparent and has been mistakenly interpreted as a soft tissue mass or enlarged lymph node.

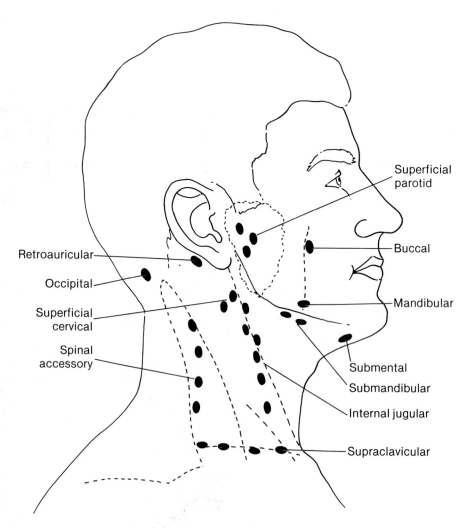

Fig. 8-10. Major lymph nodes found in head and neck region.

90

The distribution and number of lymph nodes found in the head and neck region are somewhat variable but sufficiently consistent to make general observations. So that there is continuity of information, the lymph nodes of the head, face, and neck are considered at the same time here. The terminology that is used is similar to that prepared by the International Anatomical Nomenclature Committee and published in *Nomina Anatomica*.

The lymph nodes accessible for palpation in the head and face are the occipital, retroauricular, parotid, buccal, and mandibular. They tend to have a horizontal distribution around the head (Fig. 8-10). The areas of drainage and discharge of the various nodes are listed below.

AREAS OF DRAINAGE AND DISCHARGE BY LYMPH NODE GROUPS

Occipital
Drain: Posterior scalp
Discharge: Spinal accessory nodes
Retroauricular
Drain: Adjacent scalp, posterior ear, back of external auditory meatus
Discharge: Internal jugular nodes
Parotid, superficial
Drain: Lateral and frontal scalp, lateral ear, external auditory canal, eyelids
Discharge: Superficial cervical nodes, internal jugular nodes
Parotid, deep
Drain: Parotid gland, orbit, lateral eyelids, conjunctiva, superficial parotid nodes
Discharge: Internal jugular nodes
Buccal
Drain: Medial eyelids, skin and mucous membranes of the nose and cheek
Discharge: Mandibular nodes
Mandibular
Drain: Same as buccal nodes
Discharge: Submandibular nodes

Submental
Drain: Tip of tongue, anterior floor of mouth, anterior lower gingiva, middle lower lip, chin
Discharge: Submandibular nodes
Submandibular
Drain: Submandibular salivary gland, lower and upper lip, cheeks, gingiva, teeth, anterior palatine pillar, soft palate, anterior two thirds of the tongue
Discharge: Internal jugular nodes
Superficial cervical
Drain: Parotid nodes
Discharge: Internal jugular nodes
Internal jugular
Drain: All above node groups, also directly from pharynx, tonsils, tongue, palate, larynx
Discharge: Subclavian vein right side, thoracic duct left side
Spinal accessory
Drain: Occipital nodes, retroauricular nodes, back of head, nape and lateral aspect of the neck
Discharge: Supraclavicular nodes
Supraclavicular
Drain: Spinal accessory nodes, posterior triangle, subclavicular nodes
Discharge: Joins inferior internal jugular nodes

The occipital nodes, ranging from one to three, are found along the course of the occipital artery. Usually there is only one retroauricular node, and it is located on the mastoid process. The parotid nodes are divided into the superficial and deep groups. The superficial group, varying in number from two to six, is on the surface of the parotid gland in front of and below the tragus. This group includes those that have been previously identified as the preauricular nodes. The deep group is made up of several nodes located within the parotid gland. The buccal nodes are rather inconstant and vary from none to two. When present, they are located on the buccinator muscle at the level of the angle of the mouth. The mandibular nodes are also an inconstant group. They range from none to two and are found on the lateral surface of the mandible near the inferior border and anterior to the masseter muscle.

The lymph nodes of the neck tend to have a more vertical distribution and consist of the submental, submandibular, superficial cervical, and deep cervical nodes. The submental nodes are situated between the anterior bellies of the digastric muscle and range from one to three. As many as three to six nodes may be found in the submandibular group. They are found medial to the mandible and slightly anterior to the submandibular salivary gland. At times some of these nodes are positioned on the surface of the submandibular salivary gland. The superficial cervical group consists of one to four nodes that are distributed along the external jugular vein as it passes over the upper portion of the sternocleidomastoid muscle. They probably represent a continuation of the parotid nodes.

The deep cervical group of nodes is divided into three chains: the internal jugular, the spinal accessory, and the supraclavicular. These chains form a triangle and blend together at the corners, making it difficult to determine which node belongs to which chain. The internal jugular nodes are the most important of the neck. They begin with the spinal accessory nodes near the angle of the mandible and follow the internal jugular vein down to the subclavian vein. They vary in number from 10 to 20. The spinal accessory nodes are distributed along the course of the eleventh cranial nerve and blend with the supraclavicular chain near the clavicle. The number of spinal accessory nodes varies from six to ten. The supraclavicular lymph nodes, which have also been called the transverse cervical chain, follow the transverse cervical artery. This chain joins the inferior portion of the internal jugular chain to empty into the subclavian vein on the right side and the thoracic duct on the left side. At times the nodes of the supraclavicular chain may be dispersed in the lower portion of the posterior triangle. The number of nodes ranges from six to ten.

There are two specific nodes in the internal jugular chain that require special mention because they are rather constant in location, usually larger than the others, and found with relative frequency. The jugular-digastric node is found below the posterior belly of the digastric muscle at the level of the greater horn of the hyoid bone. Because it drains the tonsil, it has also been referred to as the tonsillar node. The jugular-omohyoid node is located in the angle formed by the superior belly of the omohyoid and internal jugular vein.

Examination

Adequate access to the area is important. Clothing should be loose to allow for complete inspection and palpation. The first step is careful observation for asymmetry that may be produced by enlargement of glands or tumor masses. Inspection is facilitated by slight extension and rotation of the patient's head to the side opposite that being examined. This produces slight tension on the skin and muscles, allowing for better identification of the surface anatomy and any possible lesions.

The most useful information will be gained by thorough palpation. The entire neck should be assessed for masses and tenderness in a uniform fashion. Palpation should begin in the posterior region of the neck, moving over the lateral aspects to the anterior region. Two or three fingertips of one hand should be used in a slow, gentle, to-and-fro or rotary motion while the other hand supports or moves the head and neck for better access. Some prefer to palpate with both hands simultaneously so that one side can be compared with the other.

All areas where lymph nodes are located should be palpated. Palpation of the deep cervical chain is best accomplished by having the patient flex the head slightly to the side being examined. The fingertips of one hand should probe medial and deep to the sternocleidomastoid muscle while the other hand supports the muscle posteriorly. The entire area from the angle of the mandible to the clavicle must be examined. Again, some prefer bimanual palpation. This should be done from behind the patient, using the thumbs to support the muscle while the fingertips explore the area (Fig. 8-11).

A combination intra-extraoral (bimanual) technique of palpation (see Chapter 3) is best for investigation of the submental lymph nodes, submandibular lymph nodes, and submandibular salivary gland. Either the index or little finger of one hand should be placed intraorally on the floor of the mouth to stabilize the side being examined. Extraorally, the fingertips of the other hand should be used to palpate the tissues. The examination should begin in the midline in the submental region and move distally to the base of the tongue on one side and then the other.

Of all the structures in the neck, the normal thyroid gland is the most difficult to identify and palpate. The degree of success will vary with the experience of the examiner and the character of the neck structure. Palpation of the gland is extremely difficult in muscular and obese patients.

Palpation of the thyroid may be performed while standing either in front of or behind the patient. The posterior approach is usually easier for beginners. While standing behind the patient, the examiner places both hands on the neck. To palpate the right lobe, the fingers of the left hand gently push the thyroid cartilage toward the right side. The patient should turn and slightly flex the head to the side being examined. The fingers of the right hand locate the isthmus and then move laterally beneath the sternocleidomastoid muscle to identify the gland. Having the patient swallow water during the examination may facilitate the identification of the isthmus and gland. Both isthmus and gland move upward and then down as the patient swallows. The examination procedure is reversed for the left lobe.

Using the anterior approach, the examiner stands in front of the patient. To palpate the right lobe, the examiner's thumb or fingers of the right hand gently displace the thyroid cartilage to the patient's right. The head should be slightly flexed to the side being examined. The fingers of the left hand locate the isthmus and move left and laterally underneath the sternocleidomastoid muscle to identify the gland. As with the posterior approach, the patient's swallowing water may help in locating the isthmus and lobe. To palpate the left lobe, the procedure is reversed.

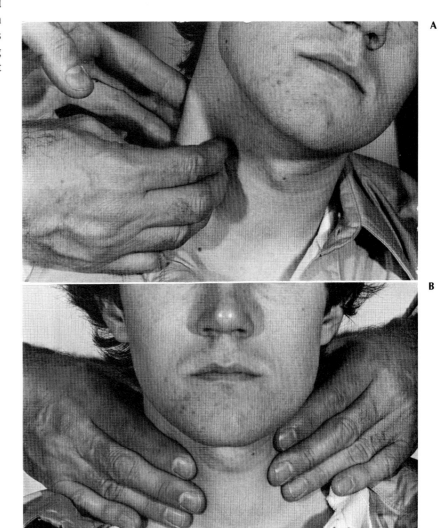

Fig. 8-11. A, Unilateral technique of palpating internal jugular nodes; palpation for nodes is deep and medial to sternocleidomastoid muscle (SCM) while supporting muscle with other hand. **B,** Bilateral technique of palpating internal jugular nodes. Lymph nodes are palpated with fingers while SCM is supported with thumbs.

Abnormalities

A large number and variety of problems can involve the neck. Only the more common lesions are considered here. A relatively complete outline of neck lesions is as follows:

LESIONS OF THE MIDDLE AND LATERAL NECK IN ORDER OF FREQUENCY

Midline neck
- Submental lymphadenopathy
- Thyroid disease
- Thyroid adenoma
- Thyroid carcinoma
- Thyroglossal tract cyst
- Dermoid cyst
- Parathyroid tumors

Lateral neck
- Lymphadenopathy
    - Acute lymphadenitis
    - Chronic lymphadenitis
    - Metastatic carcinoma
    - Primary tumor
- Epidermal cyst
- Submandibular sialolithiasis
- Submandibular tumors
- Lipoma
- Branchial cyst
- Neurogenic tumors
- Laryngocele
- Aneurysm
- Cystic hygroma
- Carotid body tumor

The consideration of neck lesions is simplified and made more practical if the lesions are divided into those that occur in the midline and those that occur in the lateral neck. Common midline lesions include thyroid disease, thyroid tumors, thyroglossal tract cyst, dermoid cyst, and submental lymphadenopathy.

Enlargement of the thyroid gland may be diffuse or nodular. Diffuse enlargements usually occur as a result of simple goiter, Graves' disease, or Hashimoto's disease (Fig. 8-12). A localized enlargement or nodule usually indicates neoplastic disease, either benign or malignant. Patients with benign lesions often report slow growth of the nodule over many years. Recent and rapid growth with-

out tenderness suggests that the nodule indicates thyroid carcinoma.

Thyroglossal tract cysts may occur anywhere along the midline, though 80% are found at or below the hyoid. They vary in size from a few millimeters to several centimeters and occasionally rupture to persist as a draining sinus. These cysts are usually asymptomatic, slowly enlarging lesions that are found in younger individuals.

The clinical features of the dermoid cyst are similar to those of the thyroglossal tract cyst, a slow-growing, painless, soft mass usually becoming apparent during the second or third decade. The dermoid cyst is found in the submental region and may produce some intraoral swelling if it is located deep in the tissue.

The submental nodes show reactive change infrequently and are palpable far less often than the submandibular nodes are. They will enlarge as a result of systemic disease and when draining rather large inflammatory lesions.

The more common swellings found in the lateral neck are the result of lymphadenopathy, salivary gland disease, epidermal cysts, lipomas, and branchial cysts. By far the most frequently palpated mass in the neck is a lymph node. When it is found, the examiner must determine whether the node is evidence of current disease or merely residual change from previous inflammatory involvement.

Cervical nodes up to 1 cm in diameter are almost always palpable in young children and are considered normal. At this age lymphoid tissue is most abundant and reactive. As chil-

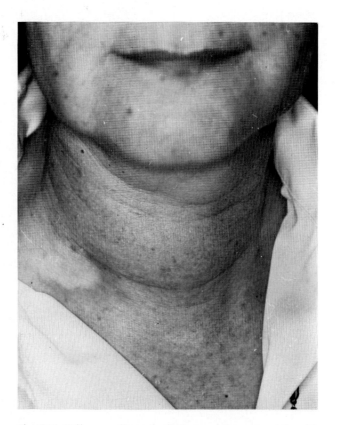

Fig. 8-12. Diffuse swelling of anterior neck because of thyroid enlargement.

dren mature, the lymphoid tissue atrophies and is not as apparent. In adults, palpable nodes are usually the sequelae of repeated episodes of involvement. In one study 53% of the adults examined had palpable nodes in the cervical or submandibular area without apparent evidence of disease.

The clinical features and distribution of involved lymph nodes help provide some insight into the nature of the problem. When lymph nodes are enlarged, they should be characterized as to the following features: size, tenderness, consistency, outline, and mobility. Determining whether a palpable lymph node is ''normal'' or enlarged is a difficult assessment to make, especially for the novice. The ability to make this distinction is gained with experience. Generally a node larger than 1 cm will be classified as enlarged. When a node is tender to palpation, this indicates that it is involved by an acute inflammatory process. The consistency of lymph nodes may range from soft to hard. Edematous nodes or those that have areas of suppuration feel soft. Previously involved nodes or those involved by a chronic disease are relatively firm. Nodes with metastatic carcinoma are ''stony'' hard. Usually the outline of a lymph node is well defined or discrete. When a disease involves several lymph nodes and the disease extends beyond their capsule, the nodes become ill defined or matted. This happens most frequently with malignant disease. Lymph nodes are generally freely movable. When a lymph node contains a tumor that extends beyond its capsule and infiltrates the surrounding tissue, the node becomes fixed.

Lymph nodes draining an area of acute infection or injury will become reactive and inflamed (acute lymphadenitis). They are enlarged, tender, soft, well defined, and movable. These nodes may undergo complete recovery, necrosis and suppuration, or fibrosis. Acute unilateral lymphadenitis occurs as a result of aphthous ulcers, acute apical periodontitis, pericoronitis, and other isolated inflammatory lesions. An acute bilateral cervical lymphadenitis is seen in herpetic gingivostomatitis, viral pharyngitis, and group A streptococcal infections. Diseases such as infectious mononucleosis, rubella, and viral hepatitis should also be suspected, though they tend to have a more generalized distribution. A distinctive feature that is usually found in patients with these diseases is enlargement of the spinal accessory nodes.

Carotid arteritis may be mistaken for an acute lymphadenitis unless the patient is examined carefully. The patient with this condition has a unilateral tenderness that involves the carotid sheath. The vascular involvement can be clearly identified with careful palpation. The tenderness may be so marked that it precludes free movement of the head.

Lymph nodes associated with healing or chronic lesions are usually less reactive and inflamed. These nodes are enlarged, less tender or nontender, firm, well defined, and movable. They decrease in size as the reactive response resolves but persist as palpable nodes because of fibrosis. Chronically involved nodes may be found because of chronic apical periodontitis, resolving cat scratch fever, or atypical mycobacterial lymphadenitis.

An enlarged cervical node may be the first and only indication of carcinoma in the head or neck region. Unfortunately, early involvement of a lymph node by metastatic tumor does not produce characteristic changes. Only after the tumor has replaced most of the node and invaded the capsule will the classic features be noted. These nodes are enlarged, nontender, hard, poorly defined, and fixed (Fig. 8-13).

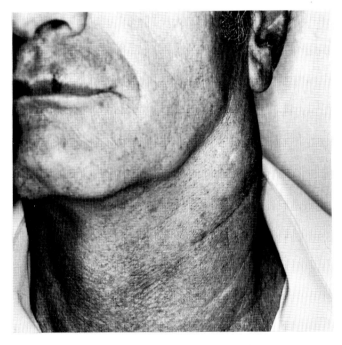

Fig. 8-13. Diffuse swelling of left neck produced by metastatic nasopharyngeal carcinoma to cervical lymph nodes.

Cervical lymph node enlargement may also be the first sign of Hodgkin's disease, lymphoma, or leukemia (Fig. 8-14). At the onset enlargement is usually unilateral, but will become bilateral with time. These nodes are enlarged, nontender, firm or rubbery, discrete, and movable at the onset but become matted and fixed as the disease progresses. Similar nodes may be found in sarcoidosis. As a general rule, any firm, nontender node that is slowly enlarging must be suspected of containing primary or metastatic tumor.

Swelling in the submandibular region associated with eating is characteristic of obstructive disease, usually caused by a sialolith. The swelling may persist from 30 minutes to hours and be quite variable as to its frequency. It may be present with each meal or may not recur for intervals of days, weeks, months, or even years. With time the gland becomes fibrotic and essentially nonfunctional. At this stage the gland is more prone to secondary infection and its accompanying symptoms of pain, swelling, and purulent discharge. Tumors occur far less frequently in the submandibular gland than in the parotid gland. The frequency of benign and malignant lesions is about equal. Since the gland is not close to the skin surface, tumors are usually not detected in early stages, and palpation of the area is important for early detection.

Epidermal cysts can occur anywhere on the neck but are found more often around the ear, especially behind or below it (Fig. 8-15). They are quite variable in size, ranging from a few millimeters to several centimeters. If the cyst is close to the surface, its contents, keratin, impart a tan yellow color to the lesion. When the cysts become inflamed they become quite large and tender.

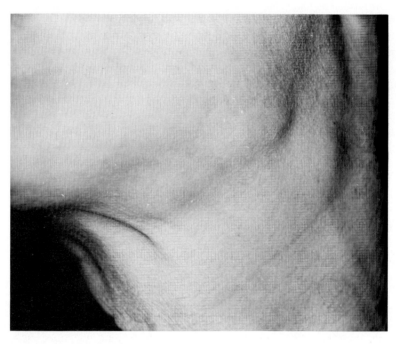

Fig. 8-14. Patient with chronic lymphatic leukemia who shows marked enlargement of submandibular and superficial deep cervical lymph nodes.

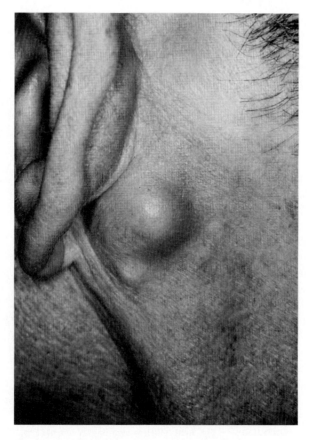

Fig. 8-15. Epidermal cyst located behind patient's ear.

The lateral and posterior surfaces of the neck are the most frequent sites for a lipoma. It begins as a subcutaneous nodule that slowly enlarges and becomes lobulated. The mass is often rubbery or compressible.

Branchial cysts usually appear as a lateral swelling in the upper third of the neck and are partially covered by the sternocleidomastoid muscle. They also occur in the submandibular area. The swelling may have been present but unnoticed for some time or have a rapid onset shortly after an upper respiratory tract infection. Its appearance may range from a deep, diffuse swelling to a superficial, well-localized lesion. At times it may also appear as a sinus.

CONCLUSION

As mentioned in the introduction, the head and neck region is a complex area that involves many structures that require significant knowledge and experience to interpret both in health and disease. This chapter considered only a few of these structures; more material is presented in subsequent chapters about the eye, ear, nose, and skin. A complete and comprehensive understanding of all this information is not readily and easily mastered. The initial effort should be directed toward developing a sound knowledge and understanding of the normal so that there is a basis for identifying the abnormal.

BIBLIOGRAPHY

De Gowin, E.L., and De Gowin, R.L.: Bedside diagnostic examination, ed. 3, New York, 1976, Macmillan Publishing Co., Inc.

Fitzpatrick, T.B., and others: Dermatology in general medicine: textbook and atlas, ed. 2, New York, 1979, McGraw-Hill Book Co.

Gorlin, R.J., and Goldman, H.M.: Thoma's oral pathology, ed. 6, St. Louis, 1970, The C.V. Mosby Co.

Gorlin, R.J., Pindborg, J.J., and Cohen, M.M., Jr.: Syndromes of the head and neck, ed. 2, New York, 1976, McGraw-Hill Book Co.

Haagensen, C.D., and others: The lymphatics in cancer, Philadelphia, 1972, W.B. Saunders Co.

International Anatomical Nomenclature Committee: Nomina anatomica, ed. 3, New York, 1966, Excerpta Medica Foundation.

9 Eye, ear, nose, and throat

EYE
Examination of the eye

The eye and its associated structures are subject to a wide variety of disorders. Some of these interfere with vision, whereas others affect only structures such as the coverings of the eyeball, the eyelids, and lacrimal apparatus and do not necessarily affect a patient's ability to see. In view of the relative frequency of eye problems and the closeness of the eye to the mouth, it is felt that the dentist should be familiar with the more common ophthalmologic problems and the methods of examining for them.

Examination of the eye may provide valuable information not only about the optic apparatus itself but also about many other body systems. The optic nerve and retina are part of the central nervous system. Retinoscopy permits the examiner to look, as it were, directly at the brain. The arterioles and venules of the retina may be readily seen and may indicate the state of the cerebral and systemic circulation. Changes in the retinal configuration may be produced in many conditions, such as hypertension, diabetes mellitus, and renal disease. Pupillary reflexes, eye movements, and the visual fields may give information about the integrity of the cranial nerves. (Half of the cranial nerves—optic, oculomotor, trochlear, trigeminal, abducent, and facial—may produce changes affecting the eye and external ocular muscles.) The actual examination of the eye should be preceded by a detailed history of any visual disturbances, pain, or discomfort in the optic area, or inflammation or swelling of the conjunctivae, lids, or lacrimal apparatus. A full eye examination will include tests for visual acuity (close and distant vision), color vision, visual fields, ocular motility, and intraocular pressure (tonometry), in addition to inspection, palpation, and retinoscopy.

Although the dentist does not normally perform a comprehensive eye examination, he should be familiar with its main features and be aware of the more common abnormalities that might be seen in dental patients. This chapter reviews the features of an eye examination and defines some of the more common terms used in ophthalmologic practice.

The eyeball and its associated structures are shown in Fig. 9-1.

Visual acuity. Visual acuity is normally tested by use of the Snellen chart or one of its modifications. These show letters or numbers, and there are charts that show varied shapes for illiterate patients. Normal visual acuity is expressed as 20/20. The letters marked 20/20 on the chart will subtend an angle of 5 minutes at the eye when the eye is 20 feet from the chart. The notation 20/40 indicates that a person will see at 20 feet what a "normal" person will see at 40 feet. The notation 20/15 implies that a person at 20 feet sees what a "normal" person will see at 15 feet.

Most people with a visual acuity of less than 20/20 probably have some refractive error correctable by the appropriate lenses. Near vision is tested by asking the patient to read type of differing sizes held at a standard distance from the eyes.

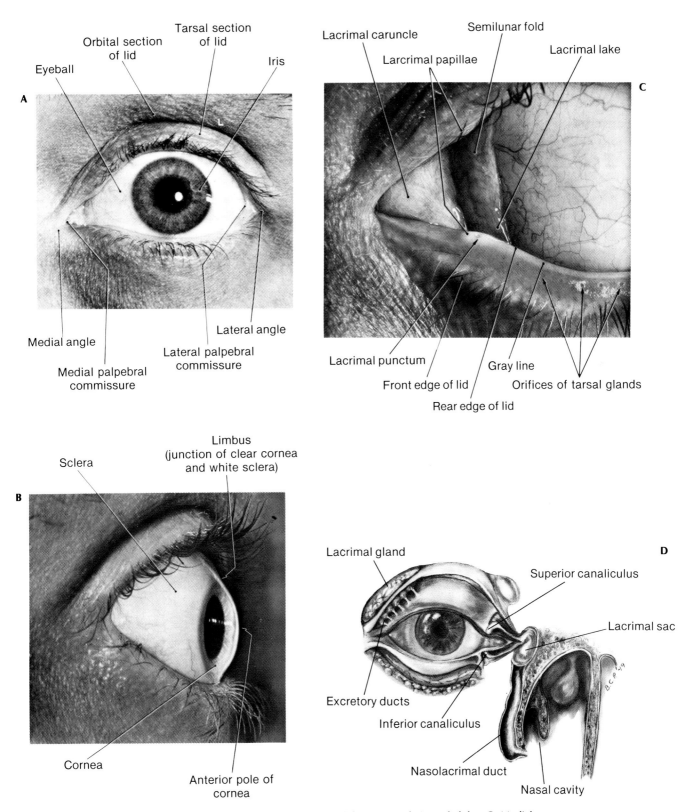

Fig. 9-1. A, Anterior view of eye and eyelids. **B,** Lateral view of globe. **C,** Medial aspect—lower eyelid slightly everted. **D,** Lacrimal drainage system. (**A** to **C** copyright Eastman Kodak Co., 1972, courtesy H.L. Gibson; **D** from Medical radiography and photography, published by Health Sciences Markets Division, Eastman Kodak Co., Rochester, N.Y.)

Color vision. Patients may be asked to match different colors or be tested to see if they can identify numbers or letters from a specially prepared dotted color picture (Ishihara's test).

Visual fields. The visual field is the area within which stimuli will produce the sensation of sight when the eye is looking straight ahead. Vascular lesions, tumors, and other abnormalities may impinge on any part of the optic pathway (from the retina back to the occipital or visual cortex) and affect the size of the visual fields. Accurate visual fields are normally mapped with a special instrument, but a satisfactory ''noninstrument'' approach is very useful in detecting gross abnormalities. Confrontation visual field examination has the examiner comparing the extent of his visual fields with that of his patient. (The assumption is that the examiner has normal visual fields!) The examiner faces the patient approximately 1 m away, covers his or her eye opposite to the one the patient is having tested (the patient's other eye is covered), and then the patient and the examiner look into each other's eyes (Fig. 9-2). The examiner brings a small object into his field of view that is easily visible from all directions. The object is held about midway between the examiner and the patient. The point at which the examiner sees the object will mark the edge of his visual field. The patient, if normal, will see the object at approximately the same time as the examiner. This technique will easily identify such defects as hemianopia (loss of half the visual field) or large scotomas (areas of deficient vision within the visual field). (See Chapter 14 for further discussion.)

Eye movements. The patient should be asked to move the eyes in all directions, and the observer should notice whether there is any abnormality in the symmetry of movement or whether the patient notices any double vision (diplopia) in a particular direction of gaze. The integrity of the orbicular muscle of the eye should also be tested by having the patient close the eyelids tightly. The significance of external ocular muscle testing is referred to later in this book in Chapter 14.

Tonometry. The intraocular pressure varies within certain limits in the normal patient. In some patients there is an increase in intraocular pressure that may give rise to the condition of glaucoma. The pressure within the eyeball may be measured by a tonometer. This consists of a small weighted device that is placed over the anesthetized cornea to take a reading of the pressure necessary to deform the cornea. Clearly, the higher the intraocular pressure, the more pressure is necessary to deform the cornea. More sophisticated techniques, such as applanation, are available for use with the slit lamp (a specialized instrument for examining the structures of the eye). These techniques also depend on deformation of the globe.

External ocular structures. The examination of the eye should be done in a clear light and may be helped by the use of a loupe. The examination should be done in a systematic way in order to avoid overlooking any particular structure.

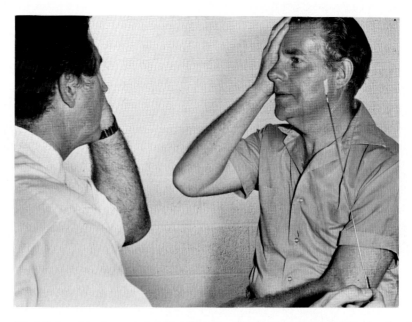

Fig. 9-2. Examiner has covered his left eye and is examining visual field of patient's left eye. Small white marker, kept in plane midway between examiner and patient, is brought into examiner's field of vision from all directions. When examiner sees marker come into view, patient, if normal, will be expected to see it at about same time.

Lids. There may be alterations in the normal anatomy of the eyelid. Entropion (inversion) of the lid usually affects the lower lid more than the upper. It is fairly common and usually unilateral. It may be seen in elderly people with decreased orbital fat and sunken eyes. When the orbicular muscle of the eye contracts without the firm support of the globe, the lid inverts. Trichiasis (the turning in of the eyelashes so that they rub on the cornea) is a serious complication of entropion, as it may cause extreme irritation of the cornea, along with inflammation, ulceration, and subsequent infection and scarring. Ectropion (sagging or eversion) of the lower lid is often bilateral and is more common in older persons. When the orbicular muscles of the eye relax, either as part of the aging process or perhaps following a facial nerve paralysis, the eyelid is "pulled" out. The lacrimal point, no longer in contact with the conjunctiva, cannot remove the tears. The patient then has marked epiphora (tearing). The full circumference of the iris is not normally seen, as the upper lid margin usually lies over the upper part of the iris. If the lid lies down at or below the level of the pupil margin, this indicates some degree of ptosis (drooping of the eyelid) (Fig. 9-3). Sometimes the sclera is exposed above the limbus (the periphery of the cornea where it joins the sclera), and this lid retraction may be evidence of a condition such as hyperthyroidism. The lids should be examined for any change in their thickness or any abnormality of their margins. Two common problems of the lids are a stye (or hordeolum) and a chalazion (literally, a hailstone). A stye is an infection of one of the sebaceous glands of the eyelids. It appears as a painful, red swelling at the lid margin. Blockage of one of the meibomian glands of the eyelid may give rise to a granulomatous reaction felt by the patient as a slightly painful, hard swelling within the lids—a chalazion. (Fig. 9-4).

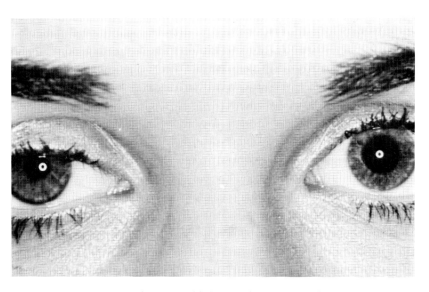

Fig. 9-3. Right upper eyelid shows mild degree of ptosis. Note that it covers much more of iris than left upper eyelid. This patient was suffering from Horner's syndrome (see Chapter 14).

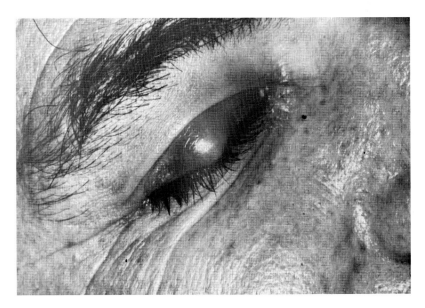

Fig. 9-4. This chalazion had been present for several weeks. It was not particularly painful, but patient felt some discomfort. He described it as if "I have a stone in my eyelid."

101

It is not infrequent for the eyelids to be the site of development of a basal cell carcinoma. This is usually a slow-growing, painless nodule. It appears with rolled borders and frequently shows a central area of umbilication that may ulcerate (Fig. 9-5). The finding of xanthelasmata (singular: xanthelasma) is not uncommon. These are intradermal deposits of lipids that are usually symmetrical and situated at the medial ends of the upper and lower eyelids (Fig. 9-6). They may grow to become large confluent masses. They do not always signify hyperlipoproteinemia, but frequently there is some elevation in the plasma levels of β-lipoprotein. The lacrimal glands secrete tears that pass across the eye and are collected through the lacrimal points and pass through the lacrimal canals, lacrimal sac, and nasolacrimal duct into the lower part of the nasal cavity. Weeping, or epiphora, may result from a blockage of any portion of the lacrimal system or from eversion of the lid margin. Occasionally an infection of the lacrimal sac (dacryocystitis) develops, and a patient may seek dental advice concerning this in the erroneous belief that it has resulted from a dental infection (Fig. 9-7).

Conjunctiva and sclera. The conjunctiva and sclera should be examined for any irregularity of their surfaces or for any discolorations. The most common discoloration is a redness caused by inflammation or infection (conjunctivitis). In very early conjunctivitis, the only finding may be an increased prominence of the conjunctival blood vessels (Fig. 9-8). Care must be taken to differentiate the redness of a superficial conjunctivitis from an inflammation that is deeper in the eye coverings, for example, scleritis or iritis. Foreign bodies frequently cause increased conjunctival vascularity and watering of the eye.

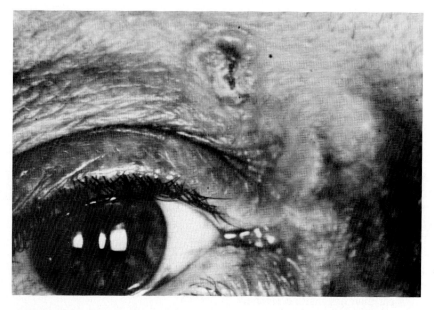

Fig. 9-5. This indurated ulcerated lesion with rolled margins and some central umbilication had been present for several months. It was discovered at routine dental examination; patient was unaware of its true nature. It was basal cell carcinoma.

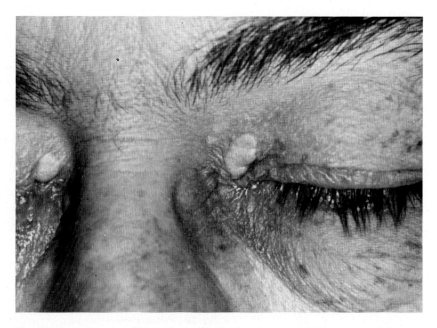

Fig. 9-6. Xanthelasmata. These slowly developing deposits of lipids were painless. Patient's only concern was their appearance.

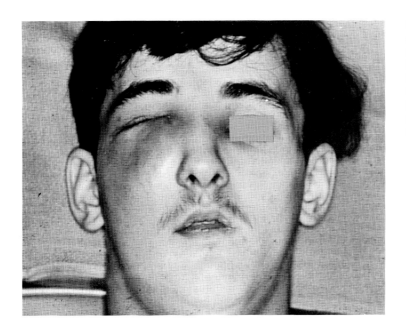

Fig. 9-7. This 18-year-old man sought advice from his dental surgeon. He had developed painful red swelling of face that had caused some closure of eyelids. Intraoral examination showed no dental or peridental pathologic condition. After further examination, diagnosis of dacryocystitis was made and condition was treated with antibiotics.

A

B

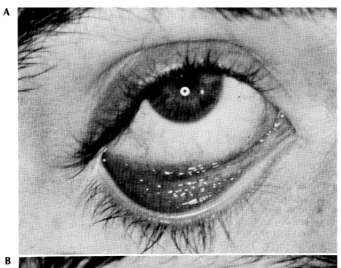

Fig. 9-8. Patient complained of some itching of eyes, more marked on left. **A,** Right eye shows little change in appearance of bulbar conjunctiva. **B,** Left eye shows some increased vascularity and injection of conjunctival blood vessels.

It may be necessary to examine the inner aspect of the upper lid. This can be done by grasping the eyelashes with the fingers of one hand and then pushing down the upper edge of the tarsal plate with a wooden stick (Fig. 9-9). This maneuver displays the inner aspect of the eyelid conjunctiva (foreign bodies may frequently lodge here). Occasionally, small fatty deposits (pingueculae) are seen on the conjunctivae at the limbus. A pterygium is an inflammatory overgrowth of the conjunctiva that may occasionally progress to the cornea and may, in some circumstances, actually cover the pupil (Fig. 9-10). A subconjunctival hemorrhage usually involves only one eye, is localized, and does not extend backward into the orbital tissues. Subconjunctival hemorrhages are painless but usually look very dramatic (Fig. 9-11). They may occur after sudden venous congestion, developing in a severe coughing or sneezing episode. They should not necessarily be considered an indication of vascular disease.

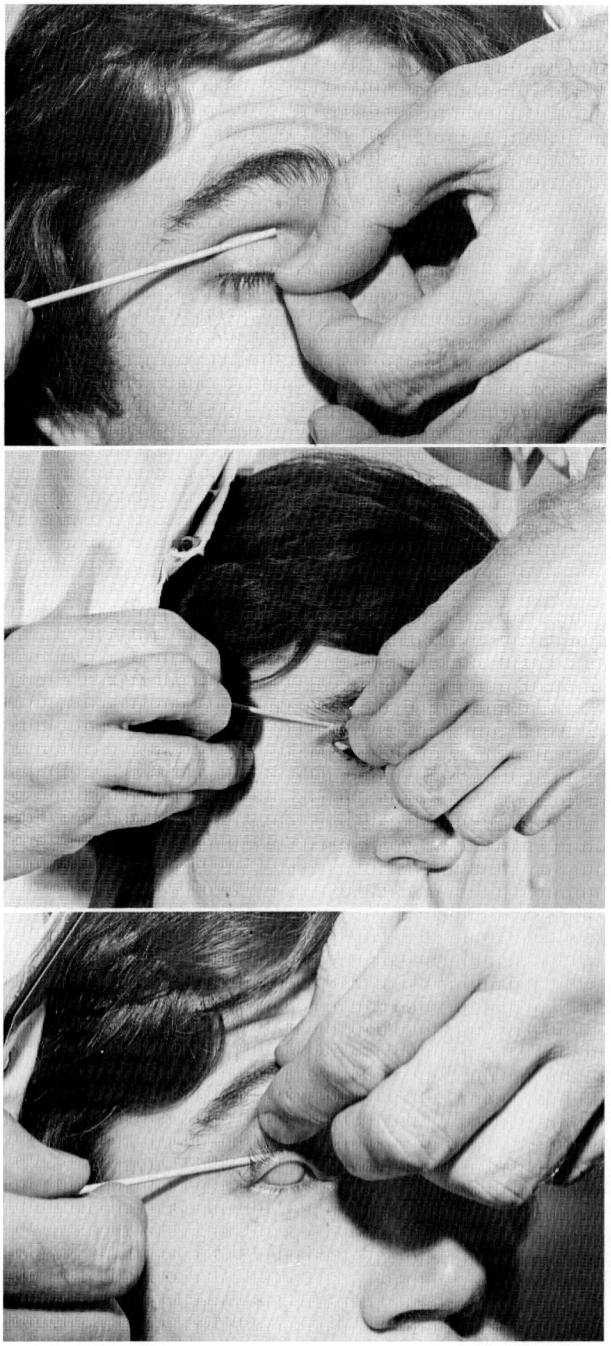

Fig. 9-9. Technique for visualizing inner aspect of upper eyelid. **A,** Lashes of upper lid are grasped firmly and wooden stick is placed against upper part of tarsal plate. **B,** Eyelid is pulled upward at same time as tarsal plate is everted. **C,** Conjunctival lining of upper eyelid can easily be seen.

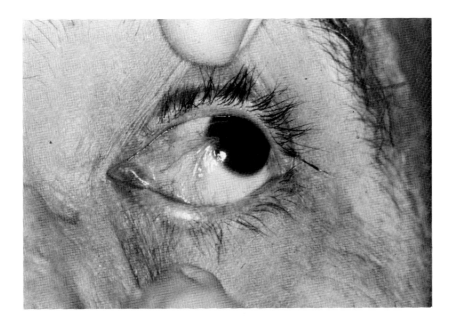

Fig. 9-10. This pterygium had been present for several months. It was painless and beginning to cross limbus. If it progressed further to cover iris and pupil, it would have to be removed.

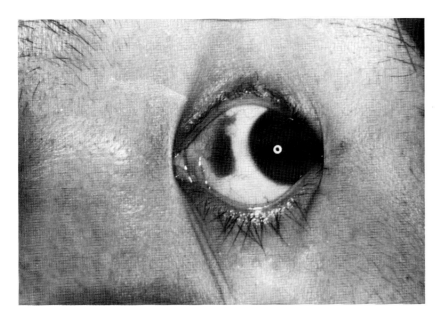

Fig. 9-11. Discrete area of subconjunctival hemorrhage is seen on medial aspect of left eye. The patient, a dental student, had experienced no pain or discomfort but had noticed development of this hemorrhagic area by accident. There was no history of trauma or of any severe bouts of coughing. Lesion resolved without treatment within 1 week.

Cornea. The cornea should be smooth and moist. It should be sensitive to light touch, and indeed this test of corneal sensitivity is one of the standard tests for determining the integrity of the trigeminal nerve. If the cornea is touched with a wisp of cotton, there should normally be a blink reflex. Corneal ulcers are generally of two types. Marginal ulcers result from a severe conjunctival infection that transgresses the corneal margin. Larger, centrally located ulcers are due to infections or result from penetration of the cornea by abrasion or a foreign body. A more superficial but indolent ulcer may be caused by herpes simplex infection (dendritic ulcer). Occasionally there is an accumulation of inflammatory exudate in the aqueous humor of the anterior chamber behind the cornea. In such cases, a hypopyon may develop, that is, a collection of exudate in the inferior angle between the cornea and the iris. The arcus senilis is a white encircling ring about 1 mm within the corneal margin. It affects only the periphery and does not interfere with sight (Fig. 9-12). As the name implies, it is more commonly seen in the elderly. Its diagnostic significance, if any, is not known. It has been reported by several workers that the premature development of an arcus senilis in a young person may presage some cardiovascular problems, but this relationship is not entirely clear.

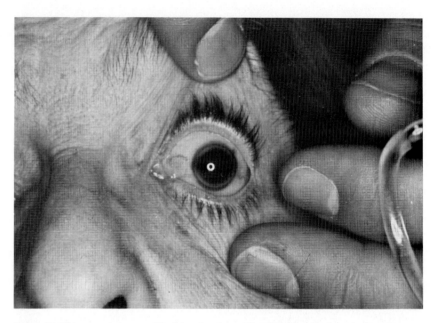

Fig. 9-12. This eye shows small white ring immediately below limbus. It does not interfere in any way with ocular function. Patient, aged 76, reported that it had slowly developed over past 10 years. An arcus senilis does not require any treatment.

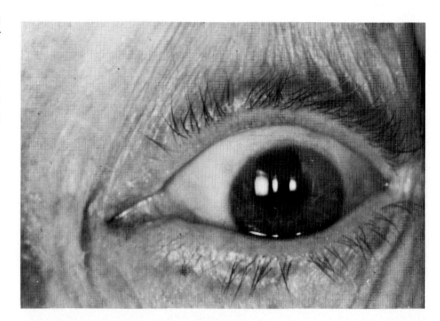

Fig. 9-13. This patient had undergone operation for removal of cataract in left eye. Resulting deformity in iris is clearly seen.

Iris and pupil. The iris and pupil should be examined closely. Normally in most people the pupillary opening is bilaterally symmetrical, although there may be some variation in up to 20% of normal individuals. Variations in pupil size are discussed briefly in Chapter 14. Occasionally a postsurgical defect in the iris will be seen after surgical removal of a cloudy lens (a cataract), as shown in Fig. 9-13.

Lens and retina. The examination of the structures within the eye, that is, the lens and retina, is normally accomplished with an ophthalmoscope (Fig. 9-14). This instrument simply provides a convenient light source with an attachment permitting lenses of varying sizes to be placed in front of the examiner's eye, enabling the examiner to see all levels of the eye and compensating for any gross irregularities in either the examiner's or the patient's refraction of light. The lens should be completely transparent. The development of an opacity within the lens (a cataract) is not an uncommon finding. Many conditions can produce such a change in the translucency of the lens. Radiation damage, direct physical or chemical trauma, metabolic disorders such as diabetes, congenital abnormalities, and senile changes may all produce cataracts.

A   B

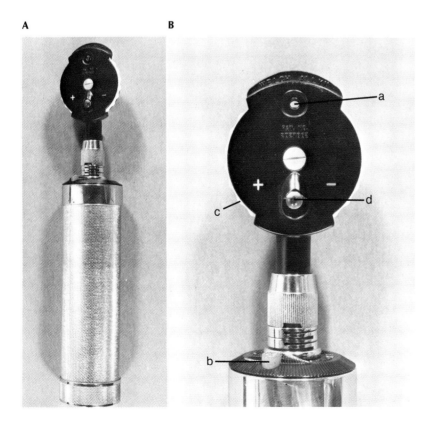

Fig. 9-14. Ophthalmoscope. **A,** Battery operated (batteries in the handle). **B,** Close-up of ophthalmoscope head shows important components: *a,* examiner looks through this aperture; beam of light is reflected by mirror or prism coincident with line of sight of observer; light can be switched on and off and its intensity changed by operation of switch *b.* Lenses of different sizes can be rotated into aperture by movement of ring, *c,* and particular lens situated in aperture is indicated at *d.* Positive or negative lens may be rotated into aperture to compensate for refraction problems in observer's or patient's eyes.

The examination of the retina requires considerable skill. A full retinoscopy by an ophthalmologist is nearly always performed when the pupils have been dilated. For the unskilled person, retinoscopy without pupillary dilatation can be very difficult and most frustrating. The fundus, as the posterior part of the retina is called, should be examined in a systematic way. First, the head of the optic nerve—the optic disc—should be identified. The margins of the disc are normally very sharp, and from the center of the disc several large blood vessels can be seen emerging, supplying the temporal and nasal aspects of the retinal field (Fig. 9-15). Lesions of the retina are normally described in terms of their size in relationship to the disc diameter; for example, a lesion may be described as being about half the diameter of the disc and $2\frac{1}{2}$ disc diameters on the temporal aspect. Blood vessels should be followed across the temporal field and special attention paid to the areas where the arteries and the veins cross. The arteries are normally slightly smaller than the veins and are usually brighter red. Hemorrhages within the disc and retina, exudates, and abnormal "nicking" at the point of crossing of an artery and vein may all be evidence of systemic diseases and should be carefully recorded.

The dentist must recognize that the examination of the eye calls for considerable experience, ability, and the use of specialized instruments, and should have no hesitation in recommending that a patient seek an ophthalmologic consultation if there is any doubt about the integrity of a patient's optical apparatus.

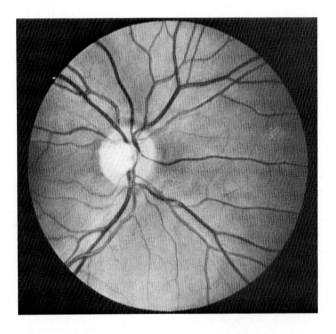

Fig. 9-15. Normal fundus, *L.* Blood vessels can be seen radiating from optic disc to nasal and temporal sides. (Courtesy Lynne Hochberg Pace, M.D.)

Diseases of the eye and dental infection

Many ophthalmologists believe that focal infection in and around the mouth may be causal or aggravating factors in such eye conditions as iritis, cyclitis (inflammation of the ciliary body), choroiditis, and uveitis. (The iris, ciliary body, and choroid form a continuous sheet along the inner wall of the cornea-sclera. The sheet is known as the *uveal tract,* and an inflammation of this tract is a uveitis.) The resolution of such inflammatory conditions after the elimination of septic oral foci has been reported many times. It is not unusual for a patient suffering from one of these ocular conditions to be referred to the dentist by the ophthalmologist with instructions to "remove teeth." The dentist should recognize the possible relationship between dental foci of infection and areas of inflammation in other parts of the body, but should not remove clinically and radiographically healthy teeth "just in case" they are responsible for an eye condition.

Only teeth that are clinically or radiographically indicated as being a focus of infection that cannot be treated in any other way should be extracted.

Eye injuries in the dental office

The dentist's eyes are frequently exposed to the risk of infection or injury resulting from salivary droplets, blood, fragments of teeth, or pieces of calculus contacting the eye. The use of plain protective eyeglasses is considered most advisable for the dentist who is not required to wear prescription glasses while treating patients. It should not be forgotten that patients, too, may suffer injuries to their eyes while receiving dental treatment. Various injuries have been reported in the professional literature. Hales[1] reported several types of ocular injury, including penetration of the globe by a dental hand instrument that fell into the patient's eye: fragments of plastic flying from a plastic tooth that was being ground and entering a patient's eye, causing corneal ulcerations; misplaced local anesthetic agents causing transient blindness and other visual problems; and a case of chemical irritation after varnish splashed into a dental assistant's eyes. He noted that "all but one [of the injuries reported] would have been prevented if the victims had been wearing their own or protective eyeglasses."

EAR

The ear is the organ of hearing and balance. It is unusual for the dentist to be involved with the diagnosis of disorders of balance, and the various tests used to determine such disorders are not discussed in this chapter. It is often necessary for the dentist to determine whether a patient is suffering from any disorder of the auditory apparatus, particularly diseases of the external and middle ear. Sometimes symptoms associated with such diseases may appear to originate in the mouth, and the patient may seek dental advice concerning them.

The examination of the ear should involve:

1. Inspection of the external ear (the auricle).
2. Examination of the external auditory canal.
3. Visualization of the tympanic membrane.
4. Testing of hearing acuity.

The examination of the auricle requires no special instruments, but an otoscope is necessary for adequate evaluation of the external auditory canal and tympanic membrane.

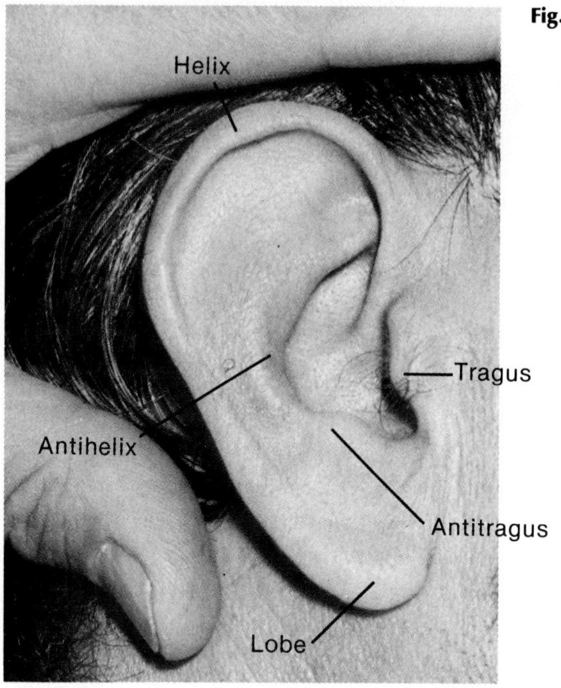

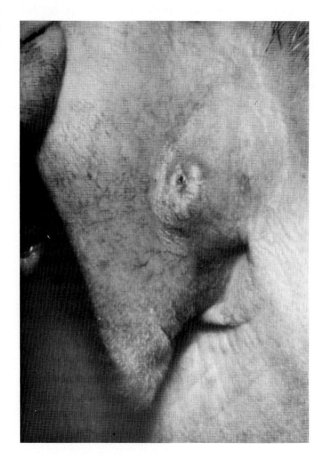

Fig. 9-16. Right auricle.

Fig. 9-17. This ulcer behind left auricle was discovered during head and neck examination conducted at initial dental appointment. Lesion resembled and was confirmed histologically to be basal cell carcinoma. (From Drinnan, A.J.: Dent. Radiogr. Photogr. **42:**11, 1969.)

The external ear

A normal auricle is illustrated in Fig. 9-16. Occasionally there are deformations of the auricle associated with maldevelopment of the jaw bones, but these are relatively uncommon. The ear should be examined for the possibility of gouty tophi and for any other abnormality of development of the epithelium covering the ear or of the underlying cartilage. A basal cell carcinoma may occasionally develop around the auricle; the one illustrated in Fig. 9-17 was discovered during a routine dental examination, the patient being unaware of its presence or nature.

External auditory canal

The examination of the external auditory canal should be conducted using an otoscope (Fig. 9-18). The auricle should be pulled gently upward, backward, and outward in order to "straighten" the external auditory canal and facilitate the examination and visualization of the tympanic membrane (eardrum), as shown in Fig. 9-19. Any particles of wax or debris in the ear canal should be removed, and special attention should be paid to the presence of any inflammatory areas. Furuncles of the external ear canal are very painful. Chronic external otitis leads to severe itching and, if there is swelling of the external auditory canal lining, perhaps to some diminution in hearing.

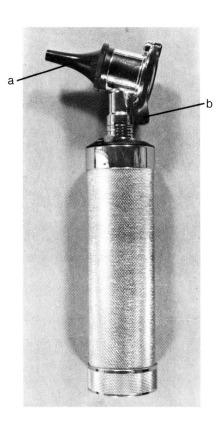

a
b

Fig. 9-18. Otoscope. Example of convenient battery-operated otoscope; handle can be easily detached from head and used with ophthalmoscope head (see Fig. 9-14); *a*, speculum—different sizes of specula can be changed easily; *b*, magnifying lens can be used to aid visualization or can be swung out of way to permit instruments to be passed through speculum into ear.

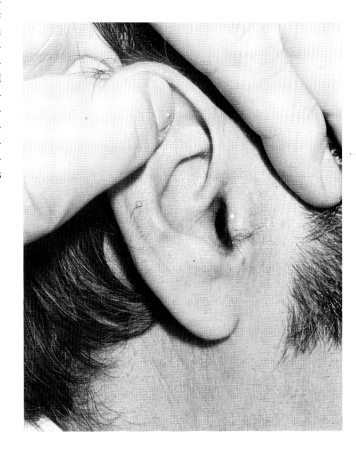

Fig. 9-19. Pulling auricle upward, backward, and outward tends to straighten out cartilaginous part of external auditory canal.

Tympanic membrane

The eardrum can normally be seen fairly easily with the otoscope if the external auditory canal is clean. It is a translucent membrane that faces downward, forward, and outward, and is normally pearly gray (Fig. 9-20). Sometimes it is not possible to see the whole drum at once, and the otoscope must be moved in several directions to visualize the whole surface. Any inflammatory changes in the drum should be noticed, and particular attention should be paid to any outward bulging of the drum, as is seen in otitis media (an accumulation of fluid within the middle ear), or any perforation of the eardrum with or without the discharge of fluid.

Testing hearing acuity

A test of hearing acuity may be made in a crude way by determining the point at which a ticking watch is heard as it is moved toward and away from a patient's ear. Sophisticated instruments are available that determine records of a patient's hearing ability (audiograms). Such tests involve presenting to a patient a wide range of sounds at different frequencies and at different levels of intensity and determining at which minimal level of intensity the patient can hear the sound. Special tests for the acoustic nerve are discussed in Chapter 14.

NOSE AND THROAT

The upper part of the respiratory tract (the nasal cavity, nasopharynx, and larynx) should be evaluated as part of a head and neck examination. The examiner should remember to include the accessory sinuses in such an examination, as they are considered "outpouchings" of the nasal cavity. The skin overlying the nose itself may show changes indicative of systemic or local diseases. The characteristic "butterfly" lesion of lupus erythematosus has been frequently described.

Fig. 9-20. Landmarks of right tympanic membrane: *a*, manubrium (handle) of malleus; *b*, umbo; *c*, long process of incus.

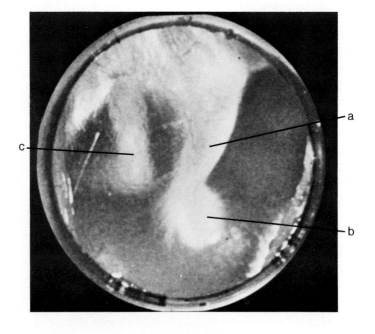

In rhinophyma the end of the nose is red and bulbous. This condition represents an overgrowth of sweat and sebaceous glands and is frequently associated with increased alcohol consumption. Basal cell carcinomas may occasionally develop on the skin of the nose, and care should be taken to evaluate any suspected lesions found in this area. Examination of the nasal fossae is conducted using a bivalve speculum (Fig. 9-21). It must be remembered that the nose runs generally anterior-posterior, rather than superior-inferior, and care must be taken that the valves of the speculum are introduced horizontally. The speculum is inserted with the blades closed, and these are then spread out vertically to give the maximal view of the nasal septum and the lateral wall of the nose with its various conchae (Fig. 9-22). Any congestion of the nasal mucosa, perforation of the septum, or discharge of exudates from the sinus openings should be looked for carefully. After repeated bouts of swelling of the nasal mucosa, a patient may develop a permanent polypoid swelling of the mucosa that may prolapse into the external nares and appear as a gray, glistening membrane, the so-called nasal polyp. Such lesions, which consist of greatly edematous, enlarged nasal mucosa, may interfere with nasal breathing and must be surgically removed. One of the polyps will occasionally prolapse posteriorly and appear in the nasal pharynx, although its point of attachment is on the nasal wall. The most common site for anterior nasal bleeding to occur is Kiesselbach's area, which is a richly vascular area of the anterior-inferior aspect of the nasal septum.

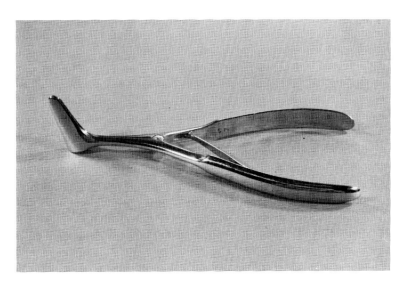

Fig. 9-21. Bivalve nasal speculum.

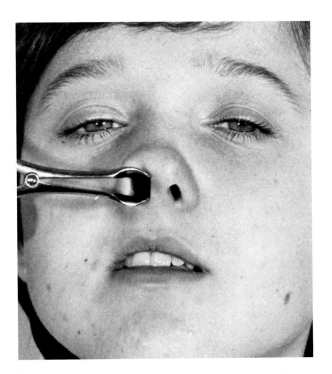

Fig. 9-22. Blades of speculum are introduced horizontally and opened vertically (this avoids painful pressure on septum). For complete visualization patient's head position must be changed. This is accomplished by using left hand to hold speculum firmly in nasal vestibule *(left or right)* and right hand to position head.

113

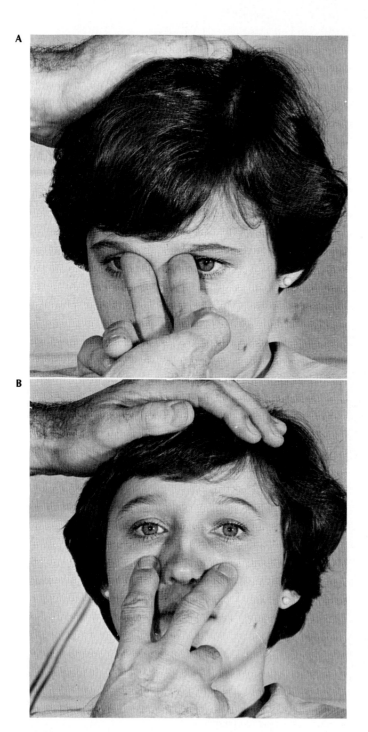

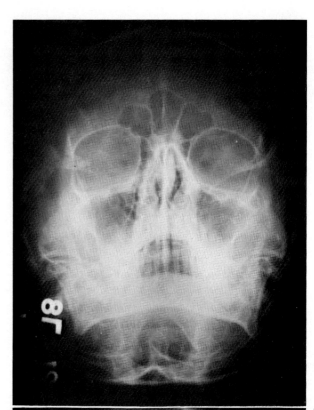

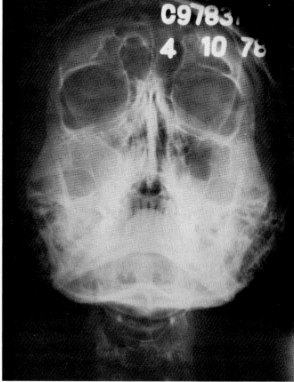

Fig. 9-23. Evaluation of sinusitis. Determining tenderness of frontal sinuses, **A,** and maxillary sinuses, **B.**

Fig. 9-24. Posterior-anterior oblique projection of face (Waters' view) radiographs show frontal and maxillary sinuses. **A,** Frontal sinuses and maxillary sinuses appear equally translucent. **B,** Right maxillary sinus has lost normal translucency.

The evaluation of chronic sinusitis should always include firm pressure over the maxillary and frontal sinuses (Fig. 9-23). Hypersensitivity in these areas frequently indicates sinusitis. Transillumination of the maxillary sinuses may be of value; the examination is conducted in a darkened room, and a light source is placed in the patient's mouth. There should normally be some moderate translucency of each of the maxillary sinuses visible through the skin of the face. In any condition in which the translucency of the sinuses is impaired by, for example, the presence of neoplastic or inflammatory material within the sinus, the air will be obliterated and the sinus translucency decreased. Although this test is occasionally of value, it is now more usual to evaluate the patency of the sinuses by radiographs, and the Waters' view (posterior-anterior oblique projection of face) is the most frequently used radiograph to display the accessory nasal sinuses (Fig. 9-24). Chronic inflammation within the maxillary sinus will occasionally produce a swelling of the mucous membrane of the sinus, and a mucocele (mucous retention cyst) may develop. Such a lesion may be found in a routine dental examination, in either an intraoral or a panoramic radiograph (Fig. 9-25). Such lesions do not necessarily require definitive treatment.

A
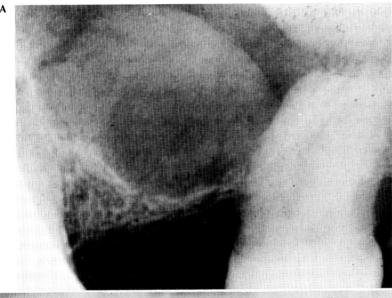

B
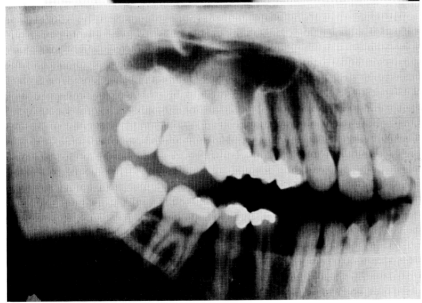

Fig. 9-25. A, Mucocele of left maxillary antrum discovered in intraoral radiograph at routine examination—no previous symptoms. **B,** Mucocele in right maxillary antrum discovered in panoramic radiograph at routine examination—no previous symptoms.

It is not unusual for patients with maxillary sinusitis to feel discomfort in their maxillary teeth. Such patients may then seek their dentist's advice concerning their facial discomfort. It is important that a dentist realize the close relationship of certain of the maxillary teeth with the maxillary sinus and avoid providing irreversible dental treatment (such as an extraction) before being certain that the patient's discomfort is "dental" rather than "nondental." The size of the maxillary sinus and the number of teeth with which it is closely related vary widely from patient to patient. However, in most patients the second maxillary bicuspid and first maxillary molar have apexes very close to the maxillary sinus floor.

Pharynx and larynx

Pharyngoscopy requires considerable experience and excellent illumination if the examiner is to be confident of seeing all areas of the pharynx and larynx. The oral pharynx (see Chapter 16 for a more detailed discussion of this subject) can usually be well visualized if a tongue blade is used to depress the tongue while the patient is asked to say "ah." The palate is elevated, and the posterior pharyngeal wall and lateral palatine tonsils can be seen easily. The size of the tonsils and the degree of development of the lymphoid tissue on the posterior pharyngeal wall and posterior third of the tongue are highly variable (Fig. 9-26). Sometimes there appears to be a considerable amount of lymphoid tissue in Waldeyer's ring, and at other times the mucosa appears very smooth and devoid of obvious lymphoid tissue. The nasal pharynx is normally examined by means of a small mirror (Fig. 9-27) that is introduced into the oral pharynx and through which the nasal pharynx and choanae (the posterior orifices of the nasal cavity) can be seen (Fig. 9-28). The pharyngeal orifice of each eustachian tube, the adenoidal tissue, and the presence of any abnormal growths, such as polyps or tumors, should be carefully looked for. The mirror should be warmed to prevent fogging.

Fig. 9-26. Hypertrophic lymphoid tissue on posterior pharyngeal wall can be seen easily; patient is saying "ah," and tongue is being depressed.

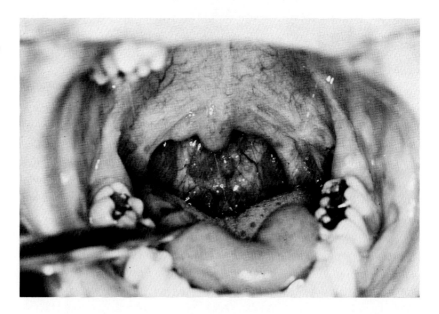

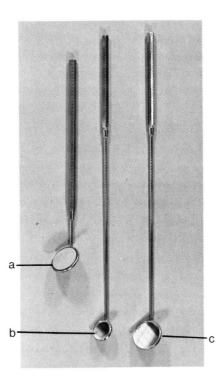

Fig. 9-27. Relative sizes of *a*, oral (dental); *b*, nasopharyngeal; and *c*, laryngeal mirrors.

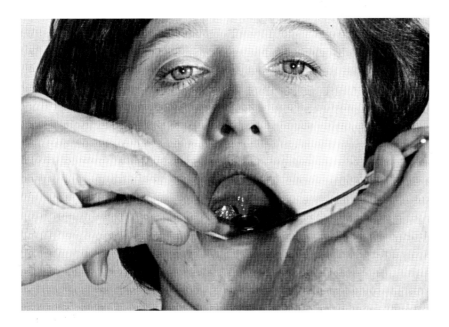

Fig. 9-28. Tongue is depressed firmly and nasopharyngeal mirror introduced into nasopharynx almost touching posterior pharyngeal wall. Care must be taken not to initiate gag reflex by stimulating posterior third of tongue or soft palate. Patient should be instructed to breathe through nose during examination.

The larynx may be examined by direct or indirect laryngoscopy. Direct laryngoscopy requires considerable skill, and it is sometimes necessary for the patient to receive a general anesthetic to obtain an adequate view of the larynx. The more usual office approach to laryngoscopy is by use of the indirect technique. A warmed laryngeal mirror (a dental mirror with an extended handle) is placed in the oropharynx. The examiner grasps the tongue with gauze, pulls it forward, and places the mirror across the soft palate in front of the uvula (Fig. 9-29). This examination may be accomplished successfully by skilled examiners without the need to resort to local anesthesia. However, sometimes it is necessary for the gag reflex to be suppressed by local anesthetic agents in order to facilitate the examination. Any abnormality of the laryngeal anatomy should be carefully noted, and the patient should be asked to phonate to determine that the vocal cords are moving symmetrically (Fig. 9-30). Mention is made in Chapter 16 of the need for the dentist to examine the posterior part of the tongue not only visually but also digitally.

REFERENCE

1. Hales, R.H.: Ocular injuries sustained in the dental office, Am. J. Ophthalmol. **70:**221, 1970.

BIBLIOGRAPHY

Ballenger, J.H.: Diseases of the nose, throat and ear, ed. 12, Philadelphia, 1977, Lea & Febiger.

Deweese, D.D., and Saunders, W.H.: Textbook of otolaryngology, ed. 6, St. Louis, 1981, The C.V. Mosby Co.

Newell, F.W.: Ophthalmology: principles and concepts, ed. 4, St. Louis, 1978, The C.V. Mosby Co.

Scheie, H.G., and Alert, D.M.: Textbook of ophthalmology, ed. 9, Philadelphia, 1977, W.B. Saunders Co.

Vaughan, D., and Asbury, T.: General ophthalmology, ed. 8, Los Altos, Calif., 1977, Lange Publishing Co.

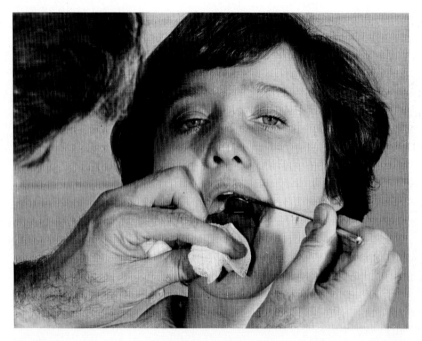

Fig. 9-29. Examiner pulls tongue forward. Mirror is placed against tip of uvula, and uvula and soft palate are pressed upward. Patient should breathe quietly through mouth, and mirror moved to visualize all parts of posterior part of tongue and epiglottis and larynx. Patient should be asked to make high-pitched "e-e-e-e". This can be facilitated by examiner's singing "e-e-e-e" along with patient. This maneuver produces movement of vocal cords.

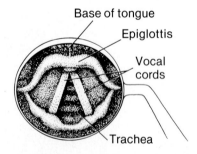

Fig. 9-30. This view of larynx, as seen in laryngeal mirror, shows main anatomic features. Vocal cords are abducted and are bilaterally symmetrical.

10   Skin

The skin is the largest organ of the body. It is of importance to the dentist, since it shares many diseases in common with the oral mucous membrane. Furthermore, skin can reflect many systemic diseases that might influence directly not only dental treatment but also the total health of the individual.

Since much of the skin is visible to the dentist at the time of examination or treatment, the short period of time required for an examination and evaluation of the skin offers an excellent opportunity to render a more complete health service to the patient.

COMPARISON OF SKIN AND MUCOSA

Oral mucous membrane (mucosa) and skin have both similarities and differences. Skin is a bit more complex than mucosa because of its additional structures and functions.

Both organs have a stratified squamous epithelial covering, but whereas skin epithelium is normally orthokeratotic, mucosal epithelium may be parakeratotic or orthokeratotic (see Fig. 6-25), depending on location. Mucosa, of course, is wet.

Fibrous connective tissue and its contents directly beneath the epithelium in skin are called the dermis and in mucosa are called the lamina propria. The dermis contains many accessory organs or appendages, such as hair follicles, smooth muscle bundles, sweat glands, and sebaceous glands. The lamina propria of the oral mucosa contains only mucous, serous, and sebaceous glands.

ANATOMY
Normal skin

The normal skin is composed of three layers (Fig. 10-1): the epidermis, the dermis, and the subcutaneous tissue, or subcutis. Epidermis, the outermost layer, is 1 to 2 mm in thickness and consists of stratified squamous epithelium that is irregularly folded, forming linear ridges or extensions, called rete ridges. The stratified squamous epithelium consists of a basal layer of cells adjacent to the connective tissue and is the germinative portion where renewal of cells takes place. Scattered among the basal cells are the cell bodies and dendritic protoplasmic extensions of melanocytes. As basal cells mature they move upward to form the spinous layer of epithelium, the thickest component of the epidermis. These cells have abundant cytoplasm and are held together by desmosomes. The outermost viable layer of the epidermis is the granular layer, a zone of compressed flattened cells containing numerous keratohyalin granules, the precursors of the epithelial product keratin. This keratin is a nonvital homogeneous layer of material that makes up the surface of the epidermis.

The second layer of the skin, the dermis, is composed of compact collagen fibroblasts, elastic fibers, and ground substance containing blood vessels and nerves. It is usually divided into two parts. The first is the papillary dermis, which is that portion intimately associated with the epithelium and its extensions, the rete ridges, and ends at or near the tips of these extensions. Below this is the reticular dermis, which contains the uppermost portion of the skin appendages. The skin appendages include the hair follicle, erector pilae smooth muscle (which on contraction causes "goose flesh"), and sebaceous glands making up the pilosebaceous apparatus. Also present are sweat glands and ducts. The sweat glands are of two types: the apocrine glands, which are localized in the nipples, the axilla, and anal-genital regions, account for an individual's characteristic odor; the eccrine glands are distributed throughout the body. The glands of the external ear and breast are modified apocrine glands.

The third layer, the subcutis, consists of more loosely arranged fat, collagen, and elastic fibers and contains the germinative portion of the hair follicle, the hair bulb and papillae, and the main portion of the parenchyma of the sweat glands.

The color of the normal skin is a combination of reds, blues, browns, and yellows, varying according to the vascularity and the presence or relative absence of oxidized or reduced hemoglobin (red and blue), melanin (brown), and the carotenes of collagen, fat, sebaceous glands, and elastic fibers (yellow).

Any increase in vascular dilatation (exercise, warmth, or embarrassment, anger, or other emotional excitability) may cause a more reddened appearance in the skin. Conversely, cold or fright may cause vascular constriction, leading to a bluish (cyanotic) or whitish (pallor) color change.

The genetic determination of quality and quantity of melanin pigmentation causes a great variation in color of skin. Exposure to ultraviolet light may increase melanin concentration and darkening of the skin. Localization of this pigment accounts for unevenness of skin color, such as freckles and brown splotches of old skin.

Any change in quality or quantity of fat, collagen, elastic fibers, or sebaceous glands may cause an increase in yellowish cast of normal skin; however, any marked departures toward a yellow color usually signifies a pathologic process.

Fig. 10-1. Normal skin, illustrating various layers and appendages.

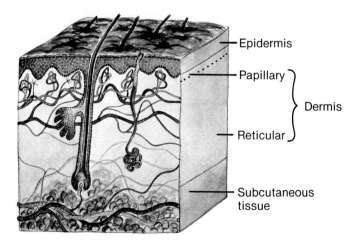

Epidermis

Papillary ⎤
⎬ Dermis
Reticular ⎦

Subcutaneous tissue

Normal skin is mobile or supple, warm, moist, and somewhat soft, but varies greatly from person to person and from one age group to another, and even from one part of the body to another. The presence of a keratin product, pores, hairs, and skin markings (furrows or wrinkles) all contribute to this texture. Softness depends on the cushioning of fat cells of the subcutis, the quality and quantity of collagen, and the amount of keratin present on the surface. Mobility of the skin depends as well on the fatty cushion of the subcutis and the collagen of the dermis and the tissue fluid (turgor). Although laxity of skin may vary with individuals, if it is excessive it may signify disease. Mobility also depends on location. Skin is generally more mobile over soft tissues and bound down over bone, but this is due (at least in part) to the fatty cushion of the subcutis. Turgor, though related to mobility, is somewhat different and represents the resistance of the skin to pressure or tension. Normal skin quickly regains its shape after deformation becasue of the fluid and elastic tissue (memory). Any increase in this time for return to normal, as in pitting edema, is abnormal.

Normal skin is warm but reflects somewhat the external environment. The surface temperature is provided by the circulation of the blood that has been warmed in the central portions of the body, largely as a by-product of energy expenditure from muscular contractions.

The moisture of the normal skin is due to the secretion of the sweat glands and sebaceous glands. This moisture may vary with external temperature and emotion. The oiliness of the skin contributes somewhat to the moist feeling. This oiliness varies markedly from individual to individual.

Skin appendages

The skin appendages (hair, nails, and sebaceous and sweat glands) are modified by hormones at puberty. The apocrine glands begin their changes somewhat early, around 6 to 7 years of age, and account for the change in smell from that of babies to children and finally to adults. Immature fine villous or lanugo hair is present over the body, but at puberty the characteristic change in male and female distribution of hair becomes obvious. The sebaceous glands mature and become larger at puberty; this becomes particularly obvious about the face.

The nails are transparent, nonvital keratin that are generally smooth and firmly adherent to the underlying nail bed, through which changes in the vasculature can be noted (such as cyanosis or anemia). Any changes in production of the keratin of the nails, such as local trauma, may produce changes in contour (ridging) or color, which are only variations of normal.

PHYSIOLOGY

The skin has protective, homeostatic, eliminatory, and sensory functions. The protective function of the skin is by virtue of its covering of epidermis, which prevents loss of fluids and electrolytes. The constant shedding of keratin, as well as the keratin itself, acts as a barrier to bacterial, viral, and fungal organisms attempting to colonize. The melanocytes of the skin prevent damage of ultraviolet light to the underlying structures. Sebum secretion by sebaceous glands also produces a deciduous and emollient protective barrier. The dermis itself is also protective in that it cushions the underlying structures from trauma.

The skin maintains homeostasis through electrolyte transfer and heat regulation by evaporation of secretions of the eccrine sweat glands. Hair in man is vestigial and has little effect in maintaining heat but is quite effective in the lower animals. The subcutis with its fat has a thermoregulatory function. The blood vessels themselves in the dermis through dilatation and constriction alter body temperature.

Elimination of electrolytes and urea and other wastes occur through the skin in the secretions of the eccrine glands.

The numerous sensory types of end organs are located in the skin and include Meissner's corpuscles, Pacini's corpuscles, and nonspecific receptors for pain and temperature. This sensory function in turn provides a protective function as well.

EXAMINATION

Examination of the skin by dentists is usually limited to the exposed portions of the body, although at times it may be important to request that specific sites normally clothed be examined. There are three primary diagnostic tools for the examination of skin: inspection, palpation, and history. Histologic diagnosis of biopsy material is also important in establishing a final diagnosis.

Since the skin is so readily accessible, and since it is confronted so often, it is easy to "look and not see." However, inspection is a most important tool for evaluation of the skin. This inspection should be carried out under good fluorescent lighting. Observation of abnormalities may require removal of makeup that is present. Inspection usually begins in the head and neck region, including the scalp, face, ears, neck, and shoulders and then extends to the arms, hands, and legs, including the nails.

The inspection should concern itself with the specific anatomic area of involvement or site. The morphologic character of the lesions, the pattern or arrangement of the lesions, and their color should be noted. Palpation aids in evaluation of texture, temperature, amount of moisture present, mobility, and turgor, and the presence or feel of any underlying masses.

History includes such things as symptoms, duration and chronology of the appearance, change or evolution, and disappearance of lesions.

Any associated conditions of exposure to injury, medication, or environment that preceded, induced, or altered the condition, the presence of other unseen lesions, other symptoms in the medical history, and prior similar or dissimilar lesions may be an exceedingly important portion of the history.

COMMON ABNORMALITIES
Color

Abnormal color changes in the skin may furnish clues to basic underlying local or systemic diseases. These abnormal colors are brown, yellow, white, red, and blue.

Brown coloration is usually due to an increase in melanin (see Chapter 5). This increase may be brought about in response to ultraviolet light stimulation or melanocyte-stimulating hormone (MSH) or by tumors of the pituitary gland or steroids similar to MSH from the adrenal glands (tumors, Addison's disease, or pregnancy). Breakdown of blood hemosiderin pigments may cause a tan discoloration in hemochromatosis. All these colorations are, of course, generalized. Local brown pigmentation may occur in melanin-producing tumors, postinflammatory hyperpigmentation (dropping of melanin into the connective tissue after epithelial disruption), and genetic disorders, such as cafe au lait spots or von Recklinghausen's neurofibromatosis.

Yellow color changes may be seen with an increased amount of bile pigment (bilirubin) as in hepatic dysfunction (jaundice), blockage of bile ducts by tumors of the head of the pancreas, or autolysis of erythrocytes in erythroblastosis fetalis.

In renal failure urochromes may show through the skin as a yellow coloration. In anemias, particularly pernicious anemia, the lack of oxygenated blood allows the yellow collagen to show through the skin. With excessive ingestion of foods high in carotene or (rarely) in cases of diabetes, myxedema, or hypopituitarism a generalized yellow color may be seen. Lipid-containing tumors or blood breakdown products such as biliverdin may cause localized yellow discoloration.

The color white is usually a relative change and is sometimes a result of a loss of melanin. It may be generalized, as in albinism, or localized, as in vitiligo, postinflammatory conditions, resolution of nevi and other melanocytic tumors, scars, and certain fungal infections, such as tinea versicolor.

A decrease in the amount of oxygenated hemoglobin may cause a whiteness or pallor, as in anemia, or a decrease in vascular profusion, as in syncope or shock; and in cases where an increase in other structures or material prevents the normal color of the blood from showing through the skin (such as edema or hyperkeratosis), a white coloration may be perceived.

Red is usually a result of increased visibility of oxygenated erythrocytes. This may be due to an increased number of erythrocytes (polycythemia) extravasation of erythrocytes (petechiae or purpura), vascular dilatation as occurs in many inflammatory diseases of the skin, fever, alcohol intake, or an increase in vessels, as in a vascular malformation or tumor.

A blue color is a result of reduced hemoglobin. This may be localized, as in a vascular tumor that predominantly contains venous blood, or when there is stasis. A generalized bluish color may be seen in anxiety, cold, heart or lung disorders, congenital metabolic defects in erythrocytes, or acquired conditions such as methemoglobinemia.

Morphology

The variety of morphologic changes seen on the skin is greater than that on the oral mucosa. However, all of the morphologic descriptions discussed in Chapter 6 can also be applied to the skin. As in oral mucosa, the skin has both primary and secondary lesions. Primary lesions are those that arise from normal skin. Secondary lesions result from a change in a preexisting lesion or abnormality. The papule, nodule, tumor, plaque, vesicle, pustule, and bulla are all elevated primary lesions that occur on the skin. In addition, the term *wheal* is used to describe a kind of lesion that is found localized and well demarcated, with a slightly raised focus of edema that appears whiter or sometimes redder than the surrounding normal skin (Fig. 10-2).

The erosion and ulcer previously described in the oral cavity may also occur on the skin as either a primary or secondary lesion.

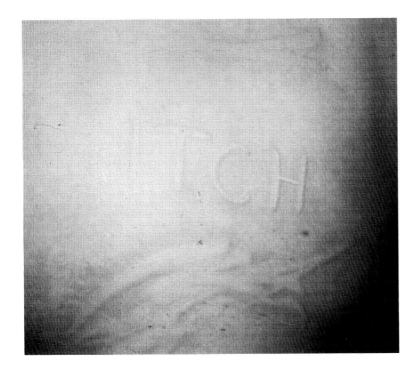

Fig. 10-2. Clinical example of wheals induced by stylus pressure in area of urticaria.

Secondary lesions that occur on the skin but not as commonly on the oral mucosa include crusts, scales, fissures, scars, and keloids. A crust is an accumulation of dried serum, blood, or pus, draining from a previous lesion, such as a vesicle or pustule (Fig. 10-3). A scale is composed of loosely attached flakes of incompletely exfoliated parakeratinized or keratinized epidermal cells (Fig. 10-4). This may occur in excessively rapid turnover of epithelium, as in psoriasis. A fissure is a narrow vertical linear crack or tear of the epidermis. This morphologic type may be seen in conditions such as athelete's foot or on the palms and soles of patients with Darier's disease. A scar is a firm, slightly depressed well-demar-

Fig. 10-3. Crust formation of dried serum from lesion of impetigo.

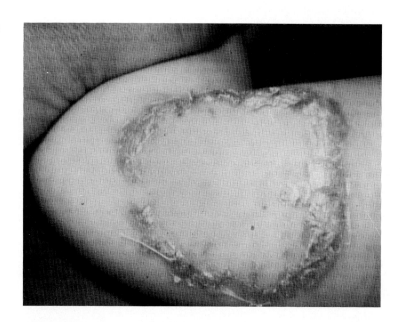

Fig. 10-4. Scale formation on lesion of psoriasis.

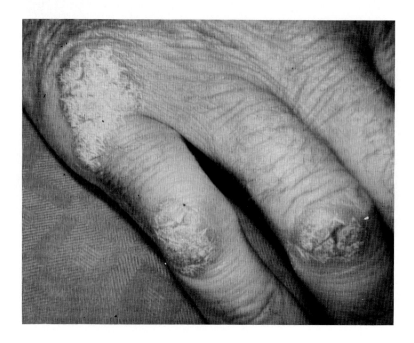

cated area that is whiter than the normal surrounding skin (Fig. 10-5). This is due to replacement of normal dermis by dense collagen fibers. In some predisposed individuals, particularly blacks, a hypertrophic raised scar may form in response to epidermal trauma, and a tumefaction of dense fibrous tissue is formed. This is called a keloid (Fig. 10-6).

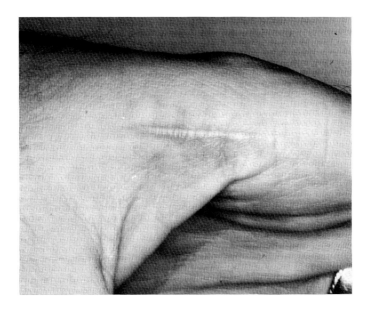

Fig. 10-5. Linear scar on hand from deep laceration.

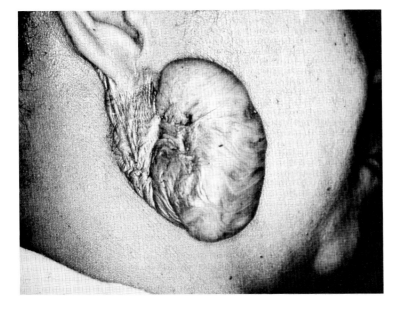

Fig. 10-6. Keloid developing after piercing of ear.

The terms *atrophy, lichenification,* and *excoriation* are also used as adjectival descriptions but not as nominative morphologic entities for certain skin lesions. Atrophy refers to a thinning of the epidermis with loss of skin markings or furrows, leaving the skin smoother and more translucent than normal. Lichenification represents the opposite of atrophy: there is thickening of the skin and an increase in the markings or furrows. Lichenification is usually seen in chronic inflammatory conditions. Excoriation refers to linear or punctate changes occurring in a pruritic (itching) lesion because of scratching (Fig. 10-7).

Patterns

Patterns of lesions, as well as morphologic type and color, are important in evaluating lesions by inspection. Some patterns are characteristic of specific diseases.

Skin lesions may be annular, that is, arranged in arches or arcs or combinations of these geometric figures. They may also be described as arciform or polycyclic (Fig. 10-8). Diseases that characteristically show these patterns include erythema multiforme, urticaria, psoriasis, and larva migrans (ringworm). A similar pattern that is more like a wavy line or snake-like configuration is described as serpiginous (Fig. 10-8). Lesions of geographic tongue often take on this appearance (see Fig. 16-112).

An iris, or target, lesion is one that appears to be composed of concentric circles (Fig. 10-9).

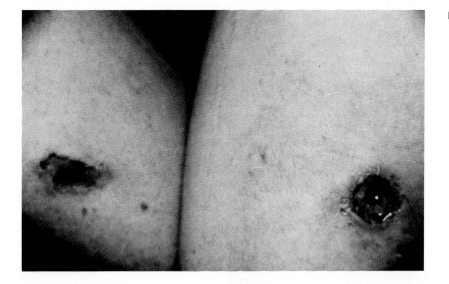

Fig. 10-7. Punctate excoriations.

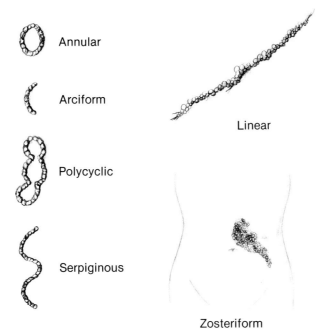

Fig. 10-8. Some common morphologic patterns that skin lesions may form.

Annular

Arciform

Polycyclic

Serpiginous

Linear

Zosteriform

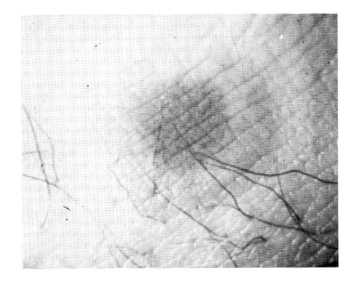

Fig. 10-9. Iris or target lesion on skin of patient with erythema multiforme.

A linear grouping of lesions may occur and is seen in lymphangitis or contact dermatitis. Linear streaks may appear within an irregular grouping, that is, one with no obvious or distinct patterns, as a result of scratching or excoriation, as often occurs in lichen planus. The linear production of skin lesions by trauma in an uninvolved area of the skin in the presence of other lesions nearby is referred to as Koebner's phenomenon (Fig. 10-10).

Zosteriform refers to groupings of lesions present in swaths in the pattern and area of a cutaneous nerve distribution (Fig. 10-11). The name comes, of course, from the classic arrangement of lesions of herpes zoster (shingles) along the course of the cutaneous sensory nerves.

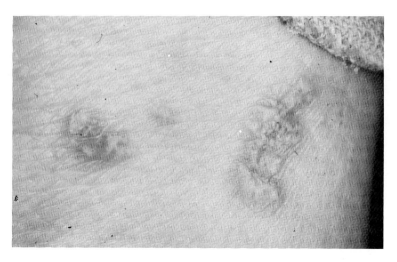

Fig. 10-10. Koebner's phenomenon: lesions of lichen planus on arm resulting from scratching previously uninvolved area of skin.

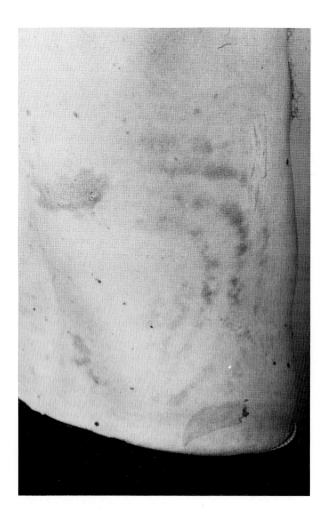

Fig. 10-11. Patient with lesions following distribution of cutaneous nerves.

Skin appendages

Abnormalities of the skin appendages, nails, and hair have specialized features and are discussed separately. Hair growth may become excessive and is referred to as hypertrichosis or hirsuitism (Fig. 10-12). This excessive growth is usually hormonal dependent, and its appearance in a female might suggest underlying tumors of the ovary or a condition called Stein-Leventhal syndrome. Hypertrichosis may be a component of some genetic syndromes and localized tumor growth, such as the bathing trunk nevus.

Alopecia, or loss of hair, may be spotty, as in alopecia areata, secondary syphilis, or aging in a male pattern (genetically determined); or diffuse, as in postpartum telogen effluvium or alopecia universalis (Fig. 10-13).

Canities, or graying of the hair, usually occurs at senescence but may occur earlier in genetically predisposed individuals.

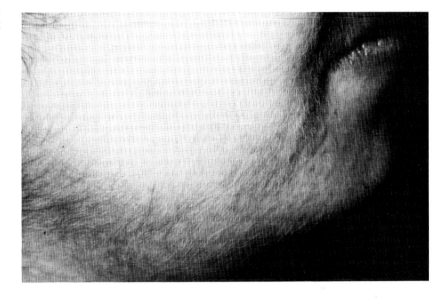

Fig. 10-12. Hirsuitism in female patient receiving high-dose steroid therapy.

Fig. 10-13. A, Spotty alopecia in patient with ectodermal dysplasia. **B,** Total alopecia in young female with ectodermal dysplasia.

A

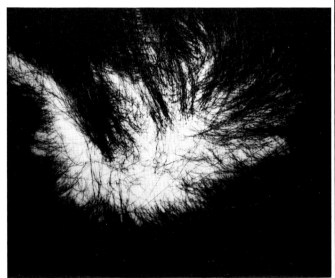

B

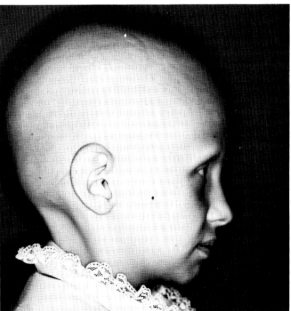

The nails reflect the past, since they are dead sheets of keratin that are produced at the rate of 0.1 mm per day from the germinative cells at the proximal portion of the nail. Disturbances in growth, local or systemic, may result in abnormalities of the keratin plate. A white change called leukonychia may result from trauma (Fig. 10-14). Transverse furrows (Beau's lines) may result from matrix growth arrest in a variety of systemic diseases or even local trauma or infection. There are typical disturbances of the nails in psoriasis and Darier's disease (Fig. 10-15).

Any inflammatory process, but particularly fungal infections, will cause periungal or paronychial swelling, erythema, and elevation of the nail plate from the nail bed (onycholysis) (Fig. 10-16). The vascular nail bed may also reflect the present status of the body in such conditions as cyanosis and anemia. Subungal vascular streaks are characteristic of Darier's disease and tumors (subungal fibromas in tuberous sclerosis). Splinter hemorrhages thought at one time to be specific for subacute bacterial endocarditis are now known to be nonspecific and may be found in a number of diseases.

Fig. 10-14. Leukonychia from trauma.

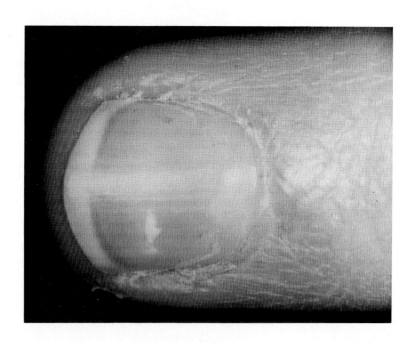

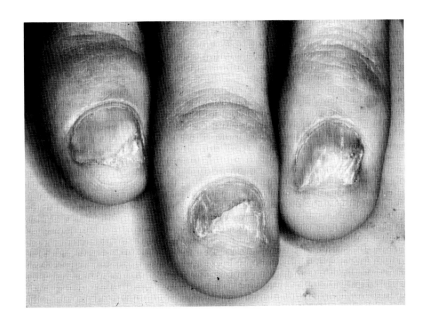

Fig. 10-15. Nail changes in patient with psoriasis.

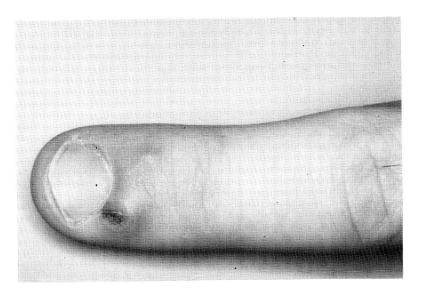

Fig. 10-16. Paronychia (herpetic whitlow).

Purpuric and vascular disorders

Since petechiae and ecchymoses result from extravasation of blood into tissue, they are signs rather than diagnoses and may result from numerous underlying diseases (see Figs. 6-24 and 16-92), including coagulation defects as occur in the hemophilias or thrombocytopenia. Infectious diseases such as Rocky Mountain spotted fever and streptococcal infections may produce petechiae and ecchymoses. The triad of adrenal hemorrhage, purpuric lesions, and septicemia, especially with meningococcemia, is called Waterhouse-Friderichsen syndrome. Similar lesions may be present in protein disturbances such as cryoglobulinemia, in autoimmune diseases such as lupus erythematosus, and reactions to toxic substances. Allergic disorders often produce a necrotizing vasculitis or angiitis, causing purpuric lesions.

The term *hemangioma of the skin* may mean a true vascular tumor, a vascular anomaly (hamartoma), or a dilatation of existing blood vessels. Large, bulky, vascular lesions resembling the usual hemangiomas seen in the oral cavity may sometimes be found on the skin but are relatively uncommon. They are called venous hemangiomas. Hemangiomas are particularly common in infants and the elderly (Fig. 10-17). Most are not associated with other systemic disorders. In infants hemangiomas often appear at or shortly after birth. Nevus flammeus, or port-wine stain, is one of the most common types. It is a capillary lesion appearing on the face as a purple or red lesion similar in color to port wine (Fig. 10-18). When this is associated with hemangiomatous involvement of the brain with ensuing epilepsy or mental retardation, it is called encephalotrigeminal angiomatosis (Sturge-Weber syndrome).

A cavernous hemangioma called a strawberry nevus (nevus vasculosus) is the other most common type of hemangioma in children. It usually undergoes spontaneous involution. A salmon patch or nuchal type of hemangioma is another common infantile vascular lesion.

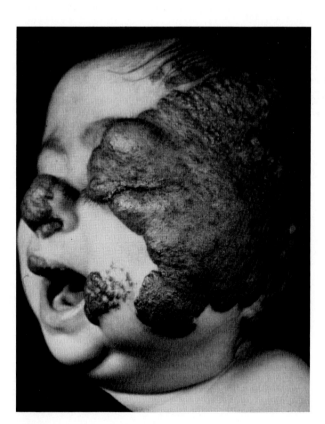

Fig. 10-17. Large facial hemangioma present at birth.

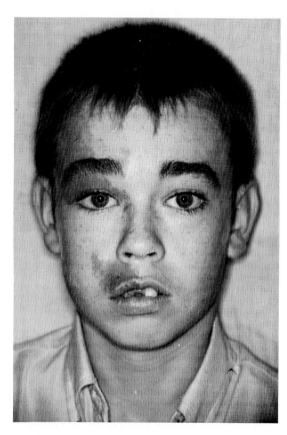

Fig. 10-18. Nevus flammeus in patient with Sturge-Weber syndrome.

In adults, various hemangiomas may be seen and include the spider hemangioma, or nevus araneosus, a small red arteriolar lesion with multiple radiating, branching, and anastomosing channels that occurs above the waist on the torso, face, and extremities and blanches on pressure. It may be found in normal people, but is more common in those with liver disease and vitamin B deficiencies (alcoholics) or in pregnant women. Cherry angiomas, small, round, slightly raised, bright red lesions, are common in adults and generally increase in number with age.

Venous stars, or venous lesions, appearing purple or blue, may be spider-like or linear, appearing most commonly on the legs in the presence of varicosities, multiple telangiectasias, or dilatation of the vessels; they may also be seen on the face and around the mouth, including the mucous membrane, as small papules or even depressed lesions in hereditary hemorrhagic telangiectasia (Rendu-Osler-Weber syndrome) (Fig. 10-19).

Lymphangiomas of the skin in the absence of congenital or other associated factors are uncommon. Diffuse lymphangiomatous involvement of the neck is seen in cystic hygroma (hygroma colli) (Fig. 10-20), and diffuse involvement of the skin is seen in Milroy's disease.

Malignant vascular lesions may occur on the skin. Lymphangiosarcoma may appear on the upper extremities after mastectomy and is known as the Stewart-Treves syndrome. Hemangiosarcoma may be seen as a solitary lesion and also as multiple smooth-surfaced purple or black nodules of the lower extremities in older individuals. This multifocal hemangiosarcoma is called Kaposi's sarcoma.

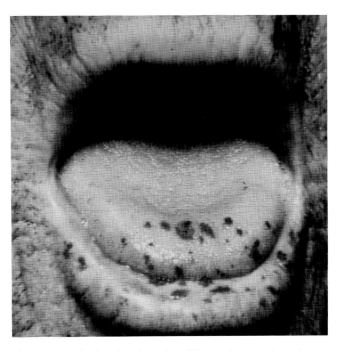

Fig. 10-19. Multiple telangiectasias of lips and tongue in patient with hereditary hemorrhagic telangiectasia.

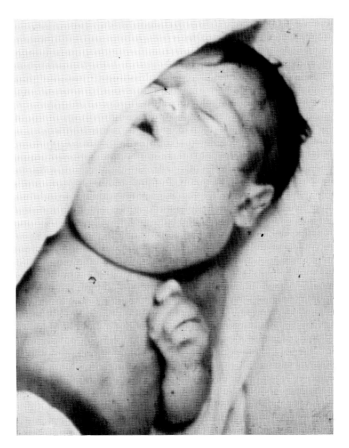

Fig. 10-20. Cystic hygroma at birth.

Pigmentation

Focal extrinsic pigmentation may be seen on the skin as a result of foreign bodies that produce localized tattoos. Materials such as graphite, pencils, or ink pens stabbed into the skin may deposit their pigmented material. Powder burns, grease gun accidents, and other explosive mishaps may introduce a variety of pigmented material into the skin, as may abrasions produced by pigmented objects. The common decorative tattoo seen in characteristic personality types may be present in a variety of unusual and usual locations. The pigments, particularly the red (cinnabar or mercuric sulfide) and green (chromium compounds), may incite an allergic inflammatory reaction of the skin. A focal grayish coloration about the face was seen when heavy metals were used in ointments and face cream. More diffuse extrinsic pigmentations may be seen in heavy metal poisoning, such as chronic bismuth or mercury ingestion.

Poikilodermatous conditions, such as result from radiation, consist of intrinsic melanin pigmentation and may be seen in exposed areas as a blotchy brown pigmentation. Pigmentation because of radiation is not as often seen as in the past since the advent of supervoltage therapy for malignancies. A generalized gray discoloration may be seen in chrysiasis, which is due to the ingestion of gold salts with exposure to sunlight; a blue gray color may be seen with argyria and with ingestion of arsenic, giving a characteristic generalized "raindrop" pigmentation. Generalized intrinsic pigmentation may be seen in Addison's disease (brown), hemochromatosis (bluish or gray), and carotenemia (yellow). Gray to silver hair and gray coloration of the skin may be seen in Chédiak-Higashi syndrome. Patients with xeroderma pigmentosum, a genetically inherited sensitivity to ultraviolet light, show inflammation, pigmentation, and eventually neoplastic changes on the skin exposed to sunlight.

Chloasma (melasma), a brown, spotty, but sometimes diffuse melanin pigmentation, may be seen as a result of external causes, such as friction or cosmetics, or internal metabolic changes, such as pregnancy, birth control pills, and endocrine imbalances. This is commonly seen about the face and neck of females.

Ephelis (ephelides, plural) is the common benign freckle seen on exposed portions of the body in light-skinned individuals. Ephelides are usually seen in children but can occur at any age. Lesions with a similar clinical appearance on unexposed portions of the body are more likely lentigines (lentigo, singular). They are benign and occur in children and adults; in the latter they are sometimes called "liver spots." The lentigo differs from freckles histologically by the presence of melanocytic hyperplasia or clear cell activity in the former.

A spotty, brown black macular, ephelis-like pigmentation around the mouth and on the palms and soles occurs in conjunction with intestinal familial polyposis in the Peutz-Jeghers syndrome (see Fig. 16-14).

A malignant form of lentigo occurs that is unrelated to the benign form. Lentigo maligna (Fig. 10-21), or melanotic freckle of Hutchinson, begins after age 40 as a light brown macule that darkens and spreads peripherally over the course of many years. It occurs most commonly on the face, but may occur in any location. Some patients may develop areas of induration and dark pigmentation that are slightly raised concomitant with an atypical change to melanocytic proliferation at the basal layer of the epidermis. Melanomas arising from this lesion are referred to as lentigo maligna melanoma and have a relatively good prognosis.

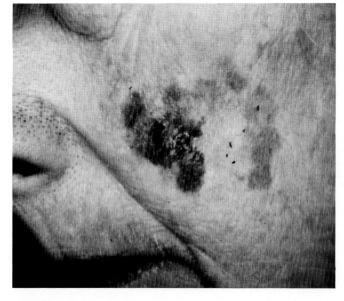

Fig. 10-21. Lentigo maligna.

Nevi

Ordinary pigmented nevi, or cellular nevi or moles, are extremely common (Fig. 10-22). Nevi usually develop during childhood after the age of 1 to 2 and may continue to develop into adulthood. The basic cell of origin is the epithelial-transformed melanocytes from the neural crest. There are three general types of nevi: junctional, intradermal, and compound. Junctional nevi are flat, brown to black pigmented lesions, predominantly on the extremities, and more common in younger people. The proliferation of melanocytes is at the junction of epithelium and connective tissue; hence the name.

In intradermal nevi, the melanocytes are transformed into nevus cells and are limited to the dermis. These nevi are rare in children, common in adults, and occur about the head and face most commonly. They may or may not show clinical pigmentation.

The compound nevus histologically shows a junctional as well as a dermal component, a combination of the features of the other two types, and clinically exhibits features between the junctional and dermal nevi. These three types of ordinary nevi are all benign. However, melanoma has been known to arise in some of them.

Since the junctional nevus shows the most cellular activity, the dermal the least, and the compound activity somewhere in between, one would suspect that their relative activity would reflect their malignant potential; and such is the case. At times, distinction between active junctional nevi and melanoma can be extremely difficult clinically as well as histologically.

Melanoma is the malignant counterpart of the benign melanocytic nevus. Although melanomas may arise from preexisting nevi, most are thought to arise de novo (Fig. 10-23). There appear to be two basic types of melanoma, the superficial spreading type and the nodular type. The superficial type appears as a predominantly macular brown lesion with darker papules within it. The pigment tends to feather out peripherally. This lesion tends to grow laterally for extended periods before deep invasion begins. It has a substantially better prognosis than the nodular type, which forms a brown or black nodular tumor and is sometimes ulcerated.

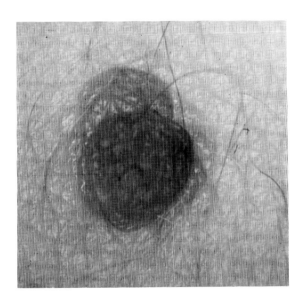

Fig. 10-22. Pigmented intradermal nevus.

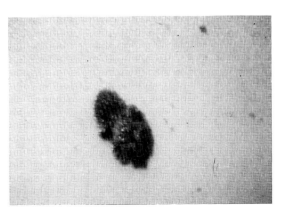

Fig. 10-23. Melanoma.

135

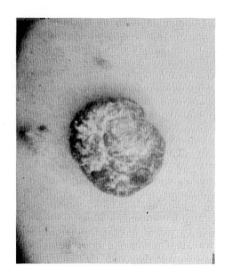

Fig. 10-24. Juvenile melanoma.

Fig. 10-25. Blue nevus.

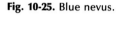

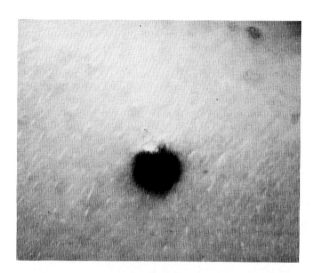

Fig. 10-26. Giant hairy nevus.

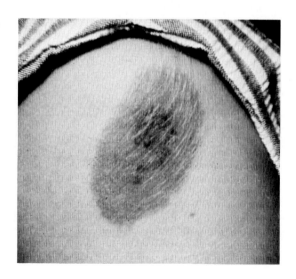

The predominant growth of the nodular type of melanoma is both upward and downward with early invasion and a poor prognosis. Dissemination of melanoma may occur by lymphatics to form satellite lesions of the skin peripherally or regional and distant node involvement. Blood-borne metastases to lungs and viscera occur frequently.

There are several other types of nevi that may be seen on the skin, one of which is a juvenile melanoma or (the name now preferred) the epithelioid and spindle cell nevus. This is a benign melanocytic tumor that may be confused microscopically with melanoma. There are criteria, however, that usually allow this important distinction. Clinically, the lesion usually appears papillary and red because of its vascularity, resembling a pyogenic granuloma, and though occurring more often in children, may occur in adults (Fig. 10-24).

Another type of nevus is the blue nevus, a discrete round or oval papule or nodule that has a smooth surface and is a steel blue, dark blue, or even blue gray or black color (Fig. 10-25). Blue nevi are more common about the face and upper extremities but may occur anywhere. They are often present at birth and may occur in adult life. They may slowly enlarge or occasionally regress. The blue nevus is composed of dermal melanocytes that have not been transformed or influenced by the epithelial cells. They actively produce melanin and are located in the lower to middle one third of the dermis. This depth modifies the brown melanin and accounts for its characteristic blue color. The blue nevus is benign, but a malignant form does exist; a rapidly growing lesion of the previously mentioned morphologic type may suggest the malignant form.

The giant hairy nevus, or bathing trunk nevus, is a congenital nevus that is brown to black with a long heavy growth of hair in the area of pigmentation (Fig. 10-26). It may be focal or may cover most of the body, sometimes in the distribution of a bathing suit. About 10% to 20% of them may undergo malignant transformation to melanoma and thus require prophylactic removal.

The halo nevus is characterized by the appearance of a conspicuous zone of peripheral depigmentation about an ordinary pigmented nevus (Fig. 10-27). They may be single or multiple; this phenomenon supposedly represents an immunologically enforced resolution of an ordinary nevus.

Bacterial dermatoses

Those diseases in which an infection is the primary cause are referred to as pyodermas.

Impetigo is one of the most common and most superficial dermatoses, causing vesiculation underneath the superficial keratin layer. It occurs primarily in children as pustules or crusted lesions on the face and other portions of the body. The cause is streptococci or staphylococci, and the condition is highly contagious (Fig. 10-28).

Ecthyma is similar to impetigo but penetrates deeper and forms larger, flat, colored crusts on the skin of the lower extremities and buttocks. It is usually caused by streptoccoci, but staphylococci may be involved.

Large, deeply inflitrating ulcerated lesions with undermined borders from streptococcal infections are called pyoderma gangrenosum.

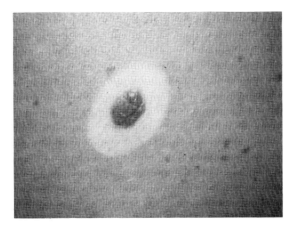

Fig. 10-27. Halo nevus.

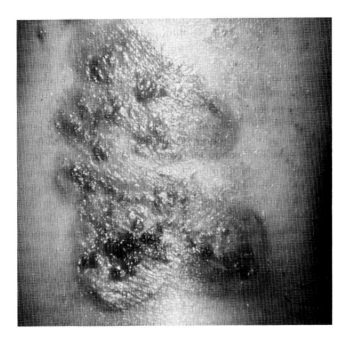

Fig. 10-28. Impetigo: May result from staphylococcus or streptococcus.

An inflammatory involvement of the pilosebaceous unit is called folliculitis and is associated with numerous disease processes, including bacteria, fungi, and even noninfectious disorders. The term is largely descriptive and clinically refers to a pustular involvement of the pilosebaceous unit.

Acne is folliculitis associated with stoppage of the follicle by a keratin plug or comedo. It is a papular, nodular, and pustular disorder occurring predominantly at puberty but at times extending into adulthood. It affects the face, neck, and upper chest and back. Bacterial involvement is secondary in this lesion. The blockage, hormonal, and genetic factors play a principal role. Acneiform lesions may be seen in steroid treatment.

A furuncle is a painful, indurated lesion, usually in relation to a hair follicle. The cause of involvement of the follicle is usually a staphylococcal infection with extension perifollicularly into the tissues to form an abscess deep in the cutis. A core may be expressed. Healing often takes place with scarring. A carbuncle is an extension of a furuncle in the cutis with the involvement of several hair follicles, resulting in numerous openings onto the surface. Extreme scarring results.

Inflammatory involvement of the sweat glands is called hidradenitis. Involvement of the apocrine glands results in hidradenitis suppurativa. It is a chronic suppurative disease caused by cocci, usually involving the axillary, genital, and inguinal regions where apocrine glands are usually found. It appears as a deep-seated tender nodule. Multiple sinus tracts and ulcerations may form, as well as cellulitis.

Acne rosacea is a chronic disease occurring on the face of adults, particularly women. A mild erythematous, telangiectatic, papular, or even pustular appearance occurs on the midface. Severe involvement with hyperplasia of the sebaceous glands in males may cause enlargement of the nose, which is called rhinophyma. The cause is probably infection.

Erysipelas is a diffuse inflammation of the skin caused by streptococci. There is redness and swelling, usually with constitutional symptoms. It may occur as a result of wounds or may be recurrent in some susceptible individuals (Fig. 10-29).

Syphilis is an extremely interesting and complex sexually transmitted disease. There are many dermatologic manifestations, including the primary lesion, the chancre. This is an indurated painless ulcer that occurs at the site of inoculation. It may be genital or extragenital. This is followed by constitutional symptoms and various combinations of secondary lesions, including a ham-colored maculopapular rash in a number of patterns, mucous patches of the mouth, alope-cia, iritis, condyloma lata (warty growths), and split papules of the oral commissures. The tertiary stage may cause gummas, large destructive ulcerated lesions with a rubbery base. Aneurysms of the ascending aorta (vascular syphilis) or encephalitis (neurosyphilis) cause mental derangement (paresis) and loss of motor function (tabes dorsalis).

Congenital syphilis may be acquired by the fetus from an infected mother. The child may develop all the stages of syphilis except the primary lesion. In addition, stigmata such as saber shins, saddle nose, Charcot's joints, Hutchinson's triad of interstitial keratitis, eighth nerve deafness, and screwdriver-shaped incisors (Hutchinson's incisors), and mulberry molars may occur (see Fig. 17-25).

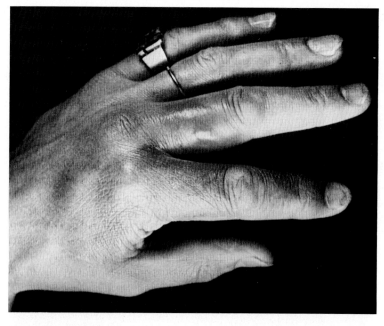

Fig. 10-29. Erysipelas.

Viral diseases

Exanthems are those viral diseases that produce a disseminated rash on the skin. Some of the more common ones are mentioned here. Measles, or morbilli, is a highly contagious viral disease transmitted by droplet infection. It occurs primarily in young children, appearing with a prodrome of fever, malaise, cough, rhinorrhea, and conjunctivitis. A characteristic rash of minute white papules with a red halo, called Koplik's spots, occurs on the buccal mucosa. This is followed by a florid erythematous maculopapular rash that begins on the head and spreads to the trunk and extremities over a 3-day period. Regression occurs with fine desquamation in reverse order of appearance after 5 to 6 days. It is normally a self-limited disease, but complications including encephalitis and death may occur.

German measles, or rubella, most often occurs in older children and young adults. The fetus is particularly susceptible and accounts primarily for the importance of this disease. Many cases are subclinical, especially in young children. Clinical infections are characterized by a generalized lymphadenopathy and mild constitutional symptoms (much less severe than with morbilli) for about 1 week before the fine maculopapular rash that spreads centrifugally within 24 hours and lasts 2 to 3 days. Adults may develop arthritis as a complication.

Acute infectious erythema, or fifth disease, clinically resembles German measles, but early in the course a flush of the cheeks (as if they had been slapped) occurs. It is probably of viral origin.

Pityriasis rosea is also probably a viral disease that begins as a "herald patch," a single oval plaque several centimeters in diameter that precedes the generalized eruption by several days or weeks. The generalized lesions are oval pink or tan plaques with a fine scale in the center and larger loose scales on the periphery, forming a collarette. Pruritus or itching may be minimal, and spontaneous regression occurs after several weeks.

Some viral exanthems, such as smallpox, chickenpox, and herpes, produce vesicles. Fortunately, variola, or smallpox, is almost of historical interest only, since it is expected that within the next few years the disease will have been eliminated through preventive vaccination. Variola is a generalized papular eruption that becomes umbilicated vesicles within 2 to 3 days. These become pustules, sometimes with a hemorrhagic base, within another 3 days, and finally crusts form. All lesions appear in the same stage at the same time. A prodromal prostrating fever, head and back pains, vomiting, and often a rash of the torso may all occur.

In contrast, varicella, or chickenpox, has no prodrome in children, though it may occur in adults, and a maculopapular rash appears over the body. Vesicles with a red halo form rapidly. These become pustular and crust. Several crops of lesions occur over several days, leaving lesions in different stages over the skin. Although usually mild and self-limited, cerebral involvement may be a serious complication (Fig. 10-30).

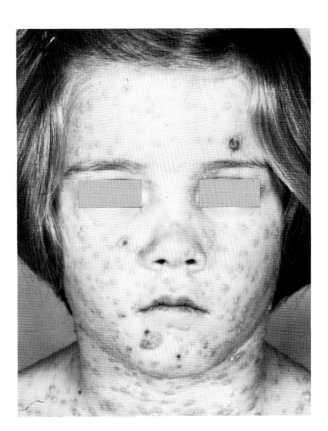

Fig. 10-30. Varicella (chickenpox).

Herpes zoster, or shingles, is caused by the varicella virus and is apparently the expression of the disease in a partially immune individual (Fig. 10-31). In adults the appearance of the lesions is heralded by a prodromal burning in the area of involvement. Within a variable period of time, a vesicular eruption occurs on an erythematous base, always unilaterally along the distribution of cutaneous sensory nerves. These vesicles rupture and crust, and after healing they often leave the patient with a postherpetic neuralgia, an intense pain of several weeks' or months' duration. The characteristic prodrome and distribution of the lesions are usually diagnostic. Smears of the vesicles of varicella or zoster show the characteristic viral cytopathogenic effect of multinucleated cells and balloon degeneration cells.

Inoculation of the varicella virus in an individual with preexisting dermatoses may result in an acute extensive eruption called eczema vaccinatum. If the herpes simplex virus is involved, the eruption is called eczema herpeticum. They are clinically indistinguishable and are referred to collectively as Kaposi's varicelliform eruption (Fig. 10-32).

Infections of herpes simplex have a peculiar clinical course in that primary infection on first exposure to the virus may be asymptomatic in most of the cases, followed by periodic recurrences in the "immune" individual. About 2% of the infections are clinically evident and are manifested by malaise, fever, lymphadenopathy, erythematous marginal gingiva, and oral ulcerations lasting 10 to 14 days. A primary infection may also involve the genitalia.

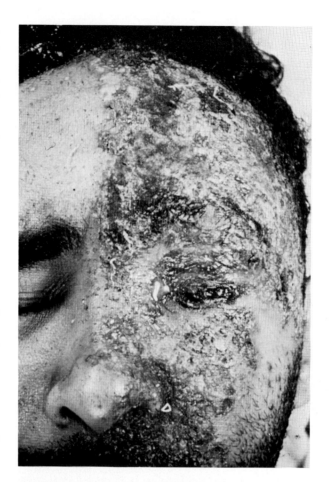
Fig. 10-31. Herpes zoster (shingles).

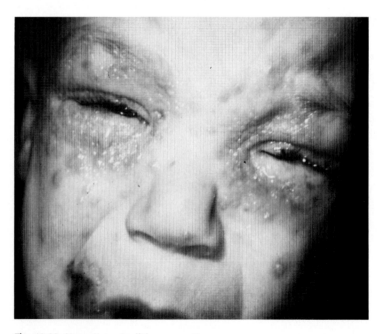
Fig. 10-32. Kaposi's varicelliform eruption.

There are two serologic types of herpes simplex infections. Type I usually involves the mouth and skin, and type II the genitalia. Periodic recurrences are manifested by painful, small, separate or coalescing vesicles that become pustular. There is exudation, crusting, and finally healing over a 1 to 2 week period. The recurrences may involve the oral cavity, lips (cold sores or fever blisters), fingers (herpetic whitlow), eyes (herpetic keratitis), glabrous skin (herpes glabiotorium), genitalia, or almost any part of the body skin (Fig. 10-33).

Some viral diseases result in tumor formation. The common wart, or verruca vulgaris, is an example of this. The lesions are single or multiple papillary keratotic growths of the skin or mucous membranes. Fingers are the most common site. Spontaneous regression is common. Verruca plana, or flat warts, also occur.

Condyloma acuminatum is a soft verrucous papule or nodule that coalesces to form a cauliflower-like mass of the genitalia and sometimes mouth. It is transmitted by sexual contact (Fig. 10-34).

Molluscum contagiosum is a virally induced tumor that is characterized by multiple, discrete, small, waxy, flesh-colored nodules with umbilicated centers from which material may be expressed. This material is composed of elementary viral bodies (Fig. 10-35).

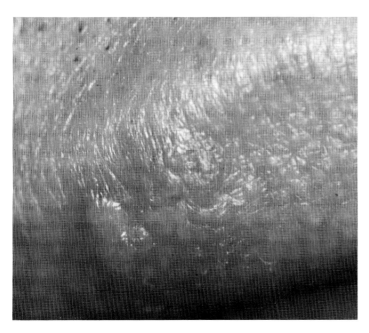

Fig. 10-33. Vesicles of early stage recurrent herpes simplex.

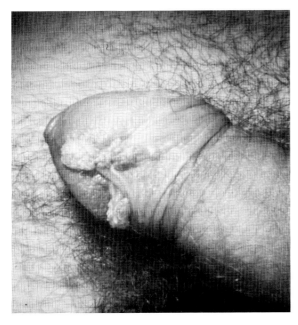

Fig. 10-34. Condyloma acuminatum.

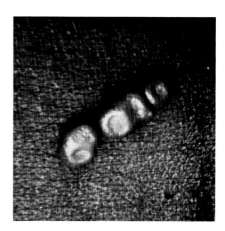

Fig. 10-35. Molluscum contagiosum.

Cysts of the skin

Milia are common cystic lesions seen about the cheeks, eyelids, and face, as well as the genitalia. They are 1 to 2 mm white firm papules appearing like seeds beneath the translucent skin. They may be congenital or may occur at any age and are asymptomatic. They are merely small epithelial-lined keratinizing cysts, similar to Epstein's pearls found in the mouths of infants (Fig. 10-36).

The epithelial, or epidermoid, cyst is one that appears as a smooth-surfaced, nonpainful, round or oval swelling beneath the skin in any part of the body. It may be soft or firm and vary from a few millimeters to several centimeters in diameter. It is an epithelial-lined cyst with a prominent granular area and contains abundant keratin. This term is synonymous with the older term, sebaceous cyst. A similar appearing lesion, which occurs most commonly on the scalp, is the pilar cyst. It is thought to arise from cells of the hair follicle, since keratinization occurs like hair, without going through the formation of keratohyaline granules (Fig. 10-37).

Dermoid cysts are usually deeply seated cysts and not often seen on the skin. They occur frequently in the midline. They are characterized by several germ layers, in other words, mesoderm and endoderm as well as ectoderm. Sebaceous glands, hair follicles with hair, bone, cartilage, muscle, intestinal epithelium, or other structures may be present.

All these cysts are benign and asymptomatic and most often produce only cosmetic problems. Expression of the contents, or cautery, is the treatment of milia, and the other types of cysts are treated by surgical removal.

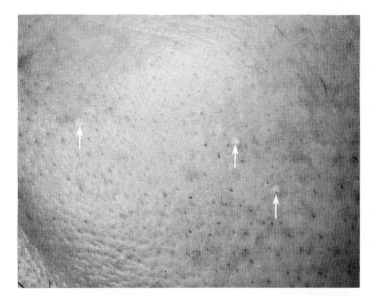

Fig. 10-36. Milia.

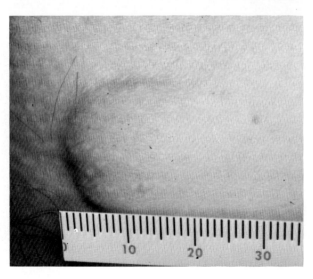

Fig. 10-37. Epidermoid cyst.

Tumors of the skin

No attempt is made here to be inclusive with the discussion of tumors of the skin because of their large number and complexity. Only the more common or more important ones are included here.

The term *nevus* (plural, nevi) is used by dermatologists as a broad definition; that is, it is considered only a mark or a spot. As previously discussed, there are pigmented, or vascular, nevi, and there are also epithe-

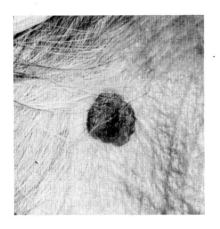

Fig. 10-38. Seborrheic keratosis.

lial nevi. The term *epithelial nevus* encompasses any nevoid condition present at birth or sometimes occuring later that involves hyperplasia of epithelial cells. This results in a keratotic rough, warty lesion of the skin. Epithelial nevi may be localized, as in sebaceous nevus of Jadassohn, or generalized in icthyosis.

Seborrheic keratoses are very common lesions developing in the fifth or sixth decade, especially on the arms, torso, and face, but they may be found in other areas. They begin as small, rough, light tan lesions and enlarge with deepening pigmentation to a brown or even black color. They may be single or multiple. The characteristic features are a "stuck-on" appearance like dirty candle wax, a soft feeling, and a greasy, scaly covering that may be rubbed off. Small multiple lesions may occur about the face in blacks, sometimes beginning in puberty, and are called dermatosis papulosis nigra. There are a variety of histologic patterns in seborrheic keratosis. It is a benign lesion (Fig. 10-38).

The actinic keratoses, also known as solar keratoses or senile keratoses, occur mostly in older persons on exposed areas (Fig. 10-39; also see Figs. 16-11 and 16-12). They appear as discrete, slightly elevated papules or plaques with an adherent scale. If the scale becomes quite thick, it may produce a fingerlike projection called a cutaneous horn (Fig. 10-40). The actinic keratoses are the skin counterpart of oral leukoplakia in that they may show histologic features running the gamut from totally benign hyperkeratosis to various degrees of dysplasia to carcinoma in situ or frank squamous carcinoma. In about one quarter of the cases of senile keratoses, carcinoma will develop.

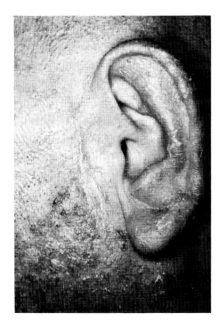

Fig. 10-39. Senile keratosis.

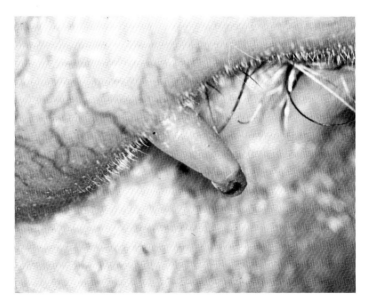

Fig. 10-40. Cutaneous horn.

Bowen's disease is a dermatologic term used for a dull red or brown, slightly thickened plaque with sharp, irregular outlines without a raised border and without infiltration. It spreads by peripheral extension (Fig. 10-41). Histologically it is carcinoma in situ. The lesion is usually a single one, but multiple ones may occur; in the latter, internal malignancy may be found in 15% to 40% of the cases. In moist areas such as the penis, vagina, and crural folds, it is called erythroplasia of Queyrat.

Most of the squamous cell carcinomas of the skin occur in sun-damaged areas. Some occur in burn scars, chronic ulcers, or areas of chronic infection. Squamous carcinoma of the skin appears as a shallow, crust-covered ulcer with a raised, indurated border (Fig. 10-42). Raised fungating lesions may sometimes be seen. Growth is slow, and metastasis occurs in only a very small percentage of the cases. Most are histologically well-differentiated lesions. A particu-lar histologic pattern, the pseudoglandular squamous carcinoma, may sometimes be seen, but the clinical appearance and evolution are essentially the same as for the other types of squamous carcinoma. Multiple squamous carcinomas may be associated with chronic arsenic ingestion.

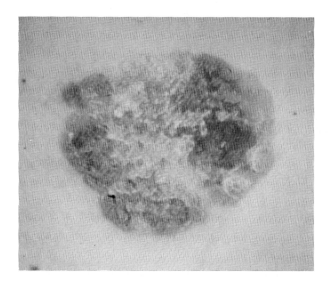

Fig. 10-41. Bowen's disease.

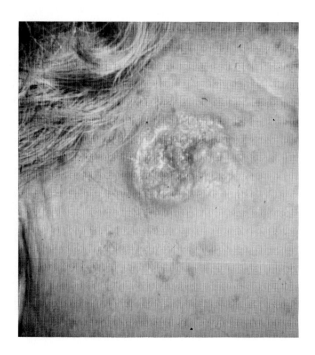

Fig. 10-42. Squamous cell carcinoma.

The keratoacanthoma can be considered as a self-healing carcinoma. It is usually single but may be multiple. Generalized multiple keratoacanthomas may be inherited. Although the keratoacanthoma resembles a carcinoma clinically and histologically, there are some distinguishing features. The classical keratoacanthoma is a dome-shaped mass with a central umbilicated core of keratinous debris (Fig. 10-43). Most occur on exposed surfaces and appear rather suddenly, reaching full size in a matter of weeks and resolving within several months without scarring.

Basal cell carcinomas, or basal cell epitheliomas, usually occur in sun-exposed areas in fair-skinned individuals. The periobital portion of the face is the most common location. In fact, if an imaginary line is drawn from the commissure of the lip to the tragus of the ear, carcinomas above the line are likely to be basal cell, and below, squamous cell. Basal cell carcinomas may appear as single or multiple lesions, generally in older adults; however, there have been some in children as well. There are several clinical types of basal cell carcinomas. The most common type begins as a small, waxy-appearing papule or nodule with overlying telangiectasia. As it increases in size it develops a necrotic center with a raised, rolled pearly border (Fig. 10-44). Some basal cell carcinomas may contain pigment and appear brown or black, simulating a melanoma. The morphea-like or sclerosing basal cell carcinoma appears as a yellow plaque or sclerotic, slightly depressed area (Fig. 10-45). Ulceration occurs late. A superficial scaling type of basal cell carcinoma also occurs.

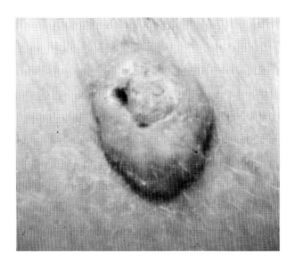

Fig. 10-43. Keratoacanthoma.

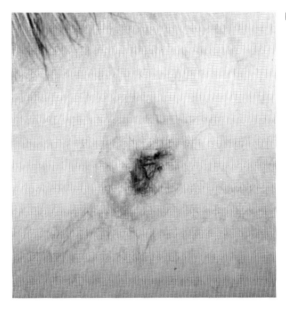

Fig. 10-44. Basal cell carcinoma.

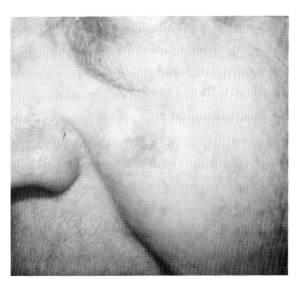

Fig. 10-45. Sclerosing basal cell carcinoma.

Multiple basal cell carcinomas in young people should prompt one to examine for multiple jaw cysts and bone abnormalities, such as frontal bossing with hypertelorism, brachymetacarpalism, bifid ribs, and sometimes pseudohypoparathyroidism, all of which are components of the basal cell nevus syndrome, or nevoid basal cell carcinoma syndrome (Fig. 10-46). This is an autosomal dominant disease with variable expressivity.

Basal cell carcinomas of all types, although locally destructive, rarely metastasize.

The skin appendage, or adnexal, tumors constitute a highly variable group of tumors of the skin. They are delineated by the structure of origin and subclassified by the portion of the structure from which the cells are derived. For example, the trichofolliculoma and trichoepithelioma are derived from the hair follicle; the apocrine hydrocystoma, cylindroma, and syringocystadenoma papilliferum are derived from the apocrine glands; and the syringoma, hidradenoma, and spiradenoma are of eccrine origin. Sebaceous adenomas also occur. These are all benign skin appendage tumors, but malignant forms derived from these structures do exist.

There are few clinical distinguishing features of these benign adnexal tumors that might be noticed by the nondermatologist. The adnexal tumors appear as single or multiple firm, oval, subcutaneous nodules.

Fibrous tumors of the skin occur. Soft, pedunculated, flesh-colored tumors or tissue tags called acrochordons occur on the neck and chest in older individuals. Other, harder fibrous lesions are classified as dermatofibromas or fibrous histiocytomas, and these appear as firm yellow or brown lesions. Multiple angiofibromas are seen in the malar area in association with mental deficiency or epilepsy, and brown and visceral tumors in an autosomal, dominantly inherited disorder called tuberous sclerosis (Bournville's disease). There are other mesodermal tumors, including lipomas, myxomas, leiomyomas, and even osteomas. The malignant counterparts of these mesodermal tumors also occur.

The calcifying epithelioma of Malherbe, or pilomatricoma, is a tumor of hair matrix that appears as a firm to hard subcutaneous nodule. It is of particular interest to the dentist, since the histology closely mimics an odontogenic tumor, the calcifying odontogenic cyst (Gorlin cyst).

Fig. 10-46. Multiple basal cell carcinomas in patient with basal cell nevus syndrome.

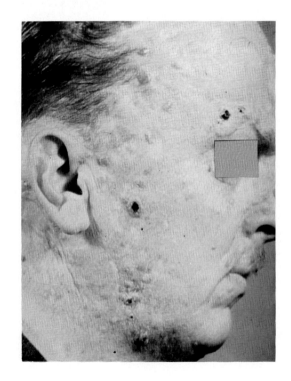

Common miscellaneous dermatoses

Allergic reactions. Eczematous dermatitis is a reaction pattern based on clinical morphologic characteristics with subtypes delineated on the basis of location and etiologic agent. Eczematous dermatitis may be associated with exogenous agents in the form of allergic contact eczematous dermatitis. Exposure to an almost unlimited number of compounds from plants, medications, and cosmetics in hypersensitive individuals results in sensitization to the substance. Subsequent exposure elicits the response, which is mediated by the cellular immune system (delayed hypersensitivity reaction). The reaction is manifested by an intense erythema followed by papules, vesicles, or bullae and edema (Fig. 10-47). Chronic lesions may result in scaling, crusting, fissuring, and lichenification. Secondary bacterial infections may modify the appearance.

Photoallergic contact eczematous dermatitis may occur following ultraviolet radiation on skin that has been subjected to certain substances, such as soaps and perfumes. Polymorphous light eruption is an eczematous reaction to ultraviolet light itself. Bacterial or fungal products may also cause eczematous dermatitis.

Endogenous agents, such as ingested drugs or metabolic or immunologic alterations, may produce the eczematous reaction pattern. In atopic dermatitis there appears to be a hereditary predeliction in addition to the etiologic factors. In infants the weeping lesions involve the head and neck region; in childhood they are drier and are seen mostly on the body and limbs; in adults any area may be involved, but the flexural areas are most frequently involved and are often lichenified.

Seborrheic dermatitis is a poorly understood condition that may start in childhood and continue through life. There is a fine papular rash with yellowish waxy scales or crusts of the scalp, face, and neck. Seborrheic dermatitis is called cradle cap in infants and in adults is often associated with baldness, dandruff, acne, and oily skin.

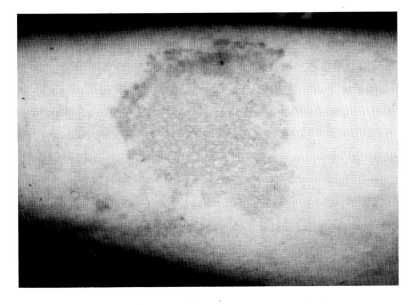

Fig. 10-47. Hypersensitivity reaction to drug.

Psoriasis is a genetically transmitted dermatosis characterized by increased activity of epithelial cells. The lesions are elevated erythematous plaques with a thick, loosely adherent scale. Removal of the scale results in small bleeding points called the Auspitz sign. Lesions may occur in the area of trauma (Köbner's phenomenon). Any area of the skin may be involved, but extensor areas, such as the elbows and knees and scalp, are most favored (Fig. 10-48). Subungual involvement causes disturbances of the nails, and arthritis is often a component of the disease.

Nummular eczema is a common eczematous lesion found frequently in mothers with new infants and in dentists. It is characterized by pruritic, vesicular lesions of the hand, particularly in the webs of the fingers. The causes are probably emotional stress and excessive washing of the hands with soap.

Neurodermatitis probably depends on a hereditary predisposition in addition to repeated trauma or scratching. Lichen simplex chronicus is an example of this type of disorder.

Xanthelasma is a focal collection of lipids within histiocytes about the eyelids. It appears as bright yellow, sharply defined, smooth-surfaced papules and plaques that may be separate or coalescent. Some individuals with xanthelasma may show plasma lipid abnormalities (Fig. 10-49; see also Fig. 9-6).

Lichen planus may be an acute or chronic disorder characterized by small flat, angular, and sometimes umbilicated papules or plaques with a violaceous color (purple polygonal papules). Often a delicate white network can be seen coursing over the surface of the papules and plaques (Wickham's striae). The lesions are variably pruritic and tend to occur on the flexor surfaces of the extremities and mucous membranes. Lesions may heal spontaneously with hypopigmentation but more often with hyperpigmentation. Annular or linear patterns may emerge, and Köbner's phenomenon is often present. The cause is unknown (see Fig. 10-10).

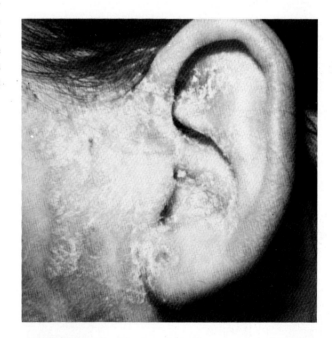

Fig. 10-48. Psoriasis.

Fig. 10-49. Xanthelasmata.

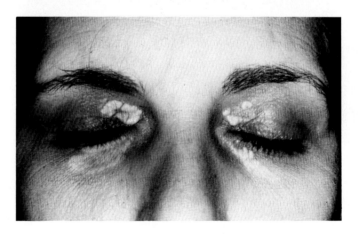

Bullous dermatoses. Erythema multiforme is an acute disorder, possibly infectious or allergic in origin, that may be precipitated by a number of factors, including drugs and herpes simplex virus. Prodromal symptoms may include upper respiratory tract infection-like symptoms followed by an eruption of red papules or macules, target lesions (concentric rings with red center and white halo, followed by a red periphery), or even blisters. Oral lesions are common, and eyes and genitalia may be involved, thus making up the Stevens-Johnson syndrome (Fig. 10-50).

Pemphigoid is an autoimmune disorder characterized by tense, large bullae with irregular outlines involving the skin. The antigen-antibody attack is at the basement membrane zone. Occasionally another disease, benign mucosal pemphigoid, or cicatricial pemphigoid, involves predominantly the mouth and eyes (Fig. 10-51).

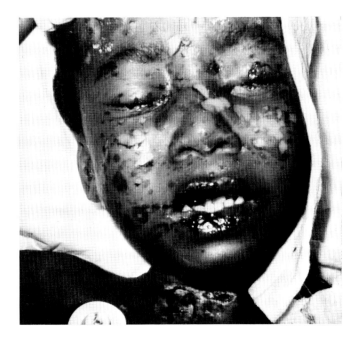

Fig. 10-50. Stevens-Johnson syndrome.

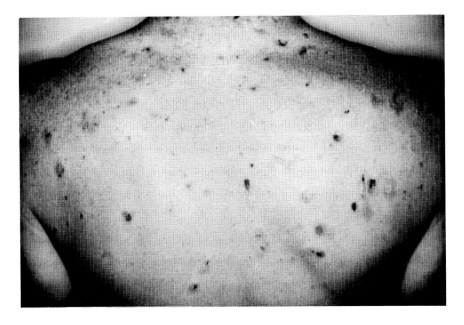

Fig. 10-51. Pemphigoid.

Pemphigus is subdivided into pemphigus vulgaris, with a variant, pemphigus vegetans, and pemphigus foliaceus, which also has an abortive form, pemphigus erythematosus. The vulgaris type is characterized by flaccid bullae that easily break. Pressure on even normal skin will elicit bulla formation (Nikolsky's sign) (Fig. 10-52). Mucous membrane lesions may be the first to appear in over half the cases. The vegetans type shows marked proliferative and vegetative lesions in response to the disease. Pemphigus foliaceus may or may not show bullae, but crusted erosions with a serpiginous border are common.

Epidermolysis bullosa is an inheritable disorder of which there are many subtypes with different modes of inheritance. There are nonscarring and scarring types that may vary from mild to occasional lesions in response to trauma, to involvement so severe that destruction of digits by scarring and death from superimposed infection may occur (Fig. 10-53).

Fig. 10-52. Pemphigus vulgaris.

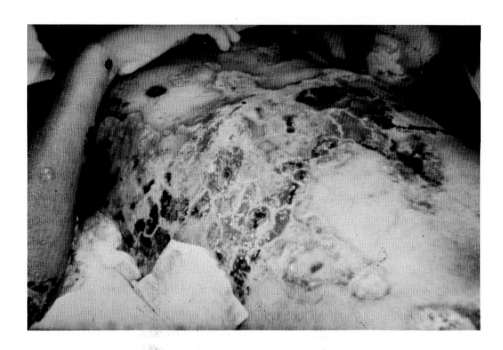

Fig. 10-53. Epidermolysis bullosa.

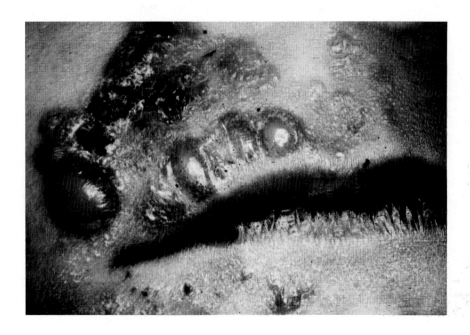

Autoimmune diseases

There are ever-increasing numbers of diseases characterized by the body's attack on itself through its immunologic defenses. Lupus erythematosus is a not uncommon autoimmune disease that occurs in young women. There is a discoid and a systemic form. The discoid type is related to the skin, whereas the systemic type involves other organs, primarily the kidney and brain.

The discoid lesions are erythematous and papular, often occurring in a "butterfly" distribution over the malar area or on the scalp. The papules become scaly, enlarge peripherally, and become atrophic in the center with accompanying hypopigmentation (Fig. 10-54). Severe disfigurement may re-sult. Antibodies have not been demonstrated in the discoid form, but some cases may change to the systemic form, which does show auto-antibodies.

Fig. 10-54. A and **B,** Lupus erythematosus.

A

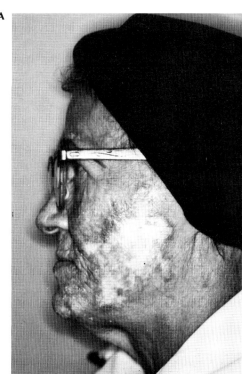

B

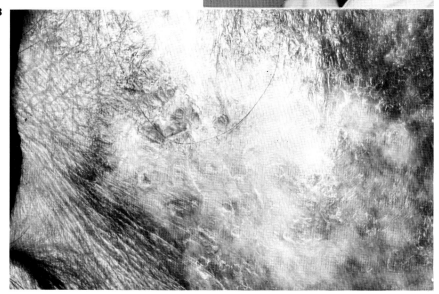

Systemic lupus erythematosus appears as chronic fatigue, accompanied by lesions similar in appearance to the lesions of discoid lupus. The joints, gastrointestinal tract, kidney, heart, lungs, and lymph nodes may be involved. Raynaud's phenomenon may occur; this is an abnormal vascular spasm on cold exposure of the digits of the hands and feet that results in cyanosis and pallor of the parts. Rewarming produces a reflex hyperemia. Raynaud's phenomenon is seen in a variety of diseases, including connective tissue disorders, cryoglobulinemia, certain intoxications, and even internal malignancy, as well as lupus erythematosus.

Dermatomyositis produces muscle soreness and weakness as one of the first symptoms. The skin lesions may include a diagnostic violaceous edema of the upper eyelids called a heliotrope, or a blotchy maculopapular telangiectatic rash (sometimes in a butterfly distribution) may occur. Periungual telangiectasia is quite characteristic of dermatomyositis as well as lupus erythematosus.

Scleroderma is a disease characterized by an increasing sclerosis of collagen. It is predominantly a disease of women that may occur in a localized (morphea) or systemic form. The localized form begins as an erythema that subsides, leaving a white, yellowish, or brown depressed, hard lesion that is bound down to the underlying tissue. It may occur in a guttate (raindrop pattern) or linear form. The linear form occurring on the facial area develops a furrow that looks like a scar from a cut and is described as coup de sabre (Fig. 10-55). Localized scleroderma may progress or sometimes regress.

The manifestations of systemic scleroderma depend on the site of involvement, but edema, Raynaud's phenomenon with ulceration of the fingertips and loss of joint mobility, loss of esophageal function, and progressive loss of renal function may occur. Loss of hair, generalized pigmentation, and widening of the periodontal membrane may occur.

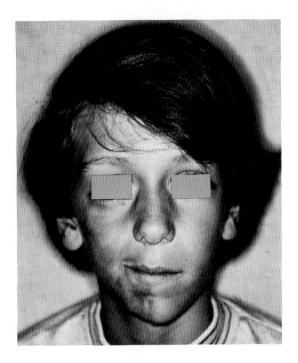

Fig. 10-55. Localized scleroderma (coup de sabre).

Dermatologic manifestations of systemic disease

Some dermatologic lesions may be markers for systemic disease. Bowen's disease has already been mentioned and is a marker for internal malignancy. Acanthosis nigricans is a brown, velvety rough change in the skin, especially in the folds of the neck, axilla, nipples, or umbilica. It may be generalized. In the absence of obesity or pubertal acanthosis nigricans, it signifies an internal malignancy.

The irregular wavy bands in a serpiginous outline resembling the grain of cut wood in erythema gyratum may signify an occult malignancy. Excessive rapid growth of the lanugo hair beginning over the face and spreading over the body may also signify a malignancy. There are other examples of dermatologic markers for internal malignancy.

Necrobiosis lipoidica diabeticorum is characterized by waxy yellow depressed lesions with a telangiectatic marking. These lesions characteristically appear on the anterior tibial area in patients with latent or overt diabetes.

There are many inherited syndromes with a marked dermatologic component, including Darier's disease (keratosis follicularis) and Ehlers-Danlos syndrome (cutis laxa), which is hyperelasticity of the skin, and anhidrotic ectodermal dysplasia (absence of sweat glands). There are, of course, many others.

Only a small number of dermatologic disorders have been mentioned in this chapter. The student interested in a more complete and thorough discussion of dermatologic diseases is referred to any of the many standard texts of dermatology.

BIBLIOGRAPHY

Bates, B.: A guide to physical examination, Philadelphia, 1974, J.B. Lippincott Co.

Degowin, E.L., and Degowin, R.L.: Diagnostic examination, ed. 3, New York, 1976, Macmillan, Inc.

Judge, R.D., and Zuidema, G.D.: Methods of clinical examination, ed. 3, Boston, 1974, Little, Brown & Co.

Lever, W.F.: Histopathology of the skin, ed. 5, Philadelphia, 1975, J.B. Lippincott Co.

Montgomery, H.: Dermatopathology, New York, 1967, Harper & Row, Publishers, Inc.

Prior, J.A., Silberstein, J.S., and Stang, J.: Physical diagnosis, ed. 6, St. Louis, 1981, The C.V. Mosby Co.

Sauer, G.C.: Manual of skin diseases, ed. 4, Philadelphia, 1980, J.B. Lippincott Co.

11   Cardiovascular system

Diseases of the cardiovascular system are some of the most common with which the dental practitioner must be familiar. An increasing number of dental patients report that they are suffering from cardiovascular diseases and may need to be evaluated physically before the provision of certain types of dental care. It is not the usual practice for the dentist to perform a complete physical examination that includes examination of the chest (lungs and heart). Nevertheless, it is important that the dentist be aware of the basic techniques of such examinations and be familiar with the more usual abnormal findings.

We realize that this chapter and the following one on the respiratory system (Chapter 12) may be considered too detailed by some and too superficial by others. We believe that these chapters present information at a level that it is reasonable to expect a modern dentist to know.

Examination of the cardiovascular system includes examination not only of the heart but also of the peripheral blood vessels, arteries, and veins. The information obtainable from the radial pulse and the significance of common variations in the pulse rate have already been discussed in Chapter 7. In this chapter the emphasis is placed on the evaluation of the heart.

The basic techniques of examining the heart have changed little over the years, but now the modern physician has an additional range of sophisticated tests available that permits him to diagnose heart disease more accurately. Cardiac catheterization, angiocardiography, phonocardiography, and echocardiography have permitted great progress to be made in diagnosing disorders of the cardiovascular system. However, evaluation of the heart by the traditional techniques of inspection, palpation, percussion, and auscultation remains the usual initial approach for most patients. In view of the frequency with which such examinations are made and the frequency of the terminology in everyday medical parlance, it is desirable to review this subject in some detail.

ANATOMY AND PHYSIOLOGY

The heart, which consists of the left and right ventricles and the left and right atria, is situated in the anterior part of the chest, with the bulk of the heart on the left side (Fig. 11-1). The term *precordium* is used to indicate the portion of the chest immediately overlying the heart. The ribs, costal interspaces, and sternum can be used as convenient landmarks, and the heart's position in relation to these landmarks can be assessed to determine whether there has been any decrease or increase in heart size or any significant shift of the heart to one side or the other.

It is possible to determine each particular rib and interspace using as a landmark the junction of the manubrium and the body of the sternum—the angle of the sternum (Louis's angle) (Fig. 11-2). The outer edge of this ridge marks the level of the second costal cartilage. The space immediately above is the first intercostal space. Superior-inferior measurements are normally indicated in terms of intercostal spaces, whereas distances from the midsagittal plane are defined as follows. The midclavicular line is a vertical line from the center of the clavicle, and the anterior, middle, and posterior axillary lines are indicated by the anterior border, the center, and the posterior border of the axilla (Fig. 11-2).

The control of the heart rate and common variations from normal have been discussed in Chapter 7. In the normal adult the heart beats approximately 60 to 80 times per minute. It beats faster after exercise and slower during sleep. During each cycle of the heartbeat, there are two phases—the systolic and diastolic phases. During systole the left and right ventricles contract and pump blood into the aorta and pulmonary arteries, respectively. During diastole the ventricles relax and refill, the atria contracting and forcing blood into the ventricles just before the start of a new systolic phase. The valves of the heart prevent reflux of blood through the mitral and tricuspid valves during systole and through the aortic and pulmonary valves during diastole.

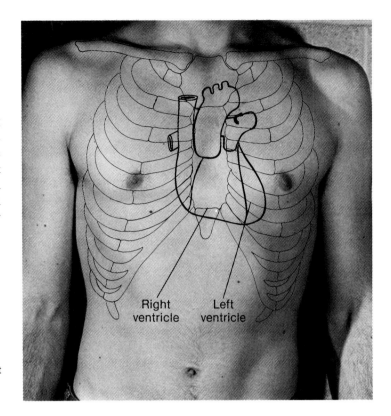

Fig. 11-1. Location of precordium. Notice that bulk of heart is on left side and right ventricle makes up most of anterior surface of heart.

Fig. 11-2. Examiner's finger is palpating sternal angle. Outer edge of this is level of second costal cartilage. Reference lines indicated are midsternal, midclavicular, and anterior axillary lines.

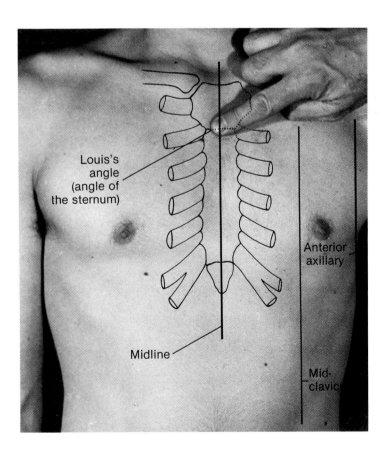

EXAMINATION
Inspection

The patient should be examined in a good light, and the observer should note whether there is any dyspnea or cyanosis and observe the shape of the chest and precordium. Particular attention should be paid to the neck veins. These communicate directly with the right atrium, and therefore the changes in atrial pressure that occur during each cardiac cycle may be detectable by observing the filling of the neck veins. The jugular venous pulse is not usually seen in the normal person until the patient is almost horizontal. It is usual to examine the jugular pulse with the patient leaning back at a 45° angle. It is important that the patient's head be relaxed; otherwise the sternocleidomastoid muscles may be tensed, making examination of the jugular vein difficult.

There is a specific form to the normal pulse wave produced in a large vein. The characteristics of this wave can be readily seen in some patients, especially those with an increased jugular venous pressure. The clinical interpretation of a jugular pulse wave requires much experience, and such an evaluation is frequently helped by the preparation of a tracing of the pulse wave.

In certain congenital heart diseases there may be obvious changes in the symmetry of the chest. Special attention should be given to the location of any pulsations. A forceful apex beat (see Palpation), such as occurs in left ventricular hypertrophy, may be readily detected on inspection. An aortic aneurysm may produce a pulsation in the upper part of the chest, and if the heart is significantly enlarged (cardiomegaly), the anterior chest wall may be seen to heave with each heartbeat. It should be remembered that a cardiac pulsation in the epigastric region may be normal in very spare people, although pulsations in this region could be due to an enlarged heart or an abdominal aneurysm.

Palpation

Palpation of the chest wall should be done in an orderly, systematic way. The right hand should be placed on the chest wall, with the middle finger lying in the fifth left intercostal space in the anterior axillary line. The apex beat should then be defined and any abnormal vibrations noted (Fig. 11-3). The apex beat has been defined as the furthest point downward and outward on the chest wall where the finger is lifted by the cardiac impulse. Occasionally, the apex beat can not be readily felt, and this is usually due to obesity or emphysema. In emphysema the anterior wall of the barrel chest lies some distance away from the surface of the heart. Occasionally a heartbeat may be impalpable in the usual area because of a pericardial effusion or, very rarely, because the heart may lie on the right side of the body (dextrocardia). The normal apex beat lies in the midclavicular line in the fifth intercostal space. It should be described in terms of its relation to a particular intercostal space and with lateral references to the midclavicular and axillary lines or the midline, for example, the fifth left intercostal space $3\frac{1}{2}$ inches from the midline. The apex beat may be displaced because the heart is displaced, and this may result from variations in the anatomy of the chest or from enlargement of the heart. Cardiomegaly may also produce changes in the character of the precordial pulsations. The apex beat is particularly forceful when there is enlargement of the heart (such as may occur in hypertension), and the forceful beat has been described as heaving or thrusting. The movement of blood within the heart may produce some abnormal vibration (a murmur), which may be so intense as to be palpable. Such vibrations are thrills. One common example is the apical thrill of mitral stenosis felt during diastole. In the condition of aortic stenosis, the thrill is felt during systole and more toward the base of the heart; that is, toward the upper sternal area. Thrills are best appreciated when the patient leans forward and holds the breath in expiration. This maneuver will reduce the size of the chest and prevent respiratory movements from interfering with the examination. Mitral stenosis thrills are usually best felt when the patient turns onto the left side. Less common cardiac anomalies may also produce thrills that have particular locations and characteristics.

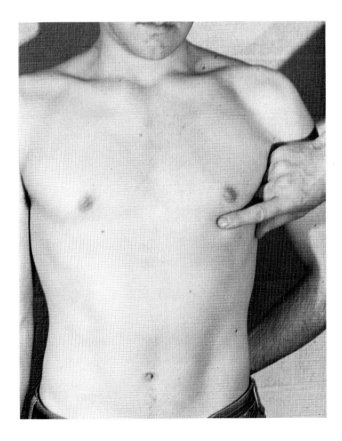

Fig. 11-3. Examiner's finger is indicating area where cardiac impulse can be felt strongest in downward and outward direction from heart—apex beat, normally midclavicular line in fifth left intercostal space.

Percussion

The technique of percussing the chest wall is described in Chapter 12. Percussion over the precordial area can usually permit the general outline of the heart to be determined. The area of cardiac dullness is best appreciated to the left of the sternum where the heart abuts the chest wall. This area of dullness may be reduced or absent in those cases of emphysema in which the chest is enlarged and barrel shaped. Enlargement of the atria and ventricles occurs in some conditions and may change the normal area of cardiac dullness. Although the skilled clinician can gain much information about the size and position of the heart by percussion, the radiograph is a much more valuable method of determining the size and location of the heart within the chest.

Auscultation

In view of the large number and styles of stethoscopes available, it seems appropriate to make a brief comment concerning this valuable diagnostic tool. Stethoscopes may have bell-shaped chest pieces or diaphragms or a combination of both (Fig. 11-4). The bell type chest piece lightly pressed against the skin is best for conducting low-pitched sounds and murmurs. The diaphragm closely applied is better for detecting high-pitched sounds or quiet murmurs.

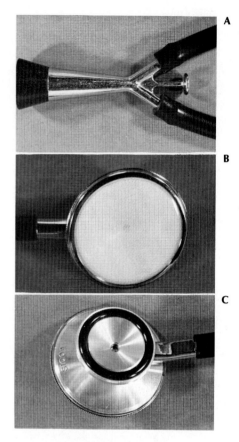

Fig. 11-4. A, Traditional bell-type stethoscope head. **B,** Diaphragm stethoscope head. **C,** Combination modified bell and diaphragm.

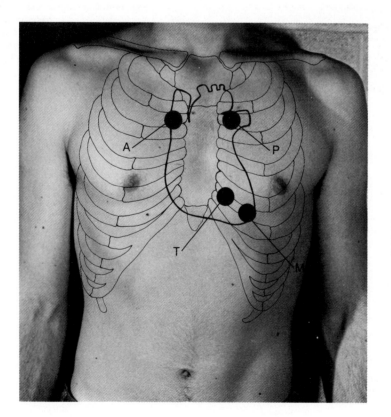

Fig. 11-5. Auscultatory areas of precordium. *M,* Mitral area; *T,* tricuspid area; *A,* aortic area; *P,* pulmonary area.

If frequent cardiac examinations are conducted, it is best to have the combination stethoscope available. It is usual to listen systematically to the various regions of the precordium, which have been identified as (1) the mitral area, which corresponds to the location of the apex beat; (2) the tricuspid area, which lies just to the left of the lower end of the sternum; (3) the aortic area, which is to the right of the sternum in the second intercostal space; and (4) the pulmonary area, which is to the left of the sternum in the second intercostal space (Fig. 11-5). It is important to remember these locations, as they are frequently used by physicians in describing the positions of abnormal sounds. Note that auscultation should not be restricted to these areas. Although generally there is a good correlation, it must be remembered that the sounds heard in a particular area do not *necessarily* originate from the valve named. The normal heart sounds heard over the precordium have been described as "lubb-dupp." The first heart sound, at the onset of ventricular systole, is produced by the closing of the mitral and tricuspid valves. The aortic and pulmonary valves open next, but these are normally inaudible movements. The closure of the aortic and pulmonary valves gives rise to the second sound. It should be recognized that the second sound has two components. The lower pressure in the right ventricle, in relation to the pressure in the left ventricle, results in a closure of the pulmonary valve just a little later than the closure of the aortic valve. After a brief interval, the mitral and tricuspid valves open inaudibly in the normal heart to prepare for the next cardiac cycle. The "splitting" of the second sound is relatively easy to hear over the pulmonary area (Fig. 11-6). Splitting is usually easily heard in children but may be difficult to hear in older adults, especially when there is a thick chest wall or emphysema. Splitting is widest during inspiration and narrowest during the expiratory phase (Fig. 11-7).

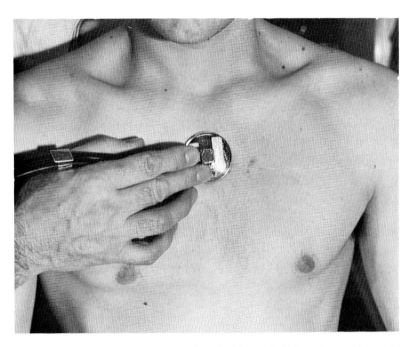

Fig. 11-6. Examiner is listening over "base" of heart. Splitting of second sound is normally heard most clearly over pulmonary area, which is slightly to patient's left of stethoscope's position as shown.

Fig. 11-7. Diagram illustrates heart sounds (S_1 and S_2) during expiration and inspiration. "Splitting" of second sound is much more readily heard during deep inspiration.

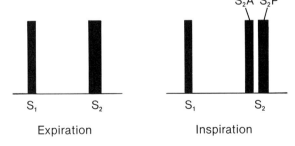

S_1 = first heart sound
S_2 = second heart sound
S_2A = second heart sound (aortic component)
S_2P = second heart sound (pulmonic component)

COMMON ABNORMALITIES

There are variations of the normal sounds that may indicate cardiac disease. These include the normal first and second heart sounds having different intensities or being abnormally split, or demonstrating a triple rhythm. Triple rhythm may be heard in normal, healthy young people, but its presence in the older patient may be a significant diagnostic sign of heart failure. The third sound has been attributed to rapid filling of the ventricle. This may occur normally in the hyperkinetic circulation of young people. In heart failure it is thought to be due to the increased atrial pressure, producing very early rapid filling of the ventricle during diastole. The third sound follows the aortic component of the second sound.

Murmurs have been described as having a blowing or musical quality. They are produced by the turbulence of the blood flowing through a narrowed or incompetent valve or through some abnormal communication channel within the heart. Not all murmurs are due to organic damage. Some may result from a rapid flow of blood through a normal valve, and such murmurs are called flow murmurs. Murmurs may also occur in large blood vessels as a result of abnormalities in the intima. Murmurs should be examined to determine the time of their occurrence within the cardiac cycle; that is, whether they are (1) systolic, (2) diastolic, or (3) throughout systole and diastole. There can be a further classification of murmurs according to whether they exist throughout the systolic phase (pansystolic) or whether they occur early on or later in the phase. Murmurs are often graded as to their intensity. Clearly, the detection and interpretation of murmurs take considerable practice. The evaluation of heart sounds, including murmurs, has been improved considerably by the introduction of phonocardiography. In this technique sounds produced by the heart can be displayed on an oscilloscope and a permanent record of the sounds produced for later evaluation. It is not necessary to explain all the varieties of abnormal heart sounds in great detail, but examples of the more common cardiac abnormalities are given.

Mitral stenosis

The mitral valve is the heart valve most commonly involved in rheumatic fever. The development of mitral stenosis, or narrowing of the valve orifice, is due to fusion of the valve cusps along their margins. The narrowing of the orifice, through which the blood flows from the left atrium to the left ventricle, produces significant changes in hemodynamics. In normal subjects the mitral valve is nearly completely closed at the end of diastole. In patients with mitral stenosis the valve tends to stay open longer in the diastolic cycle and closes suddenly and sharply when the ventricular pressure begins to rise in systole. This results in a loud first heart sound. During diastole a low-pitched murmur may be heard over the apex (Fig. 11-8). This is caused by blood passing through the narrowed mitral valve. A presystolic murmur occurs when the atrium contracts and therefore immediately precedes the first heart sound. An opening snap of the mitral valve sometimes occurs. It is heard just after the second heart sound and is a result of the high left atrial pressure that forces the mitral valve open rapidly when the ventricle relaxes at the end of systole (Fig. 11-9).

Mitral regurgitation

In mitral regurgitation the valve cusps are incompetent, and during systole a jet of blood passes from the ventricle to the atrium through the valve, producing a systolic murmur that lasts throughout the systolic phase.

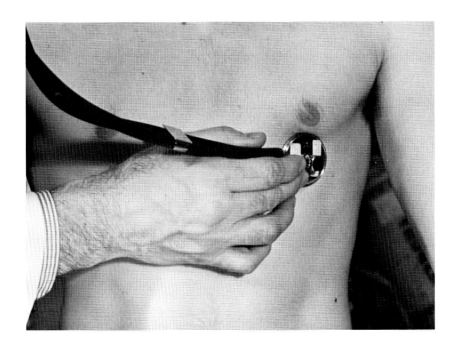

Fig. 11-8. Examiner is listening over mitral area. Diastolic murmur of mitral stenosis would normally be heard best in this area.

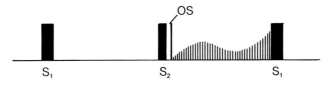

Opening snap (OS) middiastolic and presystolic murmur—mitral stenosis

Fig. 11-9. Opening snap sound immediately following S_2 is followed by middiastolic and presystolic murmur, typical of types of mitral stenosis.

Aortic stenosis

If there is some change in the cusps of the aortic valve so that there is a narrowing of the aortic orifice, a systolic murmur may develop. There is a great pressure difference between the left ventricle and aorta, and this gradient will be greatest during the middle of systole, that is, at the point of highest pressure (Fig. 11-10). Murmurs of this type are sometimes called "ejection" systolic murmurs.

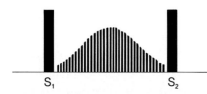

Fig. 11-10. Murmur represented here occurs between first sound and second sound, that is, during systole. Its point of maximal intensity is midsystolic. This type of murmur (heard best in aortic area) occurs with aortic stenosis. Murmur may "radiate" into neck and may be heard all over precordium.

Aortic regurgitation

If the aortic valve is incompetent, so that leakage from the aorta back to the ventricle occurs during diastole, then a murmur may be produced. Some aortic leaks may be quite significant and, for example, could result in almost half the blood passing through the aortic valve during systole to fall back into the ventricle during the diastolic phase. The heart compensates for this inefficient pumping action by increasing the stroke volume, and this may then give rise to an aortic ejection murmur, as so much blood is passing through the valve during systole. The murmur of aortic regurgitation will start with the second heart sound, that is, when the systolic phase is complete, and continue for a variable time through diastole (Fig. 11-11). It is best heard over the left sternal edge, with the diaphragm rather than the bell of the stethoscope.

Some of the congenital heart diseases, such as pulmonary stenosis, atrial septal defect (ASD), ventricular septal defect (VSD), patent ductus arteriosus, Fallot's tetralogy, and coarctation of the aorta, also produce murmurs. The evaluation of such heart conditions is often conducted with sophisticated techniques, which have been mentioned previously. However, the careful use of the stethoscope by an experienced cardiologist can still provide much valuable information about the state of the heart.

The term *functional* is sometimes used to describe murmurs that are thought to be produced by turbulent blood flow without there necessarily being any valvular damage. This term is sometimes used loosely, and care should be taken in interpreting the significance of a murmur described as functional. It is not infrequent for a patient to report to a dentist that he or she has a functional murmur and that this has not interfered in any way with the patient's general health or activities. In such cases it is appropriate for the dentist to seek medical advice concerning the true nature of the functional murmur, particularly with respect to the need for prophylactic antibiotic therapy before dental surgery. Unfortunately, it is frequently found that an undiagnosed organic condition *did* exist, and the term functional had been applied erroneously.

Fig. 11-11. This represents diastolic murmur and is produced by fall of blood back into left ventricle through incompetent aortic valve during period of ventricular relaxation (diastole).

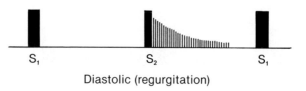

Diastolic (regurgitation)

ELECTROCARDIOGRAM

The electrocardiogram (ECG) may give important information about the health of the heart. Each time the heart contracts there are changes in electrical potential that can be recorded from the surface of the body. The electrical activity of the heart is measured by comparing two points on the body surface. Measurements are usually taken from a number of points. The electrocardiographic leads most frequently used are the standard leads:

Lead 1: right arm, left arm
Lead 2: right arm, left leg
Lead 3: left arm, left leg

Also frequently used are the unit polar or V leads in which an "exploring" electrode is placed on different positions of the chest wall. The chest positions are standard and are indicated as V_1 through V_7 (Fig. 11-12). They range from V_1 in the fourth intercostal space, just to the right of the sternum, through V_4 at the fifth left intercostal space in the midclavicular line, to V_7 in the posterior axillary line at the same horizontal level as V_4, V_5, and V_6.

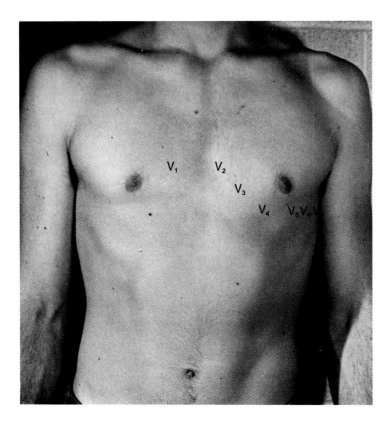

Fig. 11-12. Normal chest positions for placing "exploring" electrocardiogram electrodes are indicated. V_1, Fourth intercostal space, just to right of sternum; V_2, fourth intercostal space, just to left of sternum; V_3, midway between V_2 and V_4; V_4, fifth intercostal space in midclavicular line; V_5, anterior axillary line (same horizontal line as V_4); V_6, midaxillary line; V_7, posterior axillary line.

The standard electrocardiogram is illustrated in Fig. 11-13. The P wave is associated with atrial contraction, the QRS wave with ventricular excitation, and the T wave with ventricular recovery, that is, repolarization. Much valuable information can be gained from the electrocardiogram, including the cardiac rate and rhythm and the conduction time between atrial and ventricular contraction; and changes in the shape of the waves may give valuable information about the health of the heart muscle. Ischemic or dead heart muscle interferes with the normal electrical pattern and may change the shape of the standard waves. A myocardial infarction may be quite accurately localized by an evaluation of the changes seen in the cardiograms obtained from each of the various leads. For example, left ventricular hypertrophy will normally increase the size of the R wave in the left chest leads and increase the S wave in the right chest leads (V_1 or V_2).

The interpretation of the electrocardiogram requires considerable experience, but the dentist should be familiar with at least the basic principles of this important test.

STRESS TEST

Some patients who are suffering from coronary artery atherosclerosis may be unaware of their condition, as they may never experience any symptoms of cardiac ischemia, even during exercise. The classical pain of cardiac ischemia—angina pectoris—is thought to be produced by ischemic muscle. The heart muscle at rest has an adequate supply of blood but becomes deficient during exercise. It has been shown that ischemic changes in cardiac muscle produced during exercise, which do not cause pain, may nevertheless produce changes in the electrocardiogram. Such stress tests are now commonplace and are used frequently as part of a cardiovascular evaluation, particularly of patients with the high risk factors of coronary artery sclerosis, for example, patients who are hypertensive, obese, diabetic, or who have familial histories of cardiovascular disease.

SUMMARY

Disorders of the cardiovascular system are frequently encountered in dental practice. The dentist often seeks the advice of the patient's physician before proceeding with treatment. It is essential that the dentist be familiar with some of the more serious and common disorders, the methods of physical evaluation used to assess them, and the language used to describe the associated signs and symptoms.

BIBLIOGRAPHY

Delp, M.H., and Manning, R.T.: Major's physical diagnosis, ed. 8, Philadelphia, 1975, W.B. Saunders Co.

Prior, J.A., Silberstein, J.S., and Stang, J.: Physical diagnosis: the history and examination of the patient, ed. 6, St. Louis, 1981, The C.V. Mosby Co.

Fig. 11-13. A, Standard electrocardiographic wave form shows various components, P, Q, R, S, T. *P,* Wave of atrial depolarization; *QRS,* wave form of ventricular depolarization; *T,* wave of ventricular repolarization; (Q wave, initial deflection following P wave; R wave, upward deflection; S wave, downward deflection after R wave). **B,** Relationship of electrocardiogram to heart sounds.

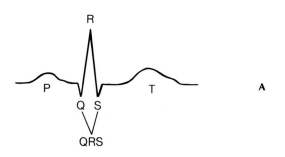

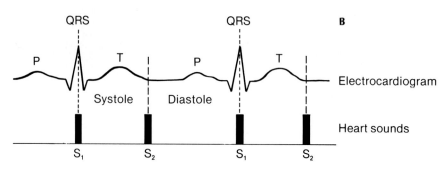

12 Respiratory system

significant number of chronically ill patients suffer from diseases of the respiratory system. Chronic bronchitis and emphysema account for much morbidity within the population, and patients with such conditions who require dental treatment involving local or general anesthesia may need to be evaluated carefully and their respiratory status determined. The importance of observing a patient's respiratory movements and some of the more common variations from the normal condition have been discussed already in Chapter 7. In this chapter an account of the more usual office techniques of evaluating the respiratory system is offered. Common terms used to describe physical findings are explained, and some of the more common manifestations of respiratory disease are discussed in detail.

ANATOMY AND PHYSIOLOGY

An understanding of the anatomy and physiology of the respiratory system is essential for the clinician who has to evaluate the respiratory status of a patient.

The upper respiratory tract consists of the nose with its accessory sinuses, the pharynx, and the larynx. The lower tract comprises the trachea, bronchial tree, and lung alveoli. The trachea lies in the midline and can be palpated in the suprasternal notch. It may be deviated to one side in certain conditions, and its position should always be established. The trachea divides into the right and left bronchi at about the level of the second costal cartilage (see Louis's angle, Fig. 11-2). The right bronchus makes less of an angle with the trachea than the left does; consequently, inhaled foreign objects are more likely to pass into the right lung than into the left. Each main bronchus divides and subdivides down to the very small bronchioles that lead into the air sacs. The right lung has three lobes and the left, two (Fig. 12-1). The pleura, the membrane covering the lungs, is in two parts. The part that covers the lung itself is the visceral pleura, whereas the parietal pleura lines the thoracic cavity. They are separated by a thin film of fluid. The lungs are normally expanded in the thoracic cavity, as there is a difference between the pressure in the respiratory passages and alveoli and the "negative" pressure between the pleural layers. The chest wall moves outward and upward during inspiration, while the diaphragm moves downward. The negative pleural pressure increases, and so the lungs expand further. The expiratory phase is largely due to a passive process that depends on the elastic recoil of the lung tissue. The vital capacity of the healthy adult lung varies from 4 to 5 L (the vital capacity is the amount of air that can be expired from the lungs by maximal expiration after maximal inspiration). Usually, under normal breathing conditions, only about 500 cc is exchanged during each respiratory cycle.

It is worth remembering that there are several mechanisms that protect the lungs from infectious agents or inflammatory agents that may be contaminating the inspired air. They include the ciliated epithelial lining of the respiratory tract, the cough reflex, and the local defenses of the lung, including the macrophages and other immune competent cells.

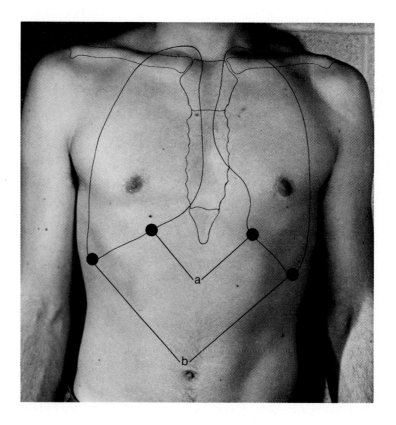

Fig. 12-1. Surface projection of lungs. Lower border is related to sixth rib at about midclavicular line, points *a,* and eighth rib at midaxillary line, points *b.* Apex of each lung rises about 3 to 4 cm above inner third of clavicle into base of neck. Posteriorly lower border of each lung is about level of spinous process of tenth thoracic vertebra, but descends during deep inspiration.

EXAMINATION

Evaluation of the respiratory system must begin with a careful history of the patient's symptoms. Attention should be paid to the presence of such factors as coughing, blood-stained sputum, chest pain on respiration, and dyspnea (see Common Abnormalities). The general examination of the patient should note whether there is any evidence of respiratory disease, such as cyanosis or finger clubbing. The examination of the respiratory system should proceed in an orderly way.

Upper respiratory tract

The techniques for evaluating the nose, pharynx, and larynx are discussed in Chapter 9.

Lower respiratory tract

The trachea should be palpated with the thumb and index finger and can be readily identified by the presence of its cartilaginous rings. The position of the trachea can be determined by placing the tip of the finger into the suprasternal notch and noting whether the trachea lies in the midline (Fig. 12-2). It should be remembered that deviation is not always due to respiratory disease but may be produced by some thyroid enlargement; consequently, the thyroid gland should always be examined as part of the upper respiratory tract examination.

Examination of the chest should include (1) noting the general configuration of the chest, (2) observing the type of respiratory movements, and (3) seeking certain signs that may indicate abnormalities within the thoracic cavity.

Inspection and palpation. The patient should be examined in good lighting, stripped to the waist, and sitting upright. The chest should be inspected from all sides and any abnormality in its shape noted. For example, patients with chronic bronchitis and emphysema frequently show barrel-shaped chests. In the normal person, the anterior-posterior diameter of the chest, relative to the lateral diameter, is approximately 5:7. In patients with emphysema, the anterior-posterior diameter approximates the lateral measurement. The chest wall itself should be observed and palpated to determine whether there are any abnormalities of the skin.

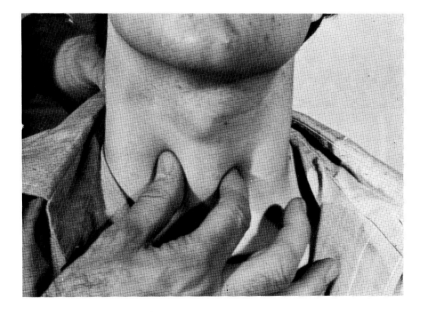

Fig. 12-2. Trachea should be identified by palpation with thumb and index finger, as shown. Tip of finger should then be placed into suprasternal notch and determination made as to whether trachea is midline.

167

It is usual for the breast to be examined at this time. Examination of the breast, including palpation of the axillary tail of the breast and the axillary glands, should be conducted in a systematic manner. The presence of any dimpling of the skin, irregular lumps within the breast substance, abnormality of the nipple, such as retraction, or abnormal discharge (blood or pus) should be investigated further.

Variations in the bony thorax should be noted, as well as any other anomalies that may be clues to diseases elsewhere; for example, spider nevi, suggesting a liver disorder. The normal respiratory rate is 14 to 18 respirations per minute. The rate may be increased in a variety of conditions, varying from anxiety to acute pulmonary infections. The depth of respiration may also be important, and variations of over- or underventilation should be noted. Chest expansion is normally bilaterally symmetrical, and a record should be made of maximal chest expansion, as measured by placing a tape measure around the chest at the level of the nipples and recording maximal inspiratory and expiratory readings in chest circumference. This is not a particularly accurate method of determining the degree of lung expansion, as in some patients breathing is primarily diaphragmatic. However, a chest expansion during inspiration of approximately 2 inches can be considered normal in the healthy adult (Fig. 12-3). A reduction in chest expansion is seen in several conditions that restrict the movement of the ribs, for example, pain resulting from a fractured rib, or lung diseases that interfere with the texture of the lung itself, for example, pulmonary fibrosis. Mention has been made in Chapter 7 that women are more likely to use the intercostal muscles than the diaphragm for breathing, whereas men rely more on the diaphragm, and their respiratory movements at rest are predominantly abdominal. Any departure from these normal modes of breathing should be examined carefully. For example, respiratory movements may be predominantly thoracic because diaphragmatic movement is inhibited by pain resulting from, say, peritoneal irritation or some disorder of the gastrointestinal tract. On the other hand, if respiratory movements are almost entirely abdominal, it may be because pleural pain or some disorder of the chest wall restricts chest expansion. Patients with severe breathing difficulties may use their accessory respiratory muscles, the sternocleidomastoid and other neck muscles, and this too should be noted.

The conduction of sounds from the vocal cords to the chest wall is affected by the state of the lungs, and much valuable information may be gained by palpating the chest in different areas when the patient is speaking (vocal fremitus). Traditionally, patients are asked to repeat "ninety-nine." The palm of the examining hand is applied flat to the chest. The vibrations detected on each side should be compared, and the examiner should realize that the vocal fremitus will be less in some areas, for example, where the heart encroaches on the lung. When part of the lung is consolidated (for example, pneumonia*) or there is a large cavity near the surface, the vocal fremitus will be increased. If a bronchus is obstructed or the lung is separated from the chest wall by, say, a pleural effusion, then vocal fremitus is diminished or absent.

Percussion. The techniques of percussion and auscultation are significant parts of the chest examination, and each has its own vocabulary. Some of the words used to describe lung examinations are in such widespread use that they are defined fully here.

---

*Pneumonia is a condition involving the lung, characterized by the presence of inflammatory exudate that obliterates the air spaces.

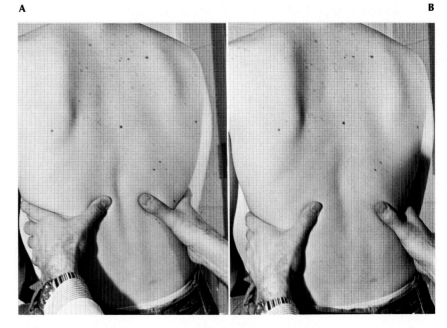

Fig. 12-3. Determination of chest movement during inspiration. **A,** Examiner's hands are placed at base of chest at point of complete expiration. Patient is then asked to take deep breath. **B,** Separation of examiner's thumbs indicates reasonable and symmetric expansion of chest cavity.

Percussion is an art that can be developed easily. It is usual for the middle finger of the right hand to be used to strike the middle phalanx of the middle finger of the left hand, placed firmly on the part of the body to be percussed (Fig. 12-4). The percussing stroke should be precise and should be no heavier than is necessary to elicit resonance. The character of the sounds produced by such percussion can vary quantitatively and qualitatively. When the air in a large cavity is set into vibration, the sound is described as having a tympanitic character. The lung, although full of air, has numerous alveoli separated by septa, and these change the character of the resonance so that it is not tympanitic. The particular resonance of the normal chest is best recognized by constant practice. Percussion should be carried out bilaterally so that the examiner can compare the quality of the sounds in comparable areas to determine whether they are identical. Generally speaking, there is symmetry, except where organs, such as the liver and the heart, interfere. As the percussing finger approaches the border of the heart, a dullness in resonance will be noted. It is possible to outline the heart by percussing this border of change in resonance (cardiac dullness). Changes in resonance may indicate some underlying lung disease. Resonance is increased when the pleural cavity contains air, as in a pneumothorax. Resonance is diminished when the pleura is thickened, when the underlying lung is more solid than usual, or when the pleural cavity contains fluid.

Auscultation. There should be a systematic examination of all areas of the chest anteriorly, laterally, posteriorly, superiorly, and inferiorly so that all areas of the lung are auscultated. The chest piece of the stethoscope should be applied flat against the skin and should not be allowed to move on the surface (Fig. 12-5). Patients should be asked to breathe with the mouth open, regularly and deeply.

Three considerations must be made at each point of the chest wall that is auscultated: (1) the character of the breath sounds, (2) the character of vocal resonance, and (3) the presence or absence of other sounds. A patient should be comfortable and completely relaxed For the bedridden patient it may be necessary for the patient to be rolled first to one side and then to the other for all parts of the chest to be examined.

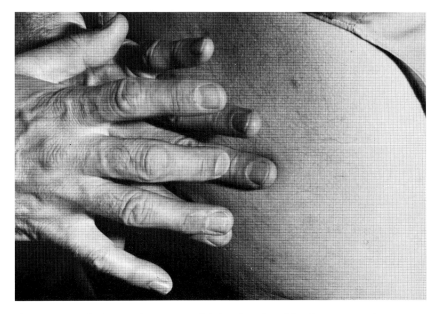

Fig. 12-4. Middle finger of examiner's left hand is placed firmly on area to be percussed. Middle finger of right hand then percusses middle phalanx of left middle finger. Percussing strokes should be precise.

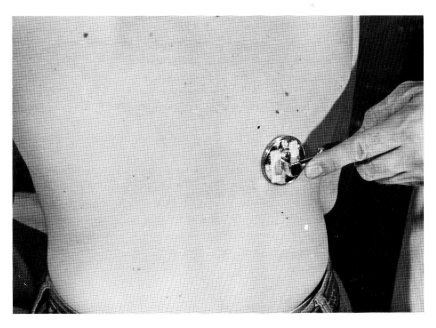

Fig. 12-5. Examiner is auscultating right lower base of lung. Notice chest piece is applied firmly and flat against skin.

Character of the breath sounds. In the normal person the passage of air in and out of normal lung tissue produces sounds of a "vesicular" type that can be heard all over the chest. Sounds produced by the passage of air through the trachea and large bronchi (bronchial breath sounds) may be heard by listening over the trachea and are not heard over normal lung tissue unless there is some disease. For example, if a lung lobe is consolidated by pneumonia, no air will enter or leave the alveoli, and no vesicular breath sounds will be heard over the affected area. However, if the bronchi are patent, bronchial sounds will be produced and conducted through them and conveyed to the chest wall.

In vesicular breathing, which is heard most easily in the axillary and infrascapular regions, the inspiratory sound is clear and audible during the whole act of respiration. The sound has been described as "rustling." The expiratory sound follows inspiration without a pause. The inspiratory sound normally lasts about twice as long as the expiratory sound.

Bronchial breathing can be heard by listening over the trachea. It should be remembered that bronchial breathing heard this way is much more intense than the bronchial breathing that might be heard over a diseased lung. The inspiratory sound tends to fade out before the end of inspiration. The expiratory sound is usually slightly more intense than the inspiratory sound and tends to be as long as, if not longer than, the inspiratory sound. Bronchial breathing can be recognized by the quality of the expiratory sound and the gap between inspiration and expiration. Prolongation of the expiratory sound is frequently heard in asthma and emphysema, and this must not be interpreted as bronchial breathing.

Breath sounds must be auscultated in various regions of the chest, comparing similar regions bilaterally. Vesicular breath sounds may be present but reduced in intensity in any of those conditions in which the air flow into that part of the lung is reduced or where some alveoli are affected and others not. Breath sounds will not be heard where there has been collapse of the lung or fibrosis. Bronchial breath sounds may be heard if there is a sound-conducting medium from the patent bronchi to the chest wall.

Vocal resonance. If the patient repeats the word "ninety-nine" and the stethoscope is moved from place to place on the chest wall, the examiner will hear, not the distinct word, but a resonant sound that will depend on the loudness of the patient's voice and on the sound conduction within his or her lungs. Each point examined on one side of the chest should be compared with the corresponding point on the opposite side. Sometimes the patient's words become clear, and this normally indicates that the lung substance has conducted the sound waves more clearly. The most usual reason for this is some consolidation of lung tissue.

Additional sounds. Disease of the lung or pleura may produce unusual sounds during respiratory movements. The examiner must be careful not to misinterpret adventitious sounds that may be produced by the shivering of a cold patient or application of the stethoscope to hairy skin! There is some confusion about the various words that are used frequently to describe adventitious sounds heard during respiratory examinations—such terms as rales, crepitations, and rhonchi. The following summarizes the definitions of some of these words.

Rale is a French word that means noise. It was used by Laennec (French physician, inventor of the stethoscope) to describe *any* added chest sound. Rale is now used interchangeably with the word *crepitation* to describe the discontinuous crackling or bubbling sounds that may be produced in the alveoli, the bronchi, or the lung cavities. They sound like the bursting of air bubbles and indicate the presence of fluid. Laennec described them as being produced "by the air forcing its way with difficulty through the sputum which the lungs are no longer able to expel." Rales have been described as being of various types, such as dry, moist, fine, or medium. The sounds may change in quantity and quality after coughing. Rales are heard in those conditions in which excessive fluid accumulates in the lung tissue, such as heart failure and diseases with inflammatory exudates. The clinician should notice the phase of the respiratory cycle in which the rales occur most loudly.

The word *rhonchi* implies wheezing. A rhonchus is a sound produced by the passage of air through the bronchi. The rhonchi may be caused by edema, spasm of the bronchial muscles, or the presence of mucous secretions within the bronchi. Coughing may clear the bronchi of mucous and reduce the number of rhonchi so the effect of coughing on the rhonchi is clearly an important feature to be evaluated by the examiner. Wheezing is a high-pitched sound, resulting from air whistling around a partial airway obstruction. It may occur with inspiration or expiration, but is usually louder during expiration. The pitch of the wheeze depends on the speed with which the air passes through the obstructed air passage. Wheezing sounds may be so loud that they can be heard without a stethoscope.

If there is some disease of the pleural lining, then *pleural friction rubs* may develop. These have been described graphically by Hippocrates, who noted that in pneumonia "the lung is congealed to the ribs and squeaks like a leather strap." A friction rub may be of varying type, louder or softer, distant or close, of low or high pitch. It must be remembered that friction rubs may also be heard over inflamed pericardium. During the respiratory movements, the visceral pleura moves greatest over the parietal pleura at the lateral and posterior bases of the lung, so pericardial friction rubs are usually best heard when they are at the base of the lung. Friction rubs may be heard during both inspiration and expiration and, of course, will disappear if the patient holds the breath. The pleural inflammation, if very painful, may cause the patient to "splint" one side of the chest, and the patient breathes superficially. In such cases, a friction rub may be missed unless the patient is forced to breathe deeply.

Conclusion

Although much valuable information can be gained about the integrity of the respiratory system by following the conventional approaches of looking, feeling, percussing, and listening, it is unusual, these days, for the examination of the respiratory system to be considered complete without radiologic studies. Although the skilled clinician can detect and localize fairly precisely areas of disease in the chest, there is no doubt that the radiograph is a more accurate method of detecting disease. For routine physical examinations, examination of the chest as described above will provide sufficient information to determine whether the patient is suffering from any serious affliction of the respiratory system.

COMMON ABNORMALITIES

Some of the more common symptoms of respiratory diseases are cough, breathlessness, and pain. Objective signs of respiratory disease, such as cyanosis and clubbed fingers, may also be seen in some patients.

Cough

A cough is probably the commonest manifestation of a respiratory disease and may result from diseases of the larynx, trachea, bronchi, or lungs. A cough may be a voluntary act or more usually a reflex response to some irritation of the respiratory mucosa. It is produced by increasing the pressure within the respiratory system against a closed glottis and then suddenly releasing the pressure. The explosive force of air produced will tend to carry the irritating matter away. The type of cough may be important in diagnosis. It may be dry or productive (producing much sputum). The former occurs when the respiratory system is irritated with little production of mucus, as during the early stages of an upper respiratory tract infection and following inhalation of noxious fumes, such as tobacco smoke. A loose cough suggests free exudate in the respiratory passage. The sudden onset of a severe bout of coughing in a patient previously free from any respiratory tract infection should always alert the examiner to the possibility of an inhaled foreign object. The time of day at which coughing is most common will also suggest a particular cause. Coughing and expectoration is common late at night and early in the morning in patients with bronchiectasis and chronic bronchitis. These two conditions are not uncommon. They are characterized by the production of bronchial mucus, diminished gas exchange, and breathing difficulties.

The quality and character of any sputum produced should always be noted, as much important information may be gained from such an observation. Purulent sputum is common in bronchitis and usually smells quite offensive. The presence of pus or blood should be noted. Yellow or green colorations (mucopus) suggest bacterial infection. In the sputum produced by asthmatic patients there are frequent "casts" of mucus originating from the bronchioles. The expectoration of blood (hemoptysis) should be evaluated with care. The amount of blood in the sputum may vary from a few streaks to almost completely blood. It is not always possible to determine whether blood that has been coughed up originated from the respiratory tract or from the gastrointestinal tract. Blood from the respiratory tract is usually frothy. That from the gastrointestinal tract is usually altered to some extent by the action of the gastric secretions and presents finely coagulated material—"coffee grounds" vomitus.

171

Breathlessness

Breathlessness, or dyspnea, sometimes referred to in medical records as SOB (shortness of breath), has been defined as an undue awareness of respiratory effort or the need to increase this effort. The feeling can be readily appreciated by people who have tried swimming for long periods under water without benefit of breathing apparatus. After a prolonged period of holding the breath, there is an almost uncontrollable desire to breathe. It takes considerable effort to inspire, and this feeling is frequently experienced by people who suffer asthma, who require particular respiratory efforts to fill their lungs with air because they have fluid or air in the pleural cavity, whose lungs are fibrosed, or who have paralysis of the respiratory muscles. The sensation of dyspnea probably results from two main areas of stimulation. One area is the receptors that are sensitive to stretching and relaxation within the chest and lungs (part of the Hering-Breuer reflex), and the second area is the receptors in the aortic and carotid arteries and the brain stem, which are sensitive to changes in blood gas tensions, for example, oxygen lack, carbon dioxide excess, or change in pH. Patients with severe dyspnea may say they have to "fight for breath." When the clinician is evaluating a complaint of dyspnea, he or she should pay particular attention to those factors that appear to provoke it. The degree of dyspnea should be assessed by determining whether the breathlessness is severe only after exercise or moderate exertion or whether it is also present during rest. Dyspnea may be due to many diseases of the lungs, pleura, or thoracic cage, to cardiac failure, or to central nervous system changes, such as alterations in blood gas levels. The diagnosis of dyspnea depends on the evaluation of each of the various organs mentioned above.

The matter of hyperventilation has been mentioned in Chapter 7. This may occur in the apprehensive dental patient and is frequently overlooked. The patient may ventilate in excess of metabolic requirements, lowering the tension of arterial carbon dioxide, which results in the development of such symptoms as paresthesia, light-headedness, and perhaps cramps.

Pain

Generally, lung tissue itself does not give rise to pain. Discomfort in breathing is nearly always a result of a condition affecting surrounding structures, especially parietal pleura. Patients may complain of a raw throat if they have acute tracheitis or bronchitis, but in conditions such as bronchopneumonia or tuberculosis, pain may be absent. When the parietal pleura is involved, pain is usually a feature. The pain may be described as sharp or cutting and may prevent sleep. The site of pain within the chest is important. It may occur in the axillary area or beneath the breasts, or in regions some distance from the chest. The parietal pleura is innervated through the intercostal nerves, which also supply the skin of the lower back and abdominal wall. Pleural pain may therefore be referred to the abdomen or lumbar regions and on occasion may give rise to a mistaken diagnosis of an abdominal disorder. Pleurisy over the diaphragm may also occasionally give rise to referred pain in the neck or shoulder. (The phrenic nerve to the diaphragm is derived from the third and fourth cervical nerves.) In nearly all cases, pleural pain is made worse on deep inspiration. Patients may therefore "guard" their respirations and breathe in a shallow way. Not all pains of this type are necessarily of pleural origin. Some may arise from musculoskeletal structures.

BIBLIOGRAPHY

Delp, M.H., and Manning, R.T.: Major's physical diagnosis, ed. 8, Philadelphia, 1975, W.B. Saunders Co.

Prior, J.A., Silberstein, J.S., and Stang, J.: Physical diagnosis: the history and examination of the patient, ed. 6, St. Louis, 1981, The C.V. Mosby Co.

13   Abdomen and gastrointestinal and genitourinary systems

This chapter is included for general information purposes. Dentists will rarely if ever have reason to perform these examinations. Knowledge of the systems is necessary because common diseases affect both the mucosae of these systems and the oral mucosa and because of the high occurrence of diseases of these systems that affect not only dental treatment but also the lives of our patients.

The examination of these systems is divided into abdominal examination and rectal-genitourinary system examination.

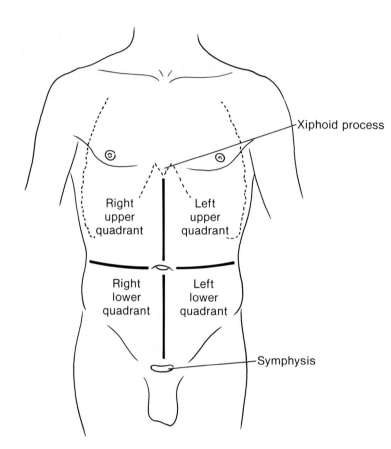

-Xiphoid process

Right upper quadrant

Left upper quadrant

Right lower quadrant

Left lower quadrant

-Symphysis

ABDOMEN
Anatomy

The abdomen is divided into sections, or quadrants, for descriptive purposes (Fig. 13-1). Supplemental divisions are also used (Fig. 13-2).

Fig. 13-1. Division of abdomen into four quadrants for descriptive purposes. Imaginary dividing lines are vertically through midline of sternum to midline of pubis and horizontally through umbilicus.

Fig. 13-2. Secondary divisions of abdomen for further descriptive purposes.

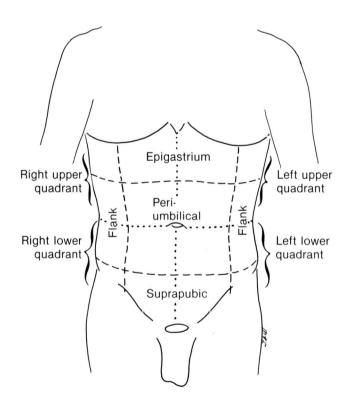

Epigastrium

Right upper quadrant

Left upper quadrant

Flank

Peri-umbilical

Flank

Right lower quadrant

Left lower quadrant

Suprapubic

The abdomen contains many organs and structures. The relationship of these to the surface anatomy is shown in Figs. 13-3 and 13-4. The organs are found in the quadrants as follows:

Upper right
  Liver
  Gallbladder
  Right kidney
  Transverse colon
Upper left
  Stomach
  Pancreas
  Spleen
  Left kidney
  Transverse colon
Lower right
  Vermiform appendix
  Right ovary
  Ascending colon
  McBurney's point (the point of tenderness in acute appendicitis—not an organ)
Lower left
  Left ovary
  Descending colon

The small intestine occupies parts of all quadrants of the abdomen. The urinary bladder, uterus in the female, abdominal aorta, and inferior vena cava are considered midline structures.

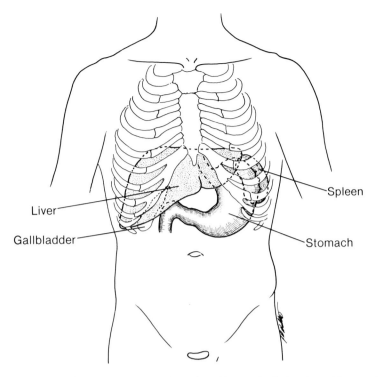

Fig. 13-3. Schematic representation of position and relative size of liver, gallbladder, stomach, and spleen.

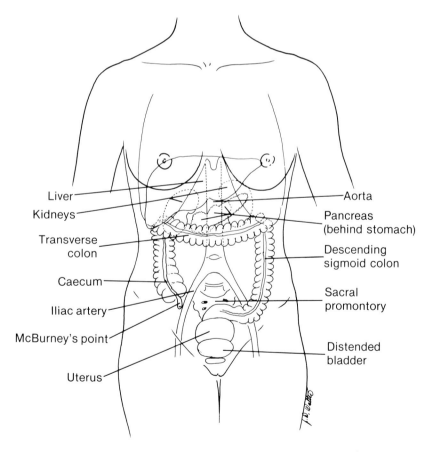

Fig. 13-4. Schematic representation of position of kidney, pancreas, colon, aorta, rectum, and bladder.

175

Examination

The technique for examination of the abdomen is as follows.

Position. The examination of the abdomen is done with the patient lying on the back (supine) on an adequate examination table. The patient needs to be draped for privacy, with the area from the xyphoid process to the pubis exposed (Fig. 13-5).

Inspection. The first part of the examination of the abdomen is observation. Inspection of the abdomen is done with the patient in the supine position. The examiner observes from above the patient and from the side.

The skin is observed, as described in Chapter 10, for the usual skin lesions and for scars, striae, and dilated veins. Scars are significant because most of them are due to abdominal operations. Striae are defined as stripes, bands, streaks, or lines distinguished by color, texture, depression, or elevation from the tissue in which they are found. Striae of the abdomen (stretch marks) are due to Cushing's disease, obesity, and pregnancies. Related superficial abdominal veins are a sign of obstruction of the abdominal vena cava, or portal vein. Cutaneous angiomas, or spider nevi of the chest or abdomen, are a frequent finding in liver disease.

The contour of the abdomen in the supine position is basically flat. Slight rounding is considered normal. Observations are made to determine if there are distortions in this normal contour. The umbilicus is observed and its position noted. The contour of the umbilicus is also noted and described as indented, flat, or protruded. Protrusion of the umbilicus is seen in increased abdominal pressure, as occurs in ascites, abdominal tumors, umbilical hernias, and pregnancy. An indented umbilicus suggests adhesion from surgery, tumors, or obesity.

Fig. 13-5. Patient in proper position and properly draped for examination of abdomen.

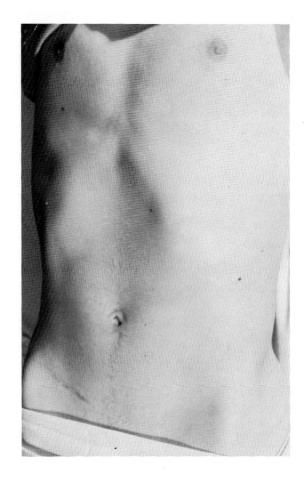

Abnormalities noted in observation of the contour may result from masses produced by enlarged organs (organomegalies) or protuberances produced by tumors or fluid retention (ascites). Ascites is the result of congestive heart failure, chronic adhesive pericarditis, cirrhosis of the liver, and some abdominal vascular obstructions. Intestine contours are visible in the extremely thin patient, whereas the abdomen is round in the obese patient. Aortic pulsations are frequently a normal finding in the epigastric region.

Auscultation. After thorough inspection, auscultation of the abdomen is performed by placing a stethoscope on each quadrant (Fig. 13-6). The normal bowel sounds are heard as clicks and gurgles that occur in varying frequencies at a rate of 5 to 34 per minute. Bruits (abnormal auscultatory sounds heard over arteries) can be heard over the abdominal aorta in patients with diseases such as aortic valve stenosis, aortic aneurysm, and arteriosclerosis. In some liver and spleen diseases, sounds of the membranes of the organs and omentum rubbing together (friction rub) may be heard over the organ.

Percussion. The procedure for percussion of the abdomen is the same as used in the other parts of the physical examination. Percussion of the abdomen is done to identify size and location of the liver and spleen, air bubbles in the stomach, and a distended bladder. Percussion over the abdominal organs produces dull sounds. Percussion over air bubbles in the stomach produces a resonant or tympanic sound. The position in the abdomen and anatomic relation of these healthy organs are demonstrated in Figs. 13-2 and 13-3.

An interesting phenomenon in ascites is the fluid wave. The fluid wave is demonstrated by placing the hand on one side of the abdomen and percussing the other side. The movement of the fluid can be felt on the side of the abdomen opposite the percussing finger.

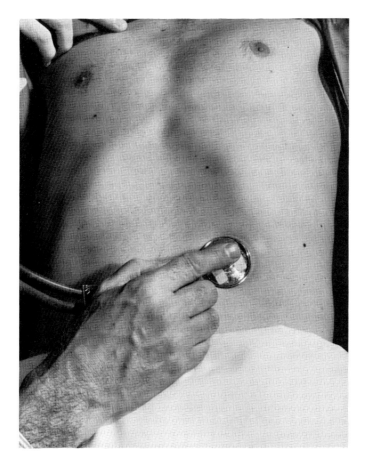

Fig. 13-6. Placement of stethoscope on upper left quadrant of abdomen for determination of abdominal sounds.

Palpation. Palpation may be the most important and revealing part of the examination of the abdomen. The surface of the abdomen is first gently palpated to determine where there are major masses or areas of tenderness. A systematic palpation of the different organs is then done. The liver is palpated by placing the hand on the upper right quadrant as demonstrated in Fig. 13-7. As the patient inhales, the hand is pressed downward toward the back and up under the rib cage. When the liver is palpated, it is frequently helpful to place the opposite hand under the flank and lift (Fig. 13-8).

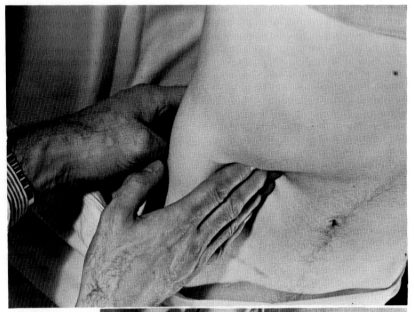

Fig. 13-7. Position and placement of hand for palpation of liver.

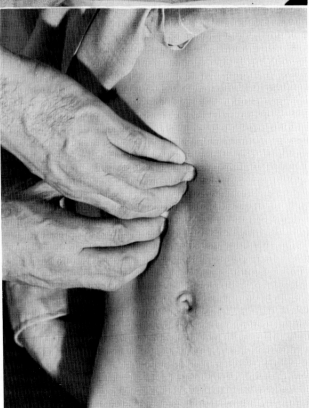

The liver is described in terms of texture, tenderness, size, and border characteristics. The normal liver is smooth, solid, and nontender with a smooth sharp border or edge. The normal liver extends only a few centimeters below the ribs (costal border).

An enlarged liver (hepatomegaly) is identified by noting the texture and tenderness of the liver and the distance it extends below the costal border. This extension is currently measured in centimeters. The old measurement of the enlargement was in fingers.

Hepatomegaly is found in hepatitis, cirrhosis, infectious mononucleosis, tumors, histiocytosis X, and lymphomas. A nodular texture is felt in cirrhosis, tumors, and lymphomas. Distinct masses may be felt when tumors are present. The liver is tender in diseases such as hepatitis and infectious mononucleosis.

The gallbladder is usually not palpable. In diseased states such as gallstones (cholelithiasis) and inflammation of the gallbladder or bile duct (cholecystitis) the gallbladder is enlarged and tender. It can be palpated at the right inferior border of the liver.

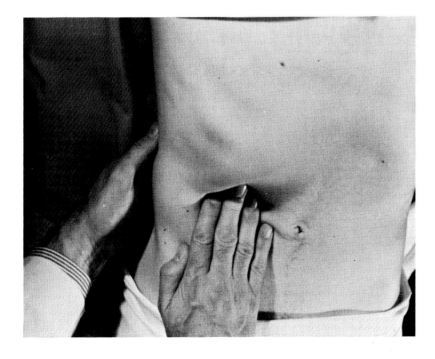

Fig. 13-8. Lifting of right flank to assist in palpation of liver.

The spleen is palpated as demonstrated in Fig. 13-9. It is frequently helpful in palpation of the spleen to lift the flank area with the nonexamining hand, shifting the spleen upward so it is more easily palpated (Fig. 13-10). The spleen is palpated to determine size, consistency, and degree of tenderness. A normal spleen can rarely be palpated and is nontender. The spleen is enlarged (splenomegaly) in blood dyscrasias, lymphomas, including all classifications of Hodgkin's disease, infectious mononucleosis, and some other viral diseases. When enlarged, the spleen is usually tender. When the examiner is palpating for the spleen, an enlarged or painful pancreas and masses or tenderness of the stomach may be encountered as an incidental finding.

The rest of the palpation of the abdomen is done to determine normal bowel positions, particularly of the transverse and descending colon, the abdominal aorta, and the stomach. Distended bladders can be palpated in the suprapubic area. The pregnant uterus can be palpated from the surface. The kidneys may on occasion be palpated using a bimanual technique. The usual examination of the kidney is accomplished by placing the left hand on the back of the seated patient below the costovertebral angle and striking it with the ulnar surface of the right hand. The patient will normally feel the blow but will not feel pain unless the kidney is tender.

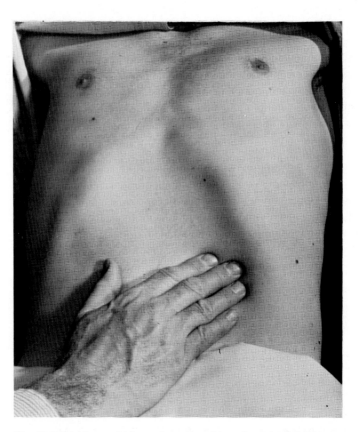

Fig. 13-9. Position and placement of hand in palpation of spleen.

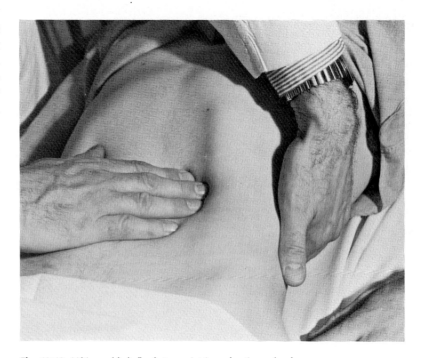

Fig. 13-10. Lifting of left flank to assist in palpation of spleen.

Diagnostic tests. The physical examination of the abdomen will reveal many disorders of the abdomen. Additional laboratory and radiographic studies are necessary to fully evaluate the abdominal organs.

Radiographs of the abdomen are frequently taken as part of a complete physical examination. These radiographs will reveal any calcified mass, large tissue masses, and radiopaque stones in the gallbladder, kidney, and urinary tract. Radiographs to outline specific organs are made with the aid of radiopaque dyes. The radiopaque material, meglumine iodipamide, is excreted by the liver in the bile. After this dye has been injected intravenously, the outline of the gallbladder, bile duct, and radiolucent stones can be identified on radiographs.

Intravenous pyelography (IVP) is performed to show the outline of the renal excretory system by intravenously injecting meglumine diatrizoate, a radiopaque material. This dye is excreted by the kidney and shows not only the outline of the kidney and urinary system but also radiolucent stones of the kidney on radiographs.

The urethra, bladder, ureter, uterus, and pelvis of the kidney are made radiopaque by the injection of radiopaque dyes directly into the urinary tract through a urethral cannula (retrograde pyelography).

The vascular system of any of the abdominal organs can be seen on a fluoroscope and sequential radiographs by injecting radiopaque dyes into the abdominal arteries (arteriography).

The gastrointestinal tract is examined radiographically by having the patient swallow radiopaque dyes (barium) to observe the functional structure of the upper intestine (upper gastrointestinal series). The evaluation is done with *fluoroscopy* so that movements of the esophagus, stomach, and intestine can be seen as the radiopaque barium is swallowed and moves through the intestinal tract. During the procedure sequential radiographs are exposed to give a permanent record. The lower gastrointestinal tract evaluation is performed after the patient's lower bowel has been evacuated of fecal material by the use of laxatives and enemas. An enema of radiopaque dye (barium enema) is given, and radiographs are taken to show the outline of the colon and lower small intestines.

RECTAL AND GENITOURINARY SYSTEMS
Anatomy

The anatomic structures of the genitourinary system are diagrammatically shown in the anatomy of the abdomen (see Fig. 13-4) and in the diagrams showing examination techniques (Figs. 13-11 through 13-14).

Examination

Male. The male genitalia are examined with the patient in a standing position. The external genitalia are inspected for asymmetries, masses, and skin lesions. The testicles and penis are gently palpated to determine if there are unusual masses. Observation of the orifice of the penis is made after gentle milking by the patient to determine if there is any discharge. To determine if the inguinal canal has been closed, a finger is gently extended along the spermatic cord up toward the abdomen (Fig. 13-11). The area is palpated to determine if any intestinal masses have protruded through the inguinal canal or abdominal wall, producing a hernia (Fig. 13-12). As the finger is inserted, the patient usually is asked to cough to determine if the pressure pushes the abdominal contents through the canal or abdominal wall.

The rectum is examined with the patient on his side. The rectum and anus are examined to determine if there are venous distensions (hemorrhoids) or other superficial lesions. A gloved, lubricated finger is inserted into the anus, and the lower intestinal tract is palpated for masses or asymmetries. The prostate gland in the male is palpated by pressure toward the bladder through the rectum.

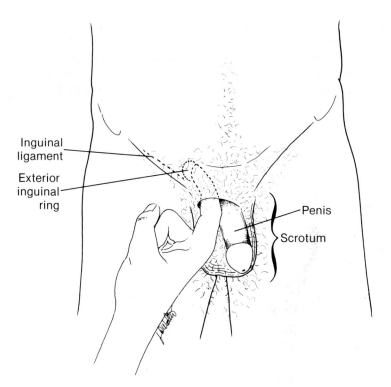

Fig. 13-11. Graphic representation of normal male genitalia and positioning of examining finger for evaluation of hernia.

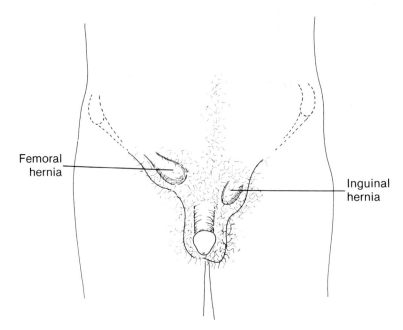

Fig. 13-12. Graphic representation of inguinal hernias.

Most complete physical examinations include a proctoscopic examination. This examination is done with the patient on a table in a kneeling position with his head down and his knees under his stomach (knee-chest position). The examination is done after the patient has used laxatives and an enema to clear the colon of fecal material. The proctoscopic examination gives a direct view of the lower portion of the colon and is important in the early detection of malignant disease of the colon.

Female. The female genitalia are examined with the patient supine with her legs spread and her knees up (lithotomy position). Frequently the legs are placed in stirrups for greater access to the area and the comfort of the patient. The external genitalia are observed for any masses, skin diseases, or asymmetries. The labia are spread with a gloved hand, and the mucosa (Fig. 13-13) is inspected for abnormalities. The urethra is viewed and observed for discharge, redness, or irritation. A gloved finger is gently inserted into the vagina, and the vagina is palpated for masses. The finger is turned toward the pubis, and the urethra is milked to determine if there is a discharge. The uterus can be palpated by placing two fingers turned upward in the vagina and the other hand on the abdomen just above the pubis (Fig. 13-14). The uterus is then palpated between the two hands (bimanual palpation). The cervix can be viewed by using a speculum to open the vagina.

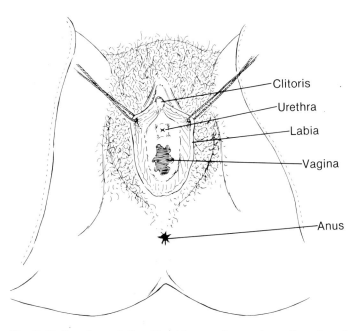

Fig. 13-13. Female genitalia with labia spread, exposing orifice of urethra and vagina.

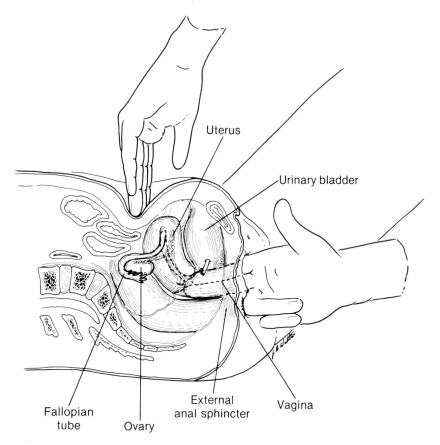

Fig. 13-14. Bimanual palpation of uterus. Internal female genitourinary structures are demonstrated.

183

Rectal examination of the female is similar to that of the male with the exception that when the rectum is palpated, the posterior wall of the vagina can be palpated, and bimanual palpation will be of some help in determining the competency of the rectal-vaginal separation. This palpation is frequently done with one finger in the vagina and one in the rectum.

Since the mucosa of the gastrointestinal and genitourinary systems is similar in many respects to the oral mucosa, there are multiple diseases that affect all areas. Some of these are listed below.

Infections
    Candida albicans
    Gonococci
    Syphilis, all stages
    Herpes simplex
Immunologic disorders
    Erythema multiforme
    Crohn's disease
    Behçet's syndrome
Malignant lesions
    Epidermoid carcinoma
    Adenocarcinoma (important because of metastases of cervical, prostate, and colon carcinoma to oral cavity)

The patient has been on an examining table for examination of the chest, heart, abdomen, and genitalia. He or she is now allowed to resume a sitting position for the neurologic examination, which is dealt with in Chapter 14.

BIBLIOGRAPHY

Bates, B.: A guide to physical examination, ed. 2, Philadelphia, 1979, J.B. Lippincott Co.

Delp, M.H., and Manning, R.T.: Major's physical diagnosis, ed. 8, Philadelphia, 1975, W.B. Saunders Co.

Prior, J.A., Silberstein, J.S., and Stang, J.: Physical diagnosis, ed. 6, St. Louis, 1981, The C.V. Mosby Co.

14 Nervous system

It is not essential that the dentist become competent to conduct a complete and definitive examination of a patient's whole neurologic system. However, the dentist should be aware of the principles of such an examination and the signs and symptoms of the more common conditions that affect the facial area.

Disorders of the nervous system may produce changes of widely varied types involving both motor and sensory components. There are several neurologic conditions that produce significant subjective and objective changes in the head and neck area, and it is frequently the dentist who is first called upon to evaluate these signs and symptoms. This chapter consists of a general review of the basic principles of evaluating the nervous system, followed by a more detailed review of the methods of evaluating the cranial nerves. Emphasis is placed on those conditions that the dentist is more likely to encounter in practice, and signs and symptoms of selected diseases are presented. For example, it is not unusual for a transient facial paralysis to follow the administration of a local anesthetic delivered before a dental procedure. Clearly, it is in the interests of the patient for the dentist to be able to evaluate such a paralysis to be certain that is is local and not just one component of a more serious condition, such as a cerebral vascular accident.

BASIC PRINCIPLES OF THE NEUROLOGIC EXAMINATION

The nervous system, containing all of its components—autonomic system, brain, spinal cord, peripheral nerves, and end organs—may be involved by conditions affecting the system generally (such as multiple sclerosis) or by diseases manifesting in very localized areas (such as traumatic avulsion of the inferior alveolar nerve during third molar surgery).

The general approach to evaluating the neurologic system is the same as that for any other body system. The evaluation should consist of a review of the patient's history followed by a detailed examination of the particular system. During the history taking special emphasis must be placed on the precise location of any areas of impaired sensation (hypesthesia), numbness, tingling, "pins and needles" pain (paresthesia), or loss of position sense. The patient should be asked about difficulty with maintaining balance, dizziness, visual disturbances, and difficulty in swallowing or speaking. Questions should be asked concerning a patient's motor functions. Conditions that affect the motor system may lead a patient to report the inability to perform fine movements with the hands, that is, such movements as buttoning a dress or shirt. (It should be noted that not all the signs or symptoms that are reviewed above necessarily indicate primary neurologic disorders; for example, an inability to cope with such maneuvers as buttoning clothes may be due to other conditions [such as rheumatoid arthritis or scleroderma] that interfere with the functioning of the fingers.)

When all the details of the patient's symptoms have been recorded, it is time to proceed to the physical evaluation of the nervous system. This should proceed in an orderly and step-wise way. The patient should be asked to walk and to demonstrate the abilities to perform various motor functions. Motor power can be tested by systematically checking the various muscle groups around the neck and limbs (Fig. 14-1). The patient should be asked to flex, extend, and rotate the joints, and any inability to do so should be noted carefully. Triceps, biceps, knee, ankle, and plantar reflexes should be evaluated, (Fig. 14-2) and the jaw jerk should be elicited (see Trigeminal Nerve).

Fig. 14-1. Testing muscle movements of upper limb. Major groups of limb muscles should be tested by having patient push or pull against examiner's hand. **A,** Subject is pushing against examiner's hand and therefore exercising triceps muscle. **B,** Subject is pulling against examiner's arm, that is, flexing muscles, and obvious contraction of biceps can be seen. Such tests of muscle function should be conducted bilaterally and generally should reveal equal muscle power.

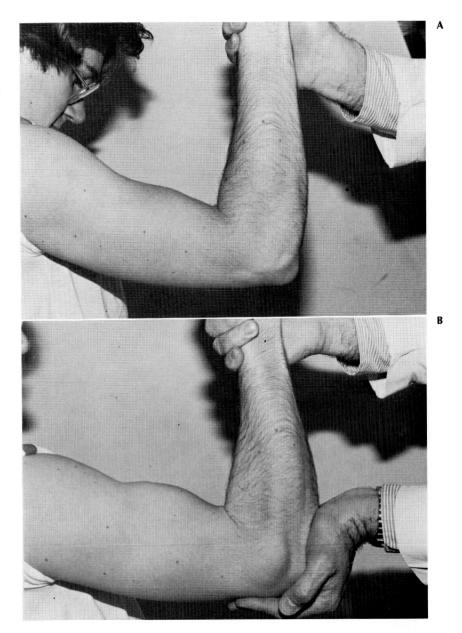

A

B

Position sense should be tested by asking the patient to touch the nose with the index finger, alternating right and left hands. This should be accomplished with the patient's eyes closed. An inability to perform this might indicate some deficiency of position sense. Similar tests can be conducted with the lower limbs by, for example, asking the patient to place the heel of one foot against the knee of the other leg and move the foot down toward the ankle. This too should be performed with the eyes closed.

Deficiencies in sensation can be detected by determining a patient's ability to perceive light touch (by touching the skin lightly with a wisp of cotton), a pin prick, pressure from a blunt instrument (for example, the head of the pin used for the pin prick test), and temperature appreciation. Special vibration sense is also determined by applying a tuning fork to various bony sites, such as the ankle, shaft of the tibia, and elbow. The interpretation of a patient's symptoms and of the various neurologic signs, motor and sensory, depends on a thorough understanding of the underlying nerve supply. If there is a very localized neurologic problem, such as, say, damage to the median nerve at the wrist, then the examiner would expect to find only those muscles innervated by the median nerve to be

paralyzed and only the skin served by that nerve to be numb. In other disorders, such as multiple sclerosis, the signs and symptoms, both motor and sensory, are varied, do not conform to any particular neurologic pattern, and do not indicate any localization of disease. The method of determining the precise location of a neurologic problem by evaluating the neurologic signs and symptoms is discussed later under the section dealing with the evaluation of the seventh cranial nerve.

The full neurologic examination, which should include an evaluation of the patient's mental status, including the ability to understand and respond to written and spoken questions, should be conducted *a capite ad calcem* (from head to foot). This evaluation requires considerable skill and experience on the part of the examiner. As previously stated, it is not suggested that the dentist perform such a complete examination, but he or she should be familiar with the principles of it. It is highly desirable that a dentist be able to conduct, understand, and interpret an examination of the cranial nerves. The following section reviews the examination of the cranial nerves in detail and illustrates problems that might be encountered in the dental office.

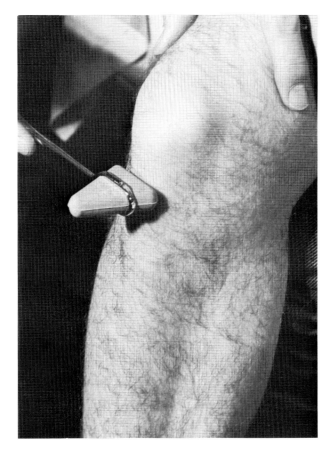

Fig. 14-2. Patella or knee jerk reflex. If patellar tendon is tapped lightly while knee is in relaxed, flexed position (for example, dangling over edge of examining table or bed), there will be upward jerk of leg at knee, caused by contraction of quadriceps. This patella reflex arc involves second, third, and fourth lumbar segments of spinal cord.

EXAMINATION OF THE CRANIAL NERVES
Olfactory nerve

Disorders of the olfactory nerve (nerve I) seldom appear as diagnostic problems to the dentist. In some cases, however, particularly those cases of severe maxillofacial trauma involving the nasal bones, it may be necessary to determine if there is any residual damage to the patient's sense of smell.

The examiner should first determine that there is no obstruction of the nasal passages. The patient, with eyes closed, is then asked to identify familiar odors, such as cloves or coffee. Each side should be tested separately by occluding the external nares.

Optic nerve

The neurologic examination of the optic nerve (nerve II) by the physician always includes an ophthalmoscopic examination. Examination of the various component structures of the eye—the cornea, iris, lens, and retina—may provide valuable evidence of local or systemic diseases. It is not practicable for the dentist to conduct such an examination regularly, as considerable experience is needed to interpret the various findings. Many important tests of ocular function, however, can be readily determined without any special instrumentation. Examination of the eye is discussed further in Chapter 9.

It must be remembered that the eye has a relatively complex nerve supply. Sensation in the conjuctiva is mediated through the fifth cranial nerve; the eye receives sympathetic and parasympathetic fibers of the autonomic system to the ciliary and iris muscles; the external ocular muscles that move the eye are innervated by the third, fourth, and sixth cranial nerves, and, of course, vision is mediated through the optic nerve itself. There are also important cross-reflex connections between both eyes, and these should be carefully evaluated.

The most usual test for optic nerve function is, of course, to determine that the patient can see with each eye. It is important to realize that a patient's vision may depend on adequate correction of refractive errors, and this possibility must be taken into consideration. One of the first tests is to determine that a patient's pupillary reflex is intact; that is, that the pupil constricts when a light is directed onto the retina. Light initiates nerve impulses from the retina, which then pass through the optic nerve and optic tract to the Edinger-Westphal nucleus (situated in the pretectal area of the midbrain). From this nucleus impulses pass back through the parasympathetic nerves to the constrictor muscles of the iris. The pupillary reflex is easily determined in the dental office by shining the dental light into the eye and noting whether there is some immediate constriction of the pupil. It is important to realize that this is a consensual reflex; in other words, if light is directed into the right eye, then it is expected that the left pupil as well as the right pupil will constrict. It is thus clearly important that the light be shown into each eye separately, that is, with the other one covered; for, if one eye were blind and the light were shown into both eyes simultaneously, then both pupils would constrict, giving the erroneous impression that each eye was intact.

The determination of the visual fields is a simple and valuable test. The patient should be asked to cover one eye and look at the examiner's nose. The examiner then moves a finger or a cotton-tip applicator in front of the patient, starting at the periphery of each quadrant of the visual field (see Fig. 9-2). The patient is asked to indicate when he or she sees the finger or applicator. This test should be performed for each eye and will reveal any gross defects in the visual field (this matter is discussed in Chapter 9). The location of such defects may give a valuable clue as to the position along the optic pathway (optic nerve to the visual cortex in the occipital area of the brain) where the problem has arisen. In Fig. 14-3, for example, a lesion interrupting the optic pathway at site *a* (the right optic nerve) will produce blindness in the right eye without having any effect on the left visual field. An involvement of the optic chiasma at site *b* by, say, a pituitary adenoma, is most likely to affect the crossing nasal fibers, so the visual field defect will be a bitemporal hemianopia. (Light from the temporal side stimulates the nasal part of the retina.) A lesion at site *c*, the right optic tract, will cause an interruption of the right uncrossed temporal fibers and the crossed nasal fibers from the left side. The resulting visual defect is a left homonymous hemianopia. It must be remembered that the temporal fibers subserve the nasal field and the nasal fibers the temporal field. Consequently, the visual defect in both the right and left eyes will be on the same side (that is, the left side) because in the right eye the temporal fibers are involved and in the left eye the nasal fibers are involved.

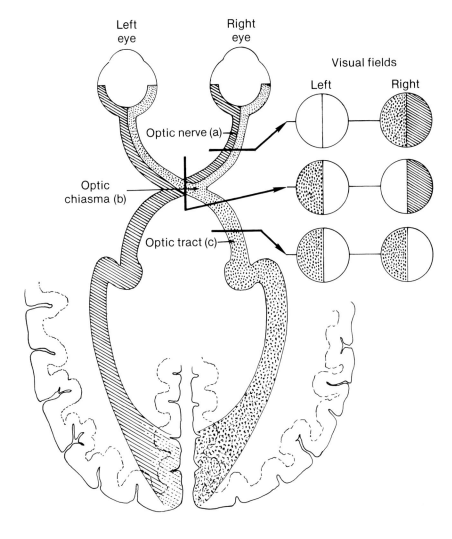

Fig. 14-3. Optic pathways from each retina back to visual cortex in occipital lobe. At optic chiasma, only fibers arising from nasal side of each retina cross to other side. Temporal fibers continue in optic pathway on same side. Lesions that interrupt continuity of optic tract will produce changes in visual fields that will provide clue as to location of lesion.

Oculomotor, trochlear, and abducent nerves

These nerves, which all supply muscles for eye movement, should be tested together. The oculomotor nerve (nerve III) is involved in the pupillary reflex, as it supplies the muscles that constrict the pupil. The finding of an intact pupillary constriction reflex suggests that the oculomotor nerves are intact. This can then be confirmed by determining whether the patient has a full range of ocular movements. The patient is asked to follow the movements of the examiner's finger as it is moved in all directions of gaze. When there is involvement of the oculomotor nerve, the patient will not be able to look up, down, or medially with the affected eye. There will be some drooping (ptosis) of the upper lid and dilatation of the pupil on the same side. The oculomotor nerve supplies the superior rectus, the inferior rectus, and the medial rectus muscles.

The trochlear nerve (nerve IV) supplies the superior oblique muscle, which pulls the eye down and out. Paralysis of this nerve will prevent the patient from looking in an inferior and lateral direction.

The abducent nerve (nerve VI) supplies the lateral rectus muscle, and paralysis of this nerve will prevent the patient from looking laterally with the involved eye. In any case of external ocular muscle paralysis, it can be expected that the patient will complain of double vision (diplopia) in the direction in which eye movement is paralyzed. It should be realized that any of these nerves to the external ocular muscles may be involved anywhere in their course from their origin in the motor cortex, during their passage through the midbrain or pons, or during their traversing of the cavernous sinus. It is important for the dentist to correlate any abnormality of eye movement with any other neurologic signs or symptoms or the presence of some other condition, such as cavernous sinus thrombosis, to determine the most likely site of the problem.*

---

*The third, fourth, and sixth nerves run in intimate relationship with the cavernous sinus. The third and fourth nerves run in the wall of the cavernous sinus, and the sixth nerve within the sinus itself. Any inflammatory condition of the sinus may interfere with the function of the nerves and lead to some paresis of the external ocular muscles with resulting diplopia.

During the examination of the ocular movements the dentist should also look for nystagmus. This is a condition in which there is an involuntary rapid movement of the eyeball that may be horizontal, vertical, or rotatory. This sign is seen in a variety of neurologic disorders and during therapy with certain drugs, such as phenytoin (Dilantin).

Mention has already been made concerning the pupillary reaction. The examiner should always note the size, shape, and equality of the pupils. For most patients it is usual for the pupils to be equal in size bilaterally (isocoria). The condition of anisocoria, or unequal pupil size, may indicate several neurologic conditions. The pupil tends to be larger in young people and to become smaller and less responsive to light in the elderly. Mention has already been made of the consensual pupillary reflex. The direct consensual pupillary reflexes should always be tested.

A 29-year-old woman visited her dentist for a routine dental examination. During the evaluation of the patient, the dentist noticed that there was some facial asymmetry. The palpebral fissures on each side of the face were not equal in size. It was also noted that there was a difference in the size of the pupils (Fig. 14-4). The patient reported that one side of her face was dry. Further questioning revealed that the patient had undergone some surgery on the right side of her neck to remove a malignant tumor. She was suffering from Horner's syndrome.

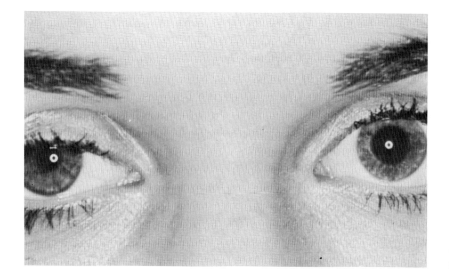

Fig. 14-4. Horner's syndrome *(right side).* Right upper eyelid is drooping, narrowing right palpebral fissure. Parasympathetic pupillary constrictor muscle is unopposed, so pupil on right side is smaller than left one. Skin of right side of face is drier than left.

The sympathetic fibers serving the head and neck, including the eyes, originate in the upper thoracic part of the spinal cord and ascend through the cervical sympathetic chain to their various end organs in association with the blood vessels of the head and neck. Occasionally, this sympathetic pathway in the neck may be involved in a process that interrupts its continuity. Such a condition may arise following surgery to the neck for removal of lymph nodes or may develop as a result of an infiltrating neoplasm that involves and obliterates the cervical sympathetic fibers. An interruption of the sympathetic impulses produces a well-recognized syndrome known as Horner's syndrome (cervical sympathetic paralysis). The features are:

1. Drooping of the upper eyelid, narrowing of the palpebral fissure, and enophthalmos. The enophthalmos (backward displacement of the eyeball into the orbit) is more apparent than real, and it appears as a result of the ptosis.
2. Pupillary constriction. The muscles supplied by the sympathetic fibers running to the eye will normally dilate the pupil. Since pupil size is a function of the balance between the pupillary constrictor muscle fibers (parasympathetic) and the pupillary dilator muscle fibers (sympathetic), the parasympathetic works, as it were, unopposed, resulting in pupillary constriction.
3. Hyphidrosis or anhidrosis of the skin of the face. The sweat glands of the facial skin are served by the sympathetic fibers. If these are nonfunctioning, the patient will have dryness of the skin, as there will be a reduction in or an absence of sweating.
4. Vascular dilatation. Loss of sympathetic tone by the muscles of the vessel walls leads to vessel dilatation. This is usually most evident in the conjunctiva.

The dentist called on to evaluate a mass in the neck should always consider the possibility of Horner's syndrome and look specifically for the components of this syndrome.

Trigeminal nerve

The trigeminal nerve (nerve V) has sensory and motor components, and each of these should be tested carefully. The trigeminal nerve has a wide area of distribution, providing the sensory nerve supply to the forehead and scalp, the skin over the face, part of the ear, the upper part of the neck, and the structures within the mouth, tongue, palate, teeth, and gingivae. Wisps of cotton should be used to touch lightly the forehead, cheeks, jaws, and upper part of the neck; any failure to respond to this stimulus might indicate anesthesia or paresthesia (altered sensation). Any difference in response to such testing on opposite sides of the face should be noted carefully. The same procedure is then followed for testing degrees of sensitivity to pin prick, to blunt pressure, and to warm and cold objects. These tests should be conducted with the patient's eyes closed. The corneal reflex is tested by observing whether the patient blinks in response to light touching of the cornea with a wisp of cotton. The efferent side of the corneal blink reflex is mediated through the facial nerve and the orbicular muscle of the eye. The integrity of the trigeminal nerve intraorally is normally evaluated only by pulp testing the teeth, although it is sometimes necessary to determine gingival and lingual sensitivity by pricking the gingivae or tongue with an explorer. The techniques for pulp testing are not discussed in this chapter. Testing the ability to taste adequately is discussed below under the seventh nerve.

The motor functions of the trigeminal nerve are examined by evaluating the movements of the muscles of mastication: the masseter, temporal, lateral, and medial pterygoids. Contraction of the masseter and temporal muscles can be evaluated by palpating these muscles when the jaws are held tightly together. The patient should be asked to open the jaw widely. It is usual for the jaw to be opened directly downward, and any deviation to the side should be noted. It should be remembered that such a deviation would not necessarily indicate a neurologic problem, as deviations in jaw movement can arise from other nonneurological conditions. The jaw jerk or maxillary reflex is tested by tapping the middle of the chin with a reflex hammer while the patient's jaw is slightly open. The normal reflex is a sudden, slight closing movement of the jaw. The tapping may be done against a tongue blade or the examiner's finger held against the chin (Fig. 14-5).

Pain from the trigeminal area is one of the most common diagnostic problems facing the dentist, who must be able to evaluate the integrity of the trigeminal nerve in both its motor and sensory functions when attempting to evaluate facial pain. One of the most severe disorders affecting the trigeminal nerve is trigeminal neuralgia, or tic douloureux. It is important to remember that between the attacks of pain of trigeminal neuralgia it is not possible to detect any neurologic sign of disease of the trigeminal system or of any other cranial nerve.

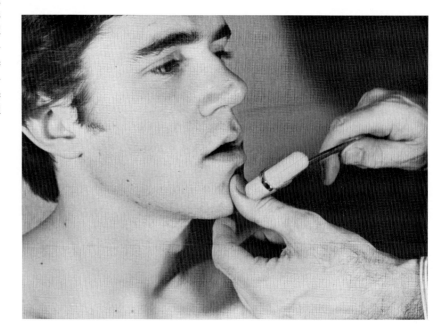

Fig. 14-5. Jaw jerk. Mouth Is held slightly open. Examiner's thumb (or tongue blade) is placed against chin and struck lightly with percussion hammer. This initiates closing action of jaw elevator muscles.

Facial nerve

It is not infrequent for a patient to develop a transient facial nerve (nerve VII) paralysis after the administration of a local anesthetic agent for a nerve block of the inferior alveolar nerve. A dentist should be well aware of the underlying neuroanatomy of the facial nerve and should be confident in being able to determine the extent of a facial nerve paralysis and the most likely cause of it. The facial nerve not only provides the innervation of the muscles of facial expression, including the orbicular muscles of the eye, but also, for part of its course, carries fibers that pass through the chorda tympani nerve and innervate the taste buds and salivary glands. Facial nerve function is tested by asking the patient to imitate the examiner, who smiles, showing the teeth. Such a smile should normally be symmetric, and, apart from the patient who has a habitual "lopsided" smile, should show equal amounts of teeth on each side.

The integrity of the orbicular muscle of the mouth is determined by asking the patient to blow the cheeks out. In the normal person this muscle should prevent any leakage of air. Another test of this muscle is to ask the patient to whistle through the lips. The orbicular muscle of the eye is then tested by asking the patient to tightly close the eyes. The strength of the eyelid muscles can be further evaluated by asking the patient to "screw" the eyelids together while the dentist attempts to open them. The patient should then be asked to wrinkle the forehead and to frown (Fig. 14-6). This last test is of particular importance for the following reasons. The peripheral fibers of each facial nerve contain fibers originating from both the contralateral and the ipsilateral sides of the brain. The ipsilateral fibers normally serve the muscles of the upper part of the face. If a patient develops a facial nerve paralysis from a central lesion (one located in the brain), such as a brain tumor or cerebral vascular accident, then it can be expected that the supranuclear fibers that arise from the affected side and cross to the other side of the body would be paralyzed, but the supranuclear fibers from the uninvolved side that serve the upper muscle fibers of their same side would be unaffected. In such circumstances, a patient, although having an obvious degree of facial paralysis on the side opposite the brain lesion, would still be able to partially wrinkle the muscles of the forehead. If, however, the facial nerve paralysis arose from some disturbance of the lower motor neuron, which carries crossed fibers and ipsilateral fibers, then there would be a total paralysis of the muscles of the face. This is obviously a most important differentiation, which must be determined by a dentist evaluating a patient who develops a facial paralysis in the dental office.

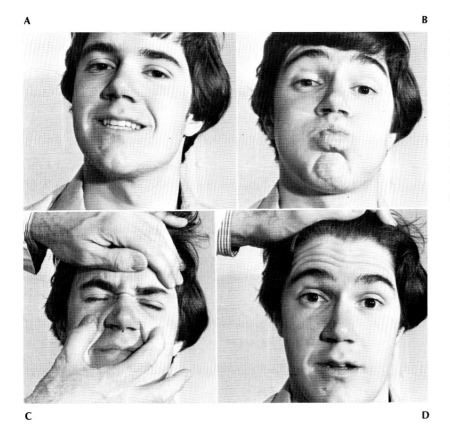

A

B

C

D

Fig. 14-6. Evaluation of facial nerve. **A,** Patient has been asked to smile, revealing "symmetric" smile, showing equal amounts of teeth on each side. **B,** Patient has been asked to blow cheeks out and orbicular muscle of mouth is clearly intact. **C,** Patient has been asked to screw eyelids together and can accomplish this in spite of examiner's attempt to hold them open. **D,** Patient has been asked to wrinkle forehead by frowning. There is symmetric frowning.

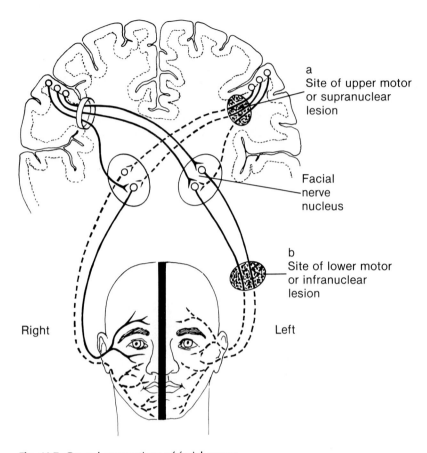

Fig. 14-7. Central connections of facial nerves.

a
Site of upper motor
or supranuclear
lesion

Facial
nerve
nucleus

b
Site of lower motor
or infranuclear
lesion

Right

Left

Fig. 14-7 illustrates the facial nerves; it should be noted that from each motor cortex there are two groups of facial nerve fibers. One group courses to the contralateral side, synapses in the facial nerve nucleus, and then passes down through the lower motor pathway to the facial muscles. A second group passes to the facial nucleus of the ipsilateral side, passing through the lower motor pathway to innervate muscles of the upper face of the same side.

The diagram also illustrates two possible sites of lesions that would affect the normal facial nerve pathway. At site *a* an upper motor lesion, or supranuclear lesion, is indicated. Such a lesion may result from, say, a brain tumor or a cerebral vascular accident. There will clearly be an interruption of those fibers that would normally pass to the contralateral side and also of the fibers that would remain on the ipsilateral side, innervating the upper part of the left side of the face. In such circumstances it should be noted that, on the right side, the facial nerve fibers that do not cross to the other side and that innervate the upper facial muscles of the right side will not be affected by the left-sided supranuclear lesion, and consequently the patient will retain some activity in the upper part of the face, that is, might be able to frown.

A lower motor neuron lesion (site *b*) will affect not only the impulses that have come from crossed fibers but also those travelling in the ipsilateral noncrossing pathway. In those circumstances the patient will have a complete paralysis, that is, no movement whatever in the muscles of the face.

A 23-year-old dental student woke one morning to find that the right side of his face felt "heavy." On looking in the mirror, he realized that the right side of his face had dropped and that he was unable to tightly close his right eye. The patient was otherwise in good health and could think of no incident that might have precipitated the facial paralysis. It was deter-

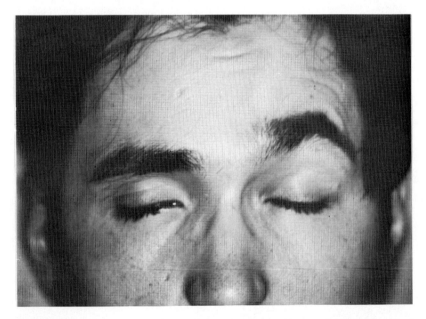

Fig. 14-8. When patient was asked to frown, he was unable to wrinkle his forehead on right side.

mined that the patient had a paralysis involving all the muscles of the right side of the face, and when the patient was asked to wrinkle his forehead, it was noted that the wrinkling was restricted to the left side (Fig. 14-8). In this particular case an electromyographic record of muscle activity in the frontalis muscle was made to confirm the diagnosis of lower motor neuron facial paralysis (Fig. 14-9).

The patient was found to have lost the sense of taste on the right side of the tongue (hemiageusia), and this suggested that the problem lay in the facial nerve canal (that part of the facial nerve course shared with the chorda tympani fibers). .

The diagnosis of Bell's palsy, an idiopathic lower motor neuron paralysis of the facial nerve, was made. No definite treatment was offered, and the patient recovered facial muscle activity within 10 days. Had the clinical examination suggested the presence of an upper motor lesion, then it would have been necessary to rule out the development of a central nervous system lesion, such as a tumor or vascular accident.

The chorda tympani nerve is tested by having the patient identify the taste of salt, sugar, or acid substances placed on the anterior part of the tongue on each side. The patient must keep the tongue protruded long enough to test the flavor. If the tongue is retracted or the patient swallows prematurely, the solution might spread to both sides of the tongue, and it might be difficult to determine the ability to taste on both sides. After each test substance, the patient should take a sip of water.

Care must be taken to determine whether a complaint of "loss of taste" is really due to a taste deficiency or whether the patient is in fact suffering a loss of smell. A patient with a deficient sense of smell will often interpret the failure to discern flavor as a lack of taste. A patient may seek a dentist's advice concerning this because of having reasoned that the taste loss may be associated with the wearing of dentures or some chronic oral inflammation. Certain abnormalities of taste and smell may occur in en-

docrine disorders and may be associated with complex metabolic changes affecting metallic ions throughout the body. In addition, certain drugs may reduce taste acuity, and bizarre gustatory symptoms may develop in some patients taking medications containing lithium. Any evaluation of

taste abnormalities must include a detailed history of the patient's general health, including a full list of any medications being taken.

The relationship between loss of taste and complete and incomplete facial nerve paralysis is shown in Table 4.

Table 4. Summary of neurologic signs produced by lesions of the facial nerve pathway located at different levels

Location of lesions	Type of paralysis	Ability to taste on affected side
Brain (supranuclear lesion)	Partial Some ability to wrinkle forehead on affected side	Normal
Facial nerve canal	Complete Lower motor pathway involement	Impaired
Extracranial course	Complete	Normal

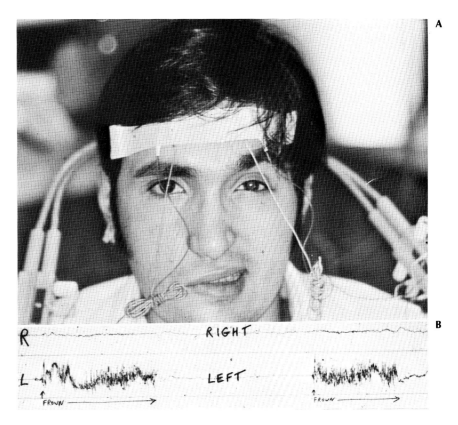

Fig. 14-9. A, Electrodes were placed over right and left frontal muscles and patient was then asked to frown; notice asymmetry of mouth. **B,** Recording of muscle activity in each muscle was made. Tracing shows clearly that on command frown there was considerable activity in left muscle, but none in right.

Acoustic nerve

The acoustic nerve (nerve VIII) is divided into two parts: the cochlear nerve and the vestibular nerve. Since special equipment is needed to examine the vestibular nerve, it is not tested routinely. The external ear canal should be observed with an otoscope to be certain that there are no gross abnormalities in or blockage of the canal. An attempt should be made to determine whether a patient has bilaterally equal hearing abilities. This can be determined by holding a ticking watch close to the patient's ear and then moving it away until the patient can no longer hear it. The maneuver should be repeated, but this time moving the watch from a distance away from the ear toward the ear. The distances from the ears at which the patient either begins to hear or ceases to hear the watch ticking should be equal bilaterally.

The ability of a patient to hear a wide range of frequencies at different intensities requires the use of a specialized instrument, and the resulting audiograms are normally taken when patients are being evaluated for deafness. A relatively simple test of determining whether deafness is due to disease of the vestibulocochlear nerve itself or merely to some problem with the conducting mechanism of the middle ear is the tuning fork test. A tuning fork, sounding strongly, should be

Fig. 14-10. Rinne's test. **A,** Vibrating tuning fork is held opposite external auditory canal. **B,** If it can be heard, it should then be placed with its base on mastoid process. Patient should then indicate whether bone conduction or air conduction is louder.

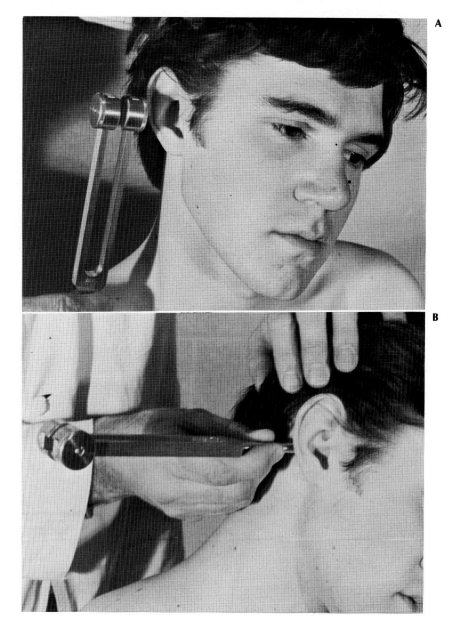

held opposite the ear. If it can be heard, it should then be placed with its base on the mastoid process in order to determine if the vibrations can be heard when conducted through the bone. If the patient hears the sound, the examiner should ask whether it is as loud as when the fork was heard through the air. Another way to determine this is to find out whether bone or air conduction permits the patient to hear the sound longer as the vibrations die out. This test is called *Rinne's test* (Fig. 14-10). Normally, air-conducted sounds are louder to the patient than those conducted through the bone. If air conduction is lost following middle ear disease or otoscle-

rosis, for example, while bone conduction remains normal, the patient will be able to hear a faint sound through the bone even though such a sound will not be heard by air conduction. Another test of auditory function is Weber's test. If a tuning fork is sounded and the end placed against the center of the patient's forehead, the patient will hear the tuning fork better on a diseased middle ear side than on a healthy one (Fig. 14-11). If, on the other hand, a patient's deafness is due to disease of the auditory nerve itself, the tuning fork will be heard only on the healthy side.

Patients may complain of "ringing in the ears" (tinnitus). The sound may be described as buzzing, hammering, or humming. The presence or absence of the symptom should always be noted, but it is often not of great diagnostic significance. The condition of hyperacusis, a condition in which even slight sounds are heard with painful intensity, may sometimes occur in paralysis of the facial nerve. Since the nerves supplying the stapedius muscle are paralyzed, there is no "dampening down" of the sound conducted through the middle ear.

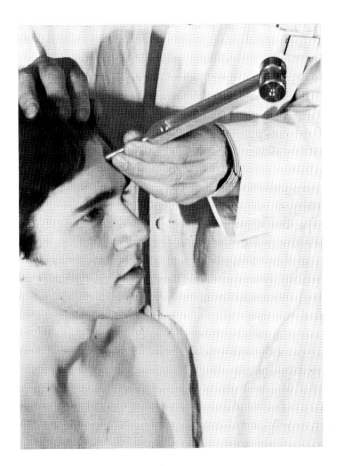

Fig. 14-11. Weber test. Sounding tuning fork is placed against center of patient's forehead. Normally, patient should hear tuning fork equally on each side.

Glossopharyngeal and vagus nerves

Nerve IX is sensory for the posterior third of the tongue and the mucous membrane of the pharynx. It also provides motor fibers for the middle constrictors of the pharynx and the stylopharyngeus muscle. It contains the taste fibers for the posterior part of the tongue. Since the ninth nerve is rarely paralyzed alone, it is usual for the ninth and tenth nerves to be tested together. Nerve X is motor for the soft palate, pharynx, and larynx. It provides sensory and motor functions for the respiratory passages, the heart, and most of the abdominal viscera. Paralysis of the vagus nerve is usually clinically obvious only through its palatine and laryngeal branches. The pharyngeal gag reflex can be tested by touching each side of the pharynx with a tongue depressor. The palatal reflex may be tested by stroking each side of the mucous membrane of the uvula. The side touched should rise. The normal function of the vagus nerve is revealed by the patient's ability to swallow and to speak clearly by symmetrical movements of the vocal cords and by symmetrical movement of the palate when the patient says "ah." Indirect laryngoscopy may reveal paralysis of one of the branches of the vagus nerve. The speech associated with paralysis of one of the vocal cords is often blurred and unintelligible.

Accessory nerve

The accessory nerve (nerve XI) is motor in function, innervating parts of the larynx and pharynx as well as the sternocleidomastoid and trapezius muscles. The integrity of the accessory nerve can easily be checked by asking the patient to shrug the shoulders against resistance (trapezius muscle action), and the sternocleidomastoid can be palpated and tested for strength when the patient moves the head against resistance.

Hypoglossal nerve

The hypoglossal nerve (nerve XII) innervates the intrinsic and extrinsic muscles of the tongue. To test the nerve, the patient should be asked to protrude the tongue as far forward as possible. The dentist should look for any lateral deviation of the tongue during this movement or for any atrophy of muscle or any tremor. The strength of the tongue may be tested by asking the patient to protrude it and move it from side to side against the resistance of a tongue depressor. Paralysis of the tongue on one side may lead to wasting of the tongue muscle on that side and will cause the tongue to protrude toward the affected side.

A 57-year-old woman was seen for a routine dental examination. It was noted that the lingual musculature on the right side of the tongue was wasted and that when the patient attempted to protrude the tongue directly forward, the tongue tip pointed to the right side (Fig. 14-12).

Fasciculation of the tongue muscle of the right side could be seen (fasciculations are spontaneous twitches of bundles of muscle fibers and may be an early sign of denervation of the muscle). No other abnormality of the cranial nerves was discovered by the dentist. The patient was referred to a neurologist for full evaluation. The diagnosis of a cerebral vascular accident involving the right hypoglossal nerve was made. The patient, apart from feeling "a change in the size of the tongue" was unaware of the onset or significance of the condition.

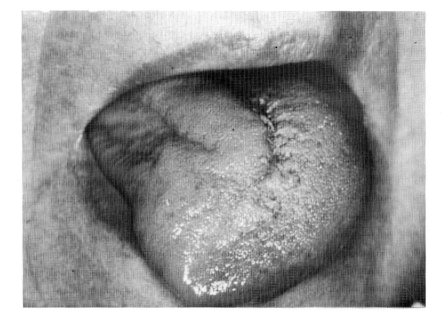

Fig. 14-12. Notice asymmetry in size of tongue. Fasciculation could be seen in right half of tongue; and when patient was asked to protrude tongue directly forward, tongue tip deviated to right.

SUMMARY

The dentist must always remember that the commonest symptom in the dental office, pain, although usually a result of dental or oral pathologic conditions, may be a signal of nondental neurologic disease. Similarly, other symptoms, such as difficulty in eating, chewing, swallowing, or speaking may arise as a result of a neurologic condition. The dentist must always be prepared to obtain a detailed history, questioning about any other possible neurologic signs or symptoms outside the head and neck area, and he or she should at least be able to conduct an examination of the 12 cranial nerves.

The following case history illustrates an example of an oral neurologic problem of a systemic disease for which the patient sought primarily his dentist's advice.

Case history

A 21-year-old man who had previously enjoyed good health sought the advice of his dentist about some numbness on the left side of his tongue. The patient described the slow onset, over the previous few weeks, of a "pins and needles" feeling on the left side of the tongue. He volunteered the information that it was similar to the feeling he had experienced after a dental injection, but stated, "I haven't been to see a dentist for ages!"

No other neurologic symptoms were reported in the head and neck area, and the functions of the cranial nerves were all examined and found to be intact. Careful questioning revealed that the man had noticed some difficulty in performing fine movements with his hands, and he reported that his legs had sometimes felt weak, a sensation that he rationalized was due to "too much exercise."

The patient was referred for a complete neurologic examination, and the diagnosis of multiple sclerosis was made.

Comment. Multiple sclerosis, or disseminated sclerosis, as its name implies, is associated with lesions that may occur in any area of the nervous system, motor or sensory. Initial symptoms are varied. Many patients first experience visual disturbances, such as blurring of vision or diplopia, whereas others may first notice irregular areas of numbness and perhaps weakness in large muscles. In this case it happened that one of the early symptoms (numbness of the tongue) caused the patient to seek dental advice. Fortunately, the dentist was able to recognize that the lingual numbness, especially in the presence of a history of muscle weakness, might indicate a more serious condition.

BIBLIOGRAPHY

Adams, R., and Victor, M.: Principles of neurology, New York, 1977, McGraw-Hill Book Co.

15   Temporomandibular joint

Disorders of the temporomandibular joint (TMJ) are frequently encountered in clinical practice. Thus, the evaluation of this area is an important part of the overall examination of the dental patient. In this context, the use of the term *temporomandibular joint* refers to much more than an isolated anatomic entity. It includes the musculature that is responsible for joint function and the neurologic mechanisms that in turn control muscle activity. The temporomandibular joint must therefore be considered as a functional system that encompasses all the anatomic, physiologic, and behavioral elements that influence it.

ANATOMY

Although a detailed description of the structure and function of the temporomandibular joint is beyond the scope of this book, a brief review of some of the most pertinent features is appropriate. It should first be recognized that the temporomandibular joint has certain unique characteristics. Its articular tissues are not composed of hyaline cartilage, as is the case in most synovial joints. In the temporomandibular joint this tissue consists of dense fibrous connective tissue with a variable number of cartilage cells that in some areas may be termed *fibrocartilage*. It has an articular disc (Fig. 15-1) that completely divides the joint into an upper and a lower compartment. The function of the joint is complex and includes a rotary or ginglymus movement that takes place in the lower compartment between the condyle and articular disc. A sliding or arthrodial movement occurs between the disc and articular eminence, that is, in the upper compartment. The normal presence of a fixed end point to jaw closure, namely the occlusion, is a unique feature and serves to influence condyle-disc position relative to the temporal bone (Fig. 15-2).

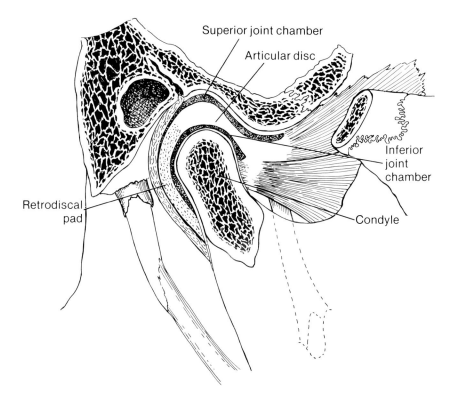

Fig. 15-1. Diagrammatic cross-section of temporomandibular joint, showing relationship of fossa, joint compartments, articular discs, muscle attachments, and condyle.

Superior joint chamber

Articular disc

Inferior joint chamber

Retrodiscal pad

Condyle

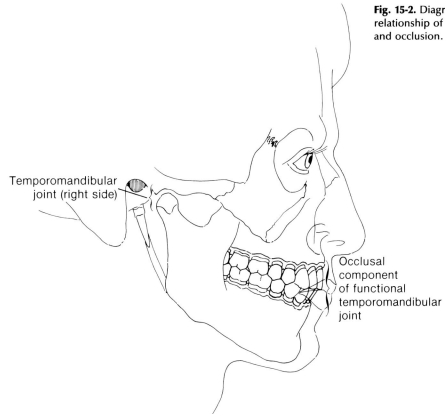

Fig. 15-2. Diagrammatic representation of relationship of temporomandibular joint and occlusion.

Temporomandibular joint (right side)

Occlusal component of functional temporomandibular joint

The muscle most responsible for condyle-disc position in relation to the articular eminence is the lateral pterygoid muscle (Fig. 15-3). It is the muscle mainly responsible for opening the mouth and for protrusion and lateral movements of the mandible. During jaw depression the digastric muscle may assist the lateral pterygoid (Fig. 15-4), particularly during rapid opening or opening against resistance. The muscles that elevate the mandible and close the mouth are much larger and more powerful than their antagonists. The masseter, temporal, and medial pterygoid muscles (Figs. 15-5 and 15-6) are powerful elevators of the mandible and can bring many pounds of force to bear on the dentition. The masseter in particular is very active during bruxism. Hyperactivity leading to hypertrophy of this muscle is frequently found in patients who chronically grind their teeth.

The activity of the muscles of mastication is influenced by that of other muscles of the head and neck. The postvertebral (scalenus group, capitus group, levator scapulae, and trapezius), sternocleidomastoid, suprahyoid (stylohyoid, digastric, mylohyoid, and geniohyoid), and infrahyoid (sternohyoid, omohyoid, sternothyroid, and thyrohyoid) muscles are among those that play a role in movement and stabilization of the head and the mandible. Thus, these muscles cannot be ignored in considering the function and dysfunction of the mandible and its joint.

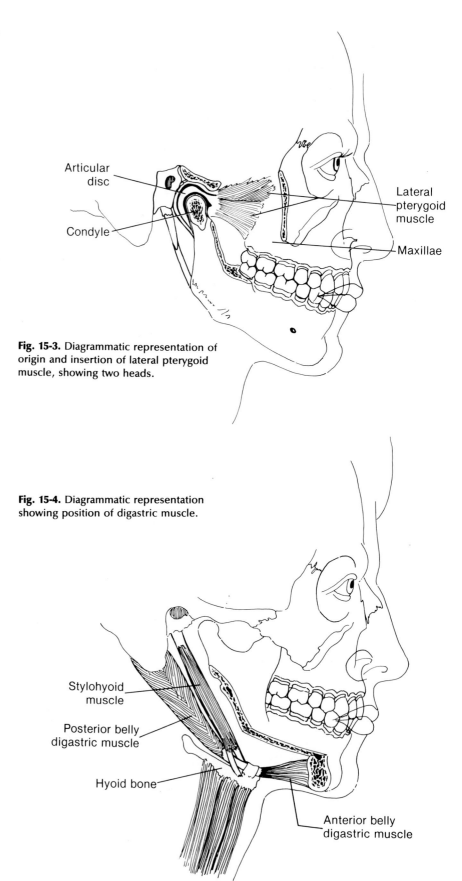

Fig. 15-3. Diagrammatic representation of origin and insertion of lateral pterygoid muscle, showing two heads.

Fig. 15-4. Diagrammatic representation showing position of digastric muscle.

The ligaments associated with the temporomandibular joint are the sphenomandibular and stylomandibular ligaments and, most important, the temporomandibular ligament (Fig. 15-7). It is the temporomandibular ligament that ultimately limits posterior movement of the condyle when the lateral pterygoid muscle is completely relaxed. Histologic, anatomic, and physiologic evidence strongly supports the conception that the condyle, with its articular disc, functions against the articular eminence and not against the depth of the mandibular fossa or against structures posterior to the condyle.

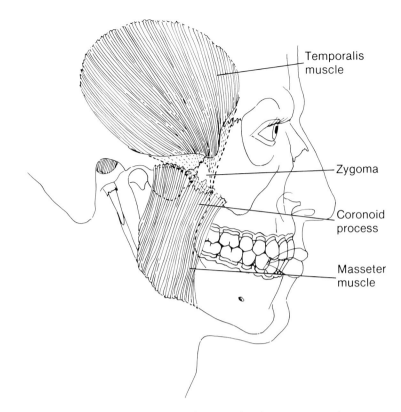

Fig. 15-5. Diagrammatic representation of temporal and masseter muscles.

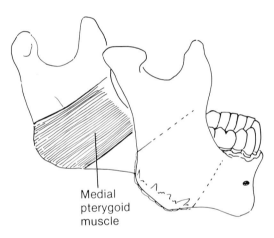

Fig. 15-6. Diagrammatic representation of position of medial pterygoid muscle.

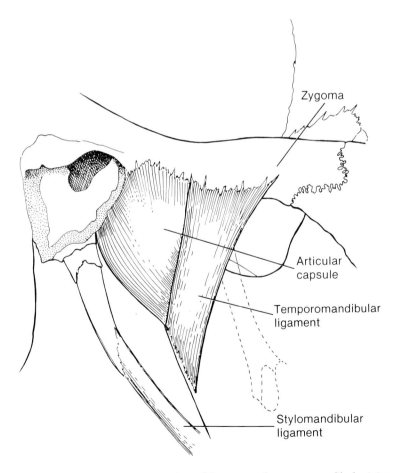

Fig. 15-7. Diagrammatic representation of ligaments of temporomandibular joint.

EXAMINATION

A complete history is important in the examination of the temporomandibular joint and associated structures. The procedures for taking a history have been described in Chapter 5. Particular emphasis is placed on the chief complaint and the patient's emotional state. The face should be observed for signs of pain and stress and for evidence of bruxism, lip biting, and other oral-facial motor behavior. Information regarding recent physical problems, medications, emotional problems, and family, social, or work-related changes in the patient's life should be explored.

The dental history also must be thorough. Information that may be related to the onset of symptoms must be included. Information of specific importance includes trauma, long dental appointments, injections of local anesthetics, oral surgical procedures, and restorative and prosthetic dentistry. Information concerning what therapeutic steps for treatment of TMJ complaints, if any, have been attempted in the past should be listed.

Questions concerning oral habits, particularly bruxism, should be asked. Negative responses to these inquiries about clenching and grinding do not mean that the patient does not have the habit. Such habits may often take place unconsciously and are frequently nocturnal.

The clinical examinations should be done in an orderly fashion and in a way that will enhance recording and, where possible, quantification of the findings. This is important because it will serve as a baseline with which therapeutic results may later be compared. It is helpful to have available a preprinted examination sheet specifically for patients with TMJ complaints. Such examination sheets usually include drawings of the face, joint, and muscles, as well as places to record interincisal openings, occlusal findings, and other appropriate data (Fig. 15-8).

Fig. 15-8. Example of extensive temporomandibular joint patient examination and questionnaire form. (From Reider, C.E.: J. Prosthet. Dent. **33:**264, 1975.)

M. TEMPOROMANDIBULAR JOINT SYMPTOMS: DATE OF ONSET_____

R L	R L	R L	R L
☐ ☐ Negative	☐ ☐ Crepitus	☐ ☐ Hypomobility	☐ ☐ Upon Awakening
☐ ☐ Acute	☐ ☐ Clicking	☐ ☐ Chronic Subluxation	☐ ☐ When Eating
☐ ☐ Episodic	☐ ☐ Popping	☐ ☐ Spontaneous Dislocation	☐ ☐ When Yawning
☐ ☐ Chronic	☐ ☐ Painful	☐ ☐ Equilibrium Distortion	☐ ☐ When Sneezing
☐ ☐ Trauma	☐ ☐ Ear Ringing	☐ ☐ Swallowing Discomfort	☐ ☐ End of Day

N. MAXIMUM OPENING (AT MIDLINE) _____ **mm.**

☐ Normal	☐ Very Restricted	☐ Acute
☐ Limited	☐ Painful	☐ Chronic

O. MANDIBULAR DEFLECTION ON OPENING:

☐ None	☐ To Right - Then Left	☐ Confluent Deflection
☐ To Right	☐ To Left - Then Right	☐ Angular Deflection
☐ To Left		

R ⊢────┼────┼────┼────┼────┼────┼────⊣ L
15 10 5 0 5 10 15 mm.

P. TEMPOROMANDIBULAR JOINT NOISE WITH MOVEMENT:

R L	R L	R L	R L
☐ ☐ Negative	☐ ☐ Crepitus	☐ ☐ Immediate	☐ ☐ Ausculative
☐ ☐ Vertical Opening	☐ ☐ Clicking	☐ ☐ Normal Range	☐ ☐ Audible
☐ ☐ Lateral Movement	☐ ☐ Popping	☐ ☐ Wide Range	☐ ☐ Very Loud

Q. TEMPOROMANDIBULAR JOINT RADIOGRAPHS:

R L	R L	R L
☐ ☐ Concentric	☐ ☐ Reduced Joint Space	☐ ☐ Flattened Condyle
☐ ☐ Condylar Protrusion	☐ ☐ Increased Joint Space	☐ ☐ Bony Lipping Condyle
☐ ☐ Condylar Retrusion	☐ ☐ Fossae Irregularities	☐ ☐ Osteoporosis

RIGHT ⌒ ⌒ LEFT

R. TEMPOROMANDIBULAR JOINT PALPATION:

R L	R L	R L	R L
☐ ☐ Negative	☐ ☐ Sore	☐ ☐ Rubbing	☐ ☐ Without Movement
☐ ☐ Laterally	☐ ☐ Painful	☐ ☐ Irregular	☐ ☐ Opening
☐ ☐ From Auditory Canal	☐ ☐ Severe Pain	☐ ☐ Popping	☐ ☐ Closing

S. MUSCULAR PALPATION:

R L	R L	R L
☐ ☐ Negative	☐ ☐ Anterior Temporal (D)	☐ ☐ Sternomastoid (H)
☐ ☐ Lateral Pterygoid (A)	☐ ☐ Deep Masseter (E)	☐ ☐ Hyoid Area (I)
☐ ☐ Medial Pterygoid (B)	☐ ☐ Superficial Masseter (F)	☐ ☐ Occipital Area (J)
☐ ☐ Posterior Temporal (C)	☐ ☐ Digastric (G)	☐ ☐ Trapezius (K)

RED: Palpation
BLUE: Symptoms

RIGHT   LEFT

T. HEADACHES AND NECKACHES:

			R L
☐ Negative	☐ Vague Location	☐ No Medication	☐ ☐ Ocular
☐ Mild	☐ Variable Location	☐ Aspirin	☐ ☐ Aural
☐ Moderate	☐ Specific Location	☐ Tranquilizers	☐ ☐ Frontal
☐ Severe	☐ Minutes	☐ Anti-Depressants	☐ ☐ Sinus
☐ Migraine	☐ Hours	☐ Muscle Relaxants	☐ ☐ Parietal
☐ Chronic	☐ All Day	☐ Narcotics	☐ ☐ Temporal
☐ Episodic	☐ Days ____	☐ Ergotamines	☐ ☐ Occipital
			☐ ☐ Neck
			☐ ☐ Shoulder Area

HEADACHES PER MONTH _____

NECKACHES PER MONTH _____

U. OCCLUSAL HABITS

☐ Negative	☐ Anterior Bracing	☐ Morning Awareness	☐ Previous
☐ Suspected	☐ Clenching	☐ Resultant Sore Mouth	☐ Episodic
☐ Patient Aware	☐ Bruxism (Gnashing)	☐ Muscle Hypertrophy	☐ Current

V. EMOTIONAL STRESS LEVEL: **CORNELL MEDICAL INDEX** _____

☐ Negative	☐ Probable	☐ Sleep Loss	☐ Anxiety
☐ Questionable	☐ Pronounced	☐ Fatigue	☐ Frustration
☐ Suspected	☐ Severe	☐ Irritability	☐ Depression

W. POSSIBLE TREATMENT SEQUENCE:

☐ ____ None	☐ ____ Occlusal Splint	☐ ____ Adrenocortical Injection
☐ ____ Preventive Counseling	☐ ____ Drug Therapy	☐ ____ Orthodontic Consultation
☐ ____ Limited Occlusal Adjustment	☐ ____ Moist Heat	☐ ____ Other TMJ Consultation
☐ ____ Occlusal Equilibration	☐ ____ Vapocoolant	☐ ____ Medical Consultation
☐ ____ Removable Prosthesis	☐ ____ Muscle Exercises	☐ ____ Neurological/Psychiatric
☐ ____ Occlusal Reconstruction	☐ ____ Local Anesthetic Injection	☐ ____ Surgical Consultation

Fig. 15-8, cont'd. For legend see opposite page.   *Continued.*

PATIENT QUESTIONNAIRE

NAME _____ SOCIAL SECURITY NO. ☐☐☐ ☐☐ ☐☐☐☐ AGE ☐☐

PLEASE CHECK ONLY ONE BOX IN EACH OF THE FOLLOWING:

13. SEX
- ☐ Male (1)
- ☐ Female (2)

14. RACE
- ☐ Caucasian (1)
- ☐ Negroid (2)
- ☐ Oriental (3)

15. MARITAL STATUS
- ☐ Single (1)
- ☐ Married (2)
- ☐ Separated (3)
- ☐ Divorced (4)
- ☐ Widowed (5)

16. EDUCATION
- ☐ Elementary (1)
- ☐ High School (2)
- ☐ Junior College (3)
- ☐ 4 Years College (4)
- ☐ Graduate School (5)

17. OCCUPATION
- ☐ Housewife (1)
- ☐ Professional (2)
- ☐ Managerial (3)
- ☐ Supervisorial (4)
- ☐ Clerical (5)
- ☐ Craftsman (6)
- ☐ Laborer (7)
- ☐ Student (8)
- ☐ Retired (9)

PLEASE ANSWER YES OR NO TO THE FOLLOWING QUESTIONS:

Yes No

18. ☐ ☐ Have you ever had orthodontic treatment?
19. ☐ ☐ Have you ever had periodontal disease (pyorrhea)?
20. ☐ ☐ Have you ever been treated for a "bad bite"?
21. ☐ ☐ Do you have extensive dental crowns and bridges?
22. ☐ ☐ Do you wear a removable partial denture?
23. ☐ ☐ Do you have missing back teeth and no replacement?
24. ☐ ☐ Have you ever been treated for problems of your jaw joint, or for facial muscle spasms?
25. ☐ ☐ Do you ever awaken with awareness of your teeth or jaws?
26. ☐ ☐ Are you aware of clenching your teeth during the day?
27. ☐ ☐ Have you ever been told that you grind your teeth during sleep?
28. ☐ ☐ Do your teeth hurt from biting?
29. ☐ ☐ Do you have any pain or soreness around your eyes, ears or other parts of your face?
30. ☐ ☐ Do you have "tension" headaches?
31. ☐ ☐ Do you ever have migraine headaches?
32. ☐ ☐ Do you frequently have neckaches or stiff neck muscles?
33. ☐ ☐ Do your jaw muscles become tired frequently?
34. ☐ ☐ Do you have difficulty in opening your mouth widely?
35. ☐ ☐ Do you have difficulty in swallowing?
36. ☐ ☐ Have you ever had arthritis?
37. ☐ ☐ Have you ever had gout?
38. ☐ ☐ Have you ever received a severe blow to the side of the head or jaw?
39. ☐ ☐ Have you ever had pain in your jaw joint?
40. ☐ ☐ Have you ever had problems with your ears, such as ringing or change of hearing?
41. ☐ ☐ Do you ever hear grating sounds from your jaw joint?
42. ☐ ☐ Do you ever hear clicking or popping sounds from your jaw joint?
43. ☐ ☐ Do you feel your bite is closed?
44. ☐ ☐ Are you presently in any pain from your jaw joint or muscles?
45. ☐ ☐ Does pain or discomfort from your jaw joint interfere with your work or other activities?
46. ☐ ☐ Are there times when you notice that this problem or pain is less or gone completely?
47. ☐ ☐ Are you afraid your problem is serious?
48. ☐ ☐ Do you feel you need treatment for this problem?
49. ☐ ☐ Do you have a problem with insomnia?
50. ☐ ☐ Do you take aspirin frequently?
51. ☐ ☐ Are you taking any tranquilizers, hypnotics, muscle relaxants or anti-depressants?
52. ☐ ☐ Do you take more than one alcoholic drink per day?
53. ☐ ☐ Do you smoke cigarettes or cigars?
54. ☐ ☐ Do you smoke a pipe?
55. ☐ ☐ Do you bite your nails, tongue or lips?
56. ☐ ☐ Do you have young children in your care?
57. ☐ ☐ Do you usually eat breakfast?

Fig. 15-8, cont'd. Patient questionnaire.

An extraoral examination always precedes the intraoral inspection. The clinician should note signs such as masseter hypertrophy, facial asymmetry, swellings, facial expressions, pain, and parafunctional habits. The patient should be asked to open as far as possible for measurement of the interincisal distance (Figs. 15-9 and 15-10). This distance is recorded, along with any evidence of lateral jaw deviation during this movement. Signs or symptoms of pain should also be noted.

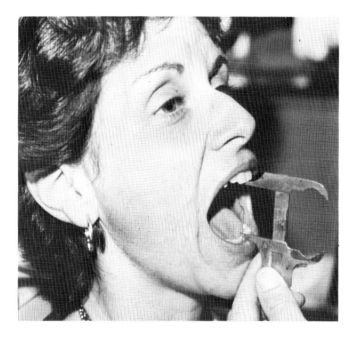

Fig. 15-9. Measurement of incisal opening with Boley gauge, showing normal opening.

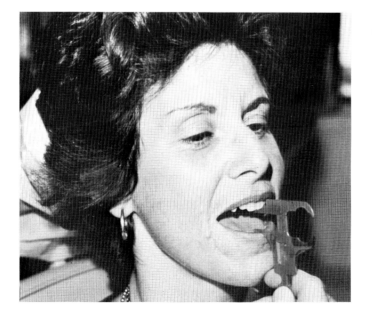

Fig. 15-10. Measurement of incisal opening with Boley gauge, showing limited motion.

The patient is asked to open and close the mouth, and the area over the lateral aspect of the temporomandibular joint is palpated in both the closed position (Figs. 15-11 and 15-12) and the open position (Fig. 15-13). Simultaneous palpation of both joint areas is the preferred method. Comparisons of condylar movement between the left and right sides are made and noted. An objective evaluation as to the presence of pain is made, and a comparison is made as to the severity between the right and left sides. Attention is given to joint sounds, vibrations, and locking or asymmetrical movements during opening and closing. The patient is then asked to move the mandible to each side with the teeth apart while bilateral palpation for condylar mobility, stimulation of pain, and crepitus or other joint vibrations is performed. A stethoscope may be used to amplify joint sounds that are palpated as vibrations. These movements of the mandible, particularly opening and closing, are repeated during bilateral intrameatal palpation (Figs. 15-14 through 15-16). This is done with the little finger in the external auditory meatus. Slight anterior pressure will yield information about condylar activity and retrocondylar pain. If placing the finger in the external ear canal produces an acutely painful reaction, otitis externa should be suspected.

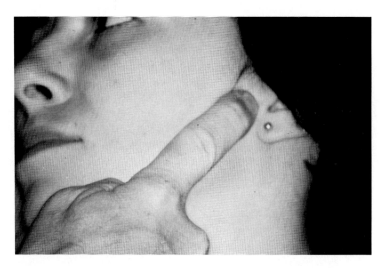

Fig. 15-11. Preauricular area for palpation of temporomandibular joint.

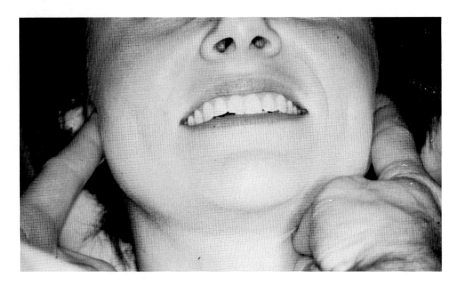

Fig. 15-12. Bilateral palpation of temporomandibular joint with patient in occlusion.

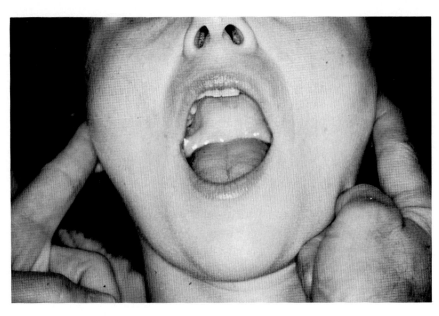

Fig. 15-13. Bilateral palpation of temporomandibular joint with patient's mouth open.

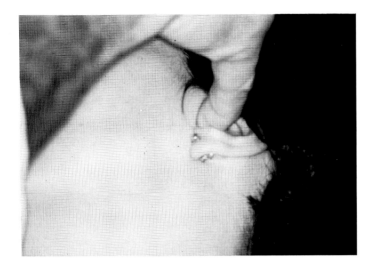

Fig. 15-14. Positioning of finger for examination of temporomandibular joint through auditory canal.

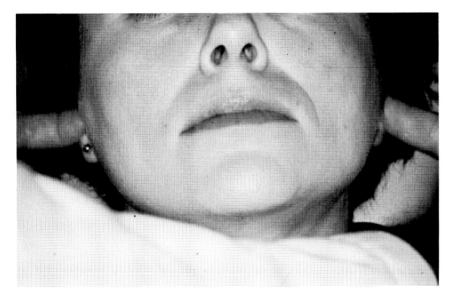

Fig. 15-15. Examination of temporomandibular joint from auditory canal bilaterally with patient in closed position.

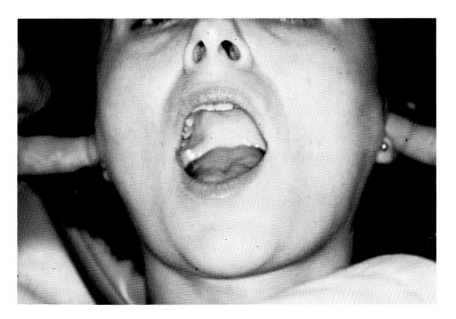

Fig. 15-16. Examination of temporomandibular joint from auditory canal with patient in open position.

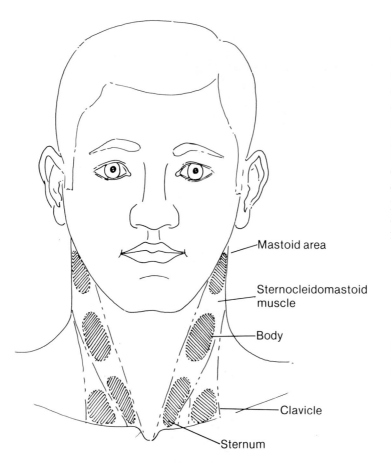

Palpation of the musculature of the head and neck is important in patients who are suspected of having TMJ disturbances. The palpation should be done in a systematic manner. A specific order of palpation is suggested (Figs. 15-17 through 15-20). Since pain and muscle tenderness are often unilateral, one side may be used as a control with which the degree of tenderness of the other side may be compared. An assessment of the location and degree of tenderness is made from information obtained by ques-

—Mastoid area

Sternocleidomastoid
muscle

—Body

Fig. 15-17. Areas to be palpated in examination of sternocleidomastoid muscle.

—Clavicle

—Sternum

Fig. 15-18. External areas to be palpated in examination of temporal, masseter, and sternocleidomastoid muscles, occipital area, and TMJ area.

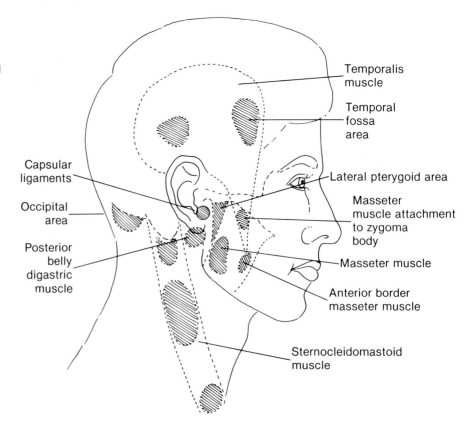

Temporalis
muscle

Temporal
fossa
area

Capsular
ligaments

Occipital
area

Posterior
belly
digastric
muscle

Lateral pterygoid area

Masseter
muscle attachment
to zygoma
body

—Masseter muscle

Anterior border
masseter muscle

Sternocleidomastoid
muscle

tioning the patient and observing the reaction to palpation. The patient's reaction is evaluated by watching the patient's eyes for movement, pupillary response (dilatation or constriction), and blinking, noting any head movement, changes in facial expression, and body movements. It is advantageous to first palpate with the jaw relaxed and again while the patient is clenching the teeth, since the latter is more likely to reveal areas of tenderness. Findings are carefully recorded on the patient's chart.

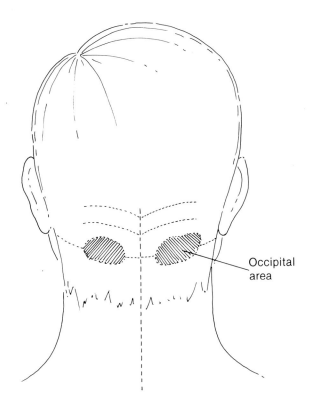

Fig. 15-19. Area to be palpated for examination of occipital area in examination of temporomandibular joint.

Occipital area

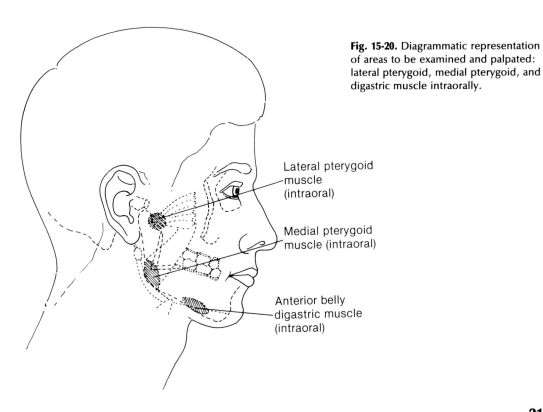

Fig. 15-20. Diagrammatic representation of areas to be examined and palpated: lateral pterygoid, medial pterygoid, and digastric muscle intraorally.

Lateral pterygoid muscle (intraoral)

Medial pterygoid muscle (intraoral)

Anterior belly digastric muscle (intraoral)

The sternocleidomastoid muscle is palpated at the points of insertion (Fig. 15-21) by pressing the muscle as it inserts on the clavicle and sternum. The body of the muscle (Fig. 15-22) is palpated by clasping the muscle between the fingers and thumb to determine if it is tender. The origin of the muscle is palpated on the mastoid process by using the fingertips (Fig. 15-23).

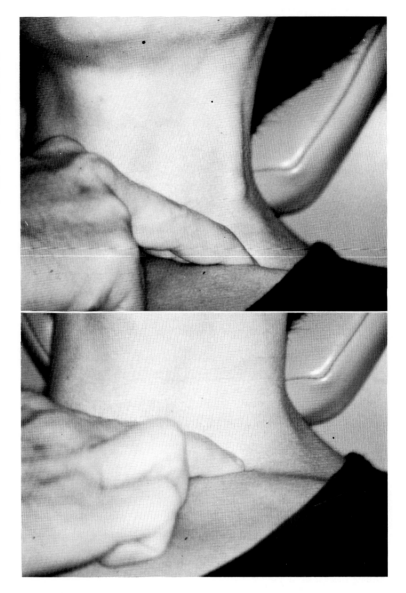

Fig. 15-21. Examination of two areas of insertion of sternocleidomastoid muscle.

Fig. 15-22. Examination of body of sternocleidomastoid muscle.

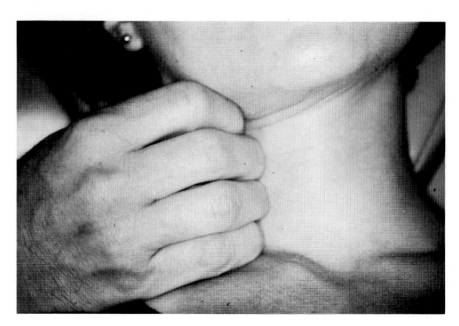

The anterior, middle, and posterior portions of the temporal muscles of both sides are palpated over the temporal fossae (Fig. 15-24). The insertion of the temporal muscle is palpated in conjunction with the lateral pterygoid.

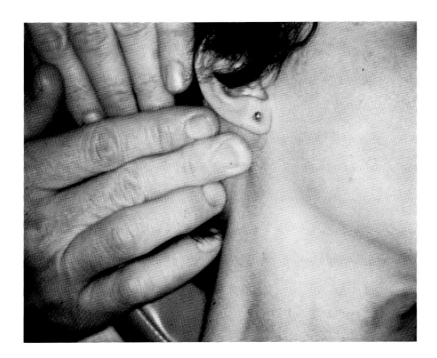

Fig. 15-23. Examination of origin of sternocleidomastoid muscle.

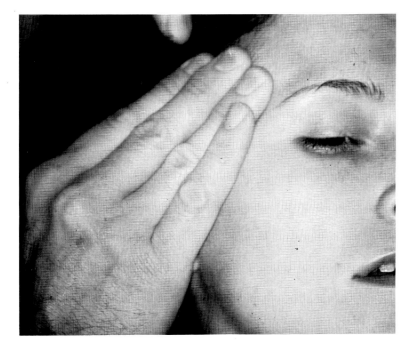

Fig. 15-24. Palpation of temporal muscle in temporal fossae.

The masseter muscle is palpated externally in the same manner. The origin, insertion, and attachment can be palpated bilaterally. The origin of the muscle is first palpated on the inferior border of the zygoma, and the body of the muscle is palpated over the ramus of the mandible (Fig. 15-25). The body of the muscle may also be examined with bidigital or bimanual palpation. Bimanual palpation is done by placing the fingers of one hand in the mouth and the fingers of the other hand on the muscle and pinching the muscle between the fingers. One side is palpated at a time (Fig. 15-26). If this operation is performed unilaterally, the same amount of pressure must be applied to each side for valid comparison of muscle tenderness. The insertion of the muscle is palpated at the inferior body of the mandible.

The medial pterygoid muscle is best palpated with the fingers of one hand under the antegonial region of the mandible while the fingers of the other hand are placed back in the floor of the mouth. The fingers of both hands are gently pressed together (Fig. 15-27). This procedure is repeated on the other side.

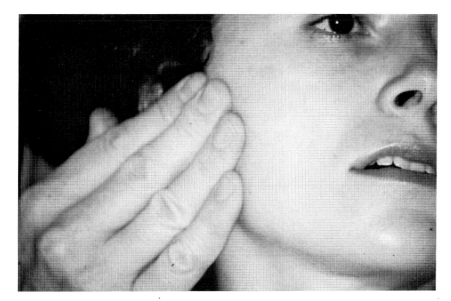

Fig. 15-25. External palpation of body and inferior border of masseter muscle.

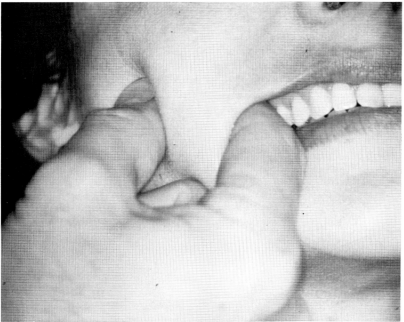

Fig. 15-26. Bidigital palpation of masseter muscle.

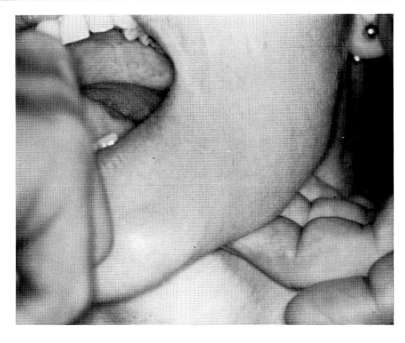

Fig. 15-27. Bimanual palpation of medial pterygoid muscle.

Both bellies of the digastric muscle are palpated. The anterior belly is palpated externally by placing pressure in the submandibular region (Fig. 15-28) or bimanually using a combined intra-extraoral approach (Fig. 15-29). The posterior belly of the digastric muscle is palpated by placing pressure in the same antegonial area as in palpation of the medial pterygoid muscle by applying pressure a little more deeply (Fig. 15-30).

The capsule and capsular ligaments are palpated by applying pressure in an inferior direction up toward the condyle (Fig. 15-31).

Fig. 15-28. External palpation of anterior belly of digastric muscle.

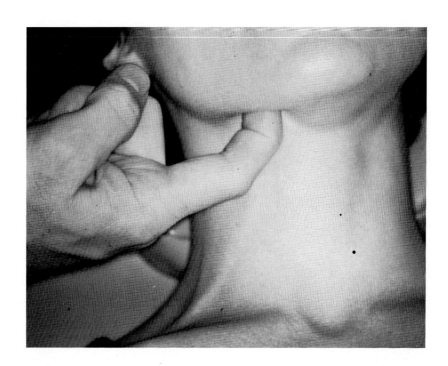

Fig. 15-29. Bimanual palpation of anterior belly of digastric muscle.

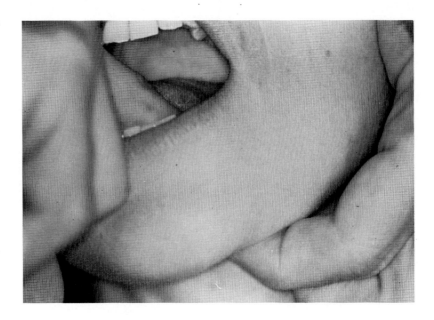

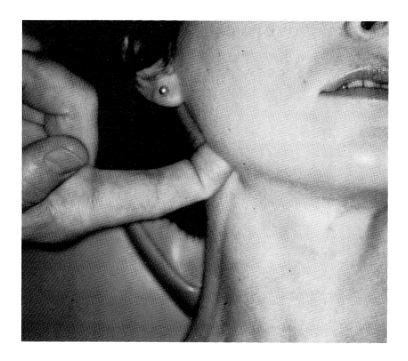

Fig. 15-30. Palpation of posterior belly of digastric muscle.

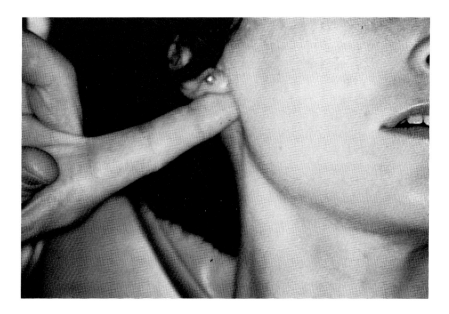

Fig. 15-31. Palpation of posterior-interior portion of joint and joint capsule.

The neck and upper back muscles are also palpated for tenderness to determine how much splinting action is being produced (Fig. 15-32). Gentle pressure is exerted with the fingers from the occipital area down the back of the neck to the shoulders.

The lateral pterygoid muscle is frequently sensitive and requires careful examination. Only the area of origin of the inferior belly of this muscle can be reached. Examination is done intraorally by placing the index finger in the upper part of the vestibule above

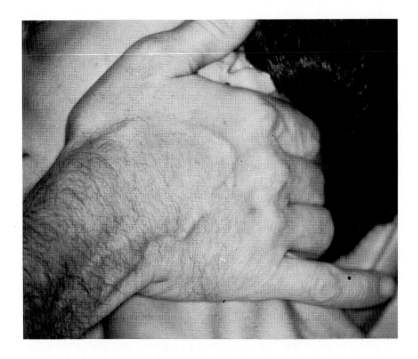

Fig. 15-32. Palpation of occipital and posterior neck region.

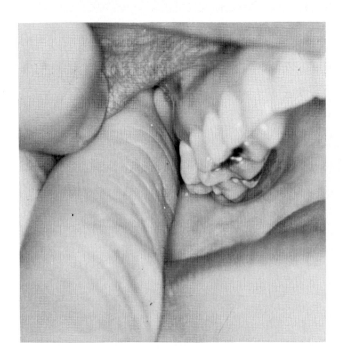

Fig. 15-33. Position of finger for palpation of lateral pterygoid muscle.

and behind the maxillary tuberosity. With the mouth only slightly open the finger is slid behind the tuberosity against the lateral pterygoid plate (Fig. 15-33). If the coronoid process prevents easy access to this area, the patient is asked to move the jaw to that side. This will move the coronoid process out of the way and permit the finger to move behind the tuberosity. Part of the tendinous attachment of the temporal muscle can also be examined at this time by palpation along the anterior border of the coronoid process (Fig. 15-34).

The hamulus and stylomandibular ligaments are palpated by slipping the first finger along the palate distal to the second molar (Fig. 15-35). This area is palpated to determine if there is an elongated hamulus or calcified stylomandibular ligament.

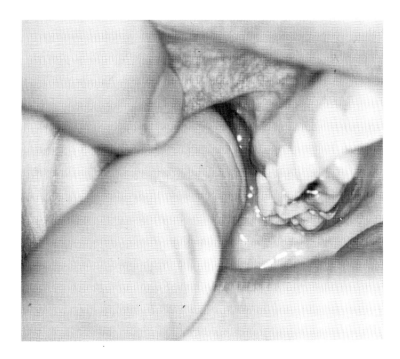

Fig. 15-34. Position of finger for palpation of insertion of temporal muscle on coronoid process.

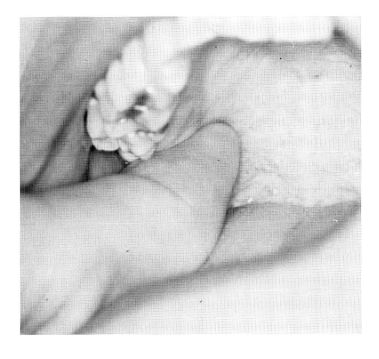

Fig. 15-35. Position of finger for palpation of hamulus and stylomandibular ligament.

The specific intraoral examination begins with an evaluation of the soft tissue. In addition to signs of overt pathologic conditions as described in Chapter 16, changes in the tissue because of function are specially looked for. Changes include evidence of lip biting, cheek biting, presence of a raised white "occlusal line" on the buccal mucosa, and scalloping on the borders of the tongue (Figs. 15-36 through 15-38). Although none of these signs may be definitive, they suggest increased oral motor behavior that may be related to the symptoms.

The dentition should be examined as described in Chapter 17 to detect pulpal disease or cracked teeth. A complete intraoral radiographic survey or panoramic radiographs with bite-wings must be included in this examination. In addition, tooth mobility and occlusal wear should be assessed, since these may strongly suggest bruxism. The radiographic signs of trauma from occlusion are also evaluated.

The periodontium also must be examined as described in Chapter 17. Particular attention is paid to detecting periodontal abscesses, food impactions, and periodontal involvement of the furcations.

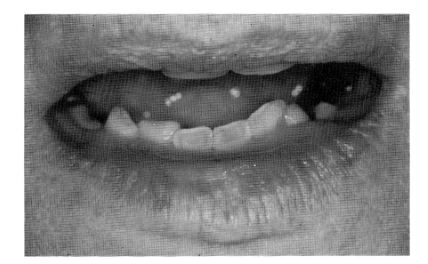

Fig. 15-36. Excessive incisal wear of teeth and lip identations produced by chewing and pressure habits.

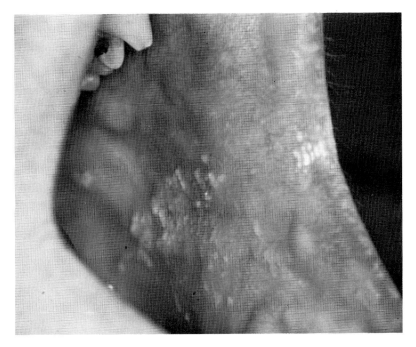

Fig. 15-37. Buccal mucosa showing roughness produced by cheek chewing.

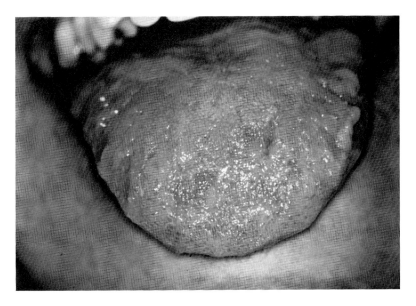

Fig. 15-38. Tongue showing scalloping produced by tongue pressure habits and chewing.

Radiographic examination

Radiographs of the temporomandibular joint are a necessary part of the examination to detect possible intracapsular problems and subcondylar fractures. The standard radiographic film used is the transcranial lateral oblique projection. Ordinarily, three exposures are made of each side: one with the mandible in rest position, one while the patient's mouth is closed in centric occlusion, and one with the mouth wide open. Both sides are compared for fossa shape and contour, condyle shape and condylar position, and mobility relative to the mandibular fossa and articular eminence (Figs. 15-39 through 15-42).

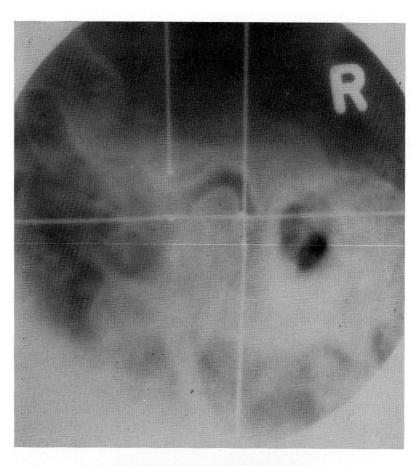

Fig. 15-39. Transcranial radiograph of right temporomandibular joint in closed position.

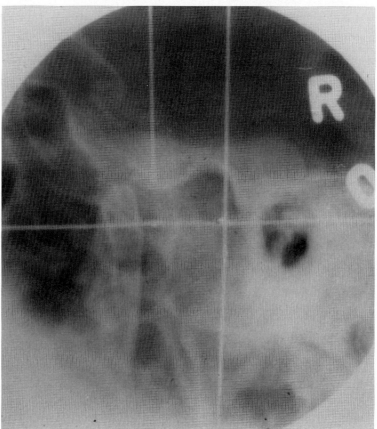

Fig. 15-40. Transcranial radiograph of right temporomandibular joint in open position.

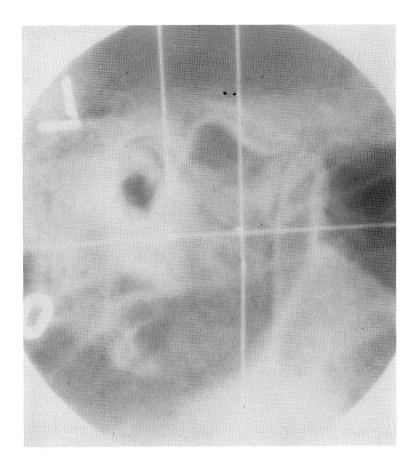

Fig. 15-41. Transcranial radiograph of left temporomandibular joint in closed position.

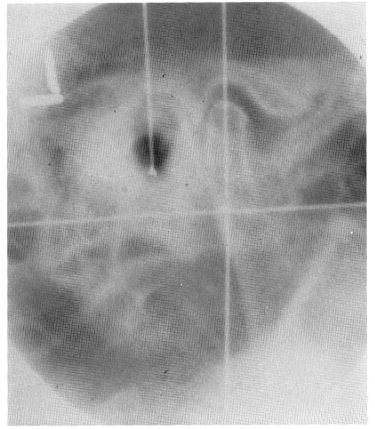

Fig. 15-42. Transcranial radiograph of left temporomandibular joint in open position.

Whether fine distinctions can be made concerning condylar shape and position is arguable, since normal variation among individuals is very great. Even standardization of a lateral oblique projection may fail to obtain an optimal image of the joint from which fine positional interpretations can be made. Since the condyle is normally twice as wide medial-laterally as it is anterior-posteriorly, an anterior-posterior full head or transorbital projection may be used to obtain a better view of condylar contour and width as well as a clearer view of the subcondylar region (Fig. 15-43).

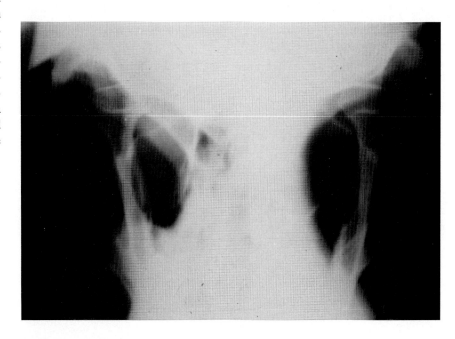

Fig. 15-43. Composite transorbital radiograph of both condyles.

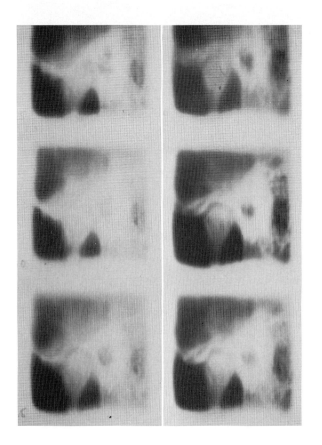

Fig. 15-44. Typical tomograms of temporomandibular joint.

224

If any of these screening radiographs leads to a suspicion of intracapsular disease, a series of tomograms should be taken. Tomography permits more accurate assessment of joint configuration, since it includes a series of radiographic "cuts" through the joint that may be collectively used to allow a three-dimensional view of the joint (Figs. 15-44 through 15-46).

It must be remembered that joint radiographs show only osseous contour and architecture. The soft articular tissues are never seen directly. Thus, degenerative joint disease, which is a breakdown of articular tissue, cannot be seen in a radiograph until later stages after osseous changes have occurred.

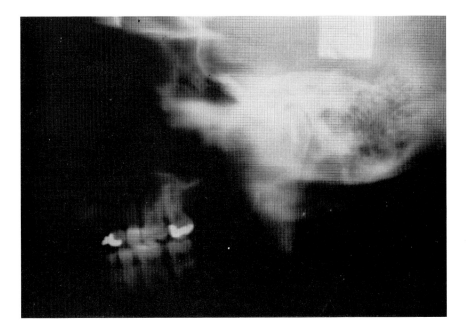

Fig. 15-45. Corrected laminography of temporomandibular joint radiograph in closed position.

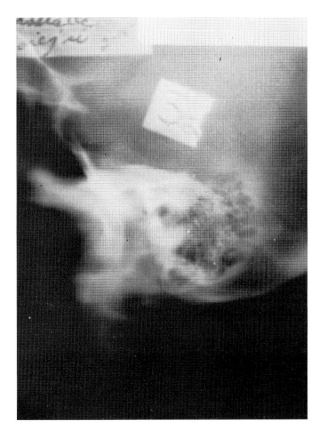

Fig. 15-46. Corrected laminography of temporomandibular joint radiograph in open position.

225

Occlusal evaluation

An examination of the occlusion is a vital part of the evaluation of any patient, particularly one with the signs or symptoms of the pain-dysfunction syndrome. The static configuration and relationships of the dentition are examined before a functional analysis of the occlusion is undertaken. This includes an assessment of arch form, tooth alignment and position, missing teeth, overbite and overjet, crossbites, and open bites, as well as occlusal relationships according to Angle's orthodontic classification system. A detailed discussion of the examination of the occlusion is given in Chapter 17.

CLASSIFICATION OF TMJ PROBLEMS

Disorders involving the temporomandibular joint may be divided into two general categories: those that involve the joint proper, that is, intracapsular problems; and those that primarily involve the neuromuscular system associated with joint movement, that is, extracapsular problems. These categories are not mutually exclusive, since intracapsular disorders may lead to hyperactivity of associated muscles, such as the so-called splinting effect by muscles in an effort to immobilize the injured joint. Likewise, chronic muscle hyperactivity or spasm may in time lead to changes within the joint itself.

Intracapsular disorders include the following:

1. Neoplasm: Usually metastatic from another primary site.
2. Developmental: Includes agenesis and hypoplasia or hyperplasia of the condyle.
3. Fracture: May be intracapsular or subcondylar.
4. Dislocation: Condyle is locked in front of the articular eminence, and the jaw cannot be closed.
5. Subluxation: Self-reducing condition in which the condyle becomes temporarily "stuck."
6. Joint sounds: Rough grating noises called crepitus or a distinct snap or click during certain movements of the condyle.
7. Arthritis: True inflammation of the joint that may be seen following trauma (traumatic arthritis), as a consequence of a generalized infection, by extension of a localized infection (infectious arthritis), or through local involvement of general rheumatoid arthritis.
8. Degenerative joint disease: Arthrosis—characterized by a breakdown of articular tissues, such as disc perforation, and leading to bizarre and uncontrolled remodeling of the osseous structures of the joint.
9. Ankylosis: Usually fibrous and may occur in the aftermath of true inflammatory arthritis, characterized by very limited jaw opening and absence of gliding movements.

Extracapsular disorders involve the musculature and associated nervous system. These are by far the most common of the problems that may affect the TMJ system. They are highly controversial because of the many contentions surrounding their causes, because of reported problems in differential diagnosis, because of lack of quantifiable data concerning pathophysiologic changes, and because a wide range of treatment modalities produce apparent remission of symptoms.

Since the work of Lazlo Schwartz,[2] the term most commonly applied to this complex of conditions has been the TMJ pain-dysfunction syndrome. More recently, the term myofascial pain-dysfunction syndrome has been used as a way of emphasizing that the problem primarily involves the musculature and its fascia and not the temporomandibular joint proper.

CARDINAL SIGNS AND SYMPTOMS OF THE PAIN-DYSFUNCTION SYNDROME

It is generally recognized that this problem involves four cardinal signs and symptoms:

1. *Pain:* Most patients who seek help do so because of pain. The pain is usually unilateral, is perceived as a dull deep ache, and is often preauricular, although reports of otalgia and other pains are quite common.

2. *Limitation of jaw movement* (trismus): Most adults should be able to open to a minimal interincisal distance of 35 mm. Patients with trismus may have various degrees of decreased opening that, with acute involvement, may permit interincisal opening of only 10 to 20 mm or less. Because of the commonly seen unilateral nature of the problem, many patients will also show a deviation of the mandible toward the affected side during opening.

3. *Joint sounds:* Epidemiologic studies have shown that clicking in the joint is very common. When it occurs without pain, the patient usually will not seek help. Crepitus or grating noises are less commonly encountered but are more bothersome and may indicate degenerative joint disease.

4. *Tenderness in one or more of the muscles of mastication:* This sign is found during palpation and may also be present in muscles other than the masticatory muscles.

Patients often complain of other symptoms along with the cardinal ones. Ear symptoms have frequently been reported, particularly otalgia. Hearing loss is sometimes mentioned, as well as dizziness and tinnitus. Such complaints often lead patients to first seek the help of an otolaryngologist for their problem. It has been shown that reported hearing loss is entirely subjective and cannot be substantiated by audiometric tests. Patients with otalgia or other ear symptoms should have their ears examined to rule out otitis externa, otitis media, or otitis interna.

Other symptoms that deserve mention include the patient's inability to bring the teeth into full comfortable occlusion, headaches, sore teeth, neck pain, and difficulty in mastication.

Data from TMJ clinics have repeatedly shown that females are four times more likely to complain of these problems than males are. However, recent epidemiologic studies in Scandinavia strongly suggest that males have symptoms as often as do females but apparently do not seek help as often and therefore do not show up in clinical data reports.

ETIOLOGY OF THE PAIN-DYSFUNCTION SYNDROME

Numerous theories and explanations have been advanced over the years to explain the causes of this problem. Each has its strong proponents. Current ideas related to etiologic factors include such things as occlusal prematurities, parafunctional activity such as bruxism, psychologic states including anxiety and depression, personality characteristics, learned behavioral patterns, unilateral jaw function, trauma, or physical stress. In a recent epidemiologic study, Helkimo[1] failed to find any predominant etiologic factor in a population sample. However, this does not mean that one factor cannot predominate in a specific patient.

In the light of our present knowledge, it seems appropriate to assume that the disorder comes about as a result of the interplay of several factors, which leads to a failure of adaptation on the part of the patient. Thus, the examination of the patient and subsequent treatment of the problem should encompass the possibility of several etiologic factors. The clinician who directs all his or her attention to a single preconceived etiologic factor will certainly achieve some success but will reduce the rate of success over time.

Despite the wide divergence of opinion concerning etiologic factors, there is one area that most clinicians and investigators generally agree on: the neuromuscular system involved in mandibular function becomes the chief target organ in the pain-dysfunction syndrome, no matter what the cause or causes. Thus, examination, diagnosis, and treatment should include strong consideration of this system during the mangement of patients with the pain-dysfunction syndrome.

TREATMENT

Specific therapy for the pain-dysfunction syndrome or for other disorders involving the temporomandibular joint is beyond the scope of this book. However, several general principles may be enumerated, particularly in regard to the pain-dysfunction syndrome:

1. Treatment should be directed toward relaxation of the musculature.
2. Treatment should include several modalities considering the probable multifactorial etiologic nature.
3. Treatment should include only reversible modalities until signs and symptoms have been relieved.
4. The decision to perform definitive nonreversible occlusal therapy should be delayed until after relief of the signs and symptoms.
5. Surgery involving the temporomandibular joint should not be done unless a specific intracapsular organic problem can be identified.

REFERENCES

1. Helkimo, M.: Epidemiological surveys of dysfunction of the masticatory system, Oral Sci. Rev. 1:54, 1976.
2. Schwartz, L.: Disorders of the temporo-mandibular joint, Philadelphia, 1959, W.B. Saunders Co.

BIBLIOGRAPHY

Blair, G.S., and others: Circular tomography of the temporomandibular joint, Oral. Surg. 35:416, 1973.

Butler, J.H., Folke, L.E., and Bandt, C.L.: A descriptive survey of signs and symptoms associated with the myofascial pain-dysfunction syndrome, J. Am. Dent. Assoc. 90:635, 1975.

Coin, C.G.: Tomography of the temporomandibular joint, Dent. Radiogr. Photogr. 47:23, 1974.

Coin, C.G.: Tomography of the temporomandibular joint, Medical Radiogr. Photogr. 50:26, 1974.

Ermshar, C.B.: Anatomy and neuroanatomy. In Morgan, D.H., Hall, W.P., and Vamvas, S.J.: Diseases of the temporomandibular apparatus: a multidisciplinary approach, St. Louis, 1977, The C.V. Mosby Co.

Gelb, H.: Clinical management of head, neck and TMJ pain and dysfunction: a multi-disciplinary approach to diagnosis and treatment, Philadelphia, 1977, W.B. Saunders Co.

Greene, C.S., and others: The TMJ pain-dysfunction syndrome: heterogeneity of the patient population, J. Am. Dent. Assoc. 79:1168, 1969.

Isaac, H.K., and Bean, L.R.: Simple techniques for radiographing the condyle, J. AM. Dent. Assoc. 81:691, 1970.

Morgan, D.H., Hall, W.P., and Vamvas, S.J.: Diseases of the temporomandibular apparatus: a multidisciplinary approach, St. Louis, 1977, The C.V. Mosby Co.

Reider, C.E.: Development of a simplified system for clinical evaluation of occlusal interrelationships. I. Acquisition of information, J. Prosthet. Dent. 33:264, 1975.

Reider, C.E.: The interrelationship of various temporomandibular joint examination data in an initial survey population, J. Prosthet. Dent. 35:299, 1976.

Rosenberg, H.M.: Laminagraphy: methods and application in oral diagnosis, J. Am. Dent. Assoc. 74:88, 1967.

Scott, A.J. III: TMJ dysfunction: principles of clinical examination implants, J. Prosthet. Dent. 37:550, 1977.

Shields, J.M., Clayton, J.A., and Sindledecker, L.D.: Using pantographic tracings to detect TMJ and muscle dysfunctions, J. Prosthet. Dent. 39:80, 1978.

Thomson, H.: Mandibular joint pain symptoms, signs and diagnosis, Rev. Belge Med. Dent. 21:79, 1966.

Yale, S.H.: Radiographic evaluation of the temporomandibular joint, J. Am. Dent. Assoc. 79:102, 1969.

16   Oral cavity

The oral cavity shares many features in common with other mucosally bounded cavities, but because of the dentition and its supportive tissues the oral cavity is a unique part of the body in both structure and function.

The oral cavity can be considered to have two broad categories of tissue that can manifest disease: (1) the soft tissues that are analogous to other mucosal cavities with the surfacing epithelium and underlying connective tissue, musculature, and glands; and (2) the osseous tissues that are similar to other bones but unique in containing the odontogenic apparatus.

It is only natural for the oral cavity to reflect systemic diseases as well as unique problems associated with the dentition and periodontium. The accessibility of the oral cavity therefore lends itself as a unique showcase of health and disease. The dentist, being the oral cavity specialist, is therefore in a unique position to detect early changes in the oral tissues that may indicate systemic or oral diseases.

To evaluate the oral cavity, the examiner must have a thorough knowledge of the anatomy and physiology of the oral tissues. Knowledge of histology adds a great dimension to understanding and correlating structural and functional changes that may represent normal variations or disease. Anatomically, the oral cavity contains all the basic tissue elements found anywhere in the body.

The oral cavity, for the purposes of this book, is divided into the following sites:

Lips
Labial mucosa
Buccal mucosa and vestibular sulcus
Gingiva and alveolar mucosa
Palate
Fauces and pharynx
Tongue
Floor of mouth

The oral cavity (Fig. 16-1) is the oval-shaped space bounded anteriorly by the lips, laterally by the cheeks, superiorly by the palate, and inferiorly by the floor of the mouth. It communicates externally through the opening between the lips and internally with the pharynx through the fauces or tonsillar pillars.

The oral cavity is subdivided by the alveolar processes and the teeth into the oral cavity proper and the oral vestibule. The oral cavity proper is the space enclosed within the alveolar processes and the teeth. The oral vestibule is divided into a posterior and an anterior section (Fig. 16-2). The anterior vestibule exists only with the lips closed (Fig. 16-3).

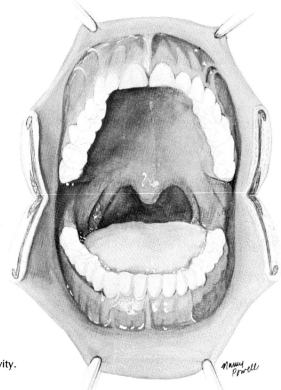

Fig. 16-1. Content and boundaries of oral cavity.

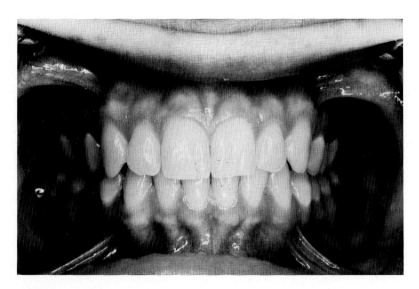

Fig. 16-2. Normal posterior vestibule of oral cavity.

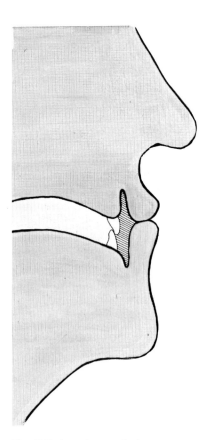

Fig. 16-3. Anterior vestibule.

LIPS
Anatomy

The lips are two highly sensitive, mobile folds composed of skin, muscle, glands, and mucous membrane. They surround the oral orifice and form the anterior boundary of the oral cavity (Fig. 16-4). The upper lip begins under the nose and extends laterally toward the cheek to the nasolabial sulcus. This depression begins just lateral to the nose and passes downward, lateral to the corner of the mouth, or commissure. The lower lip is bounded inferiorly by the prominent groove, the labiomental sulcus, which tends to deepen with age. Laterally the lower lip may have no distinct border, simply merging with the skin of the cheek.

Fig. 16-4. Tissues of lips.

With increasing age a furrow, the labiomarginal sulcus, usually develops at or close to the commissure and passes in a convex arch toward the lower border of the mandible (Fig. 16-5).

The upper and lower lips are joined at the corners of the mouth, the commissures, by a thin connecting fold well visible when the mouth is opened.

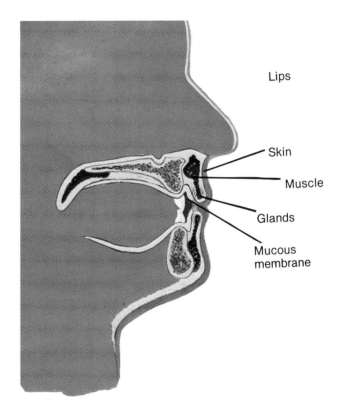

Fig. 16-5. *a,* Nasolabial sulcus; *b,* labiomental sulcus; *c,* labiomarginal sulcus.

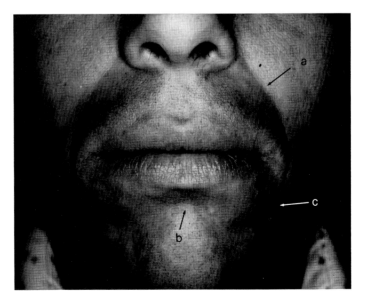

The skin of the lips ends in a sharp, sometimes elevated line. The transitional zone between the skin and mucous membrane is known as the red or vermilion zone. The vermilion zones end at an imaginary wet line where the lips touch the labial surfaces of the anterior teeth when the lips are closed lightly (Fig. 16-6).

The texture of the lips is normally smooth, soft, and resilient, with minimal fissuring in the young individual. With advancing age and environmental influences, fissuring, roughness, and thickness increase (Fig. 16-7).

The color of the vermilion zone of the lips is a unique human characteristic. The surface epithelium is non-keratinized, thin, and hence more translucent. The proximity to the surface of the connective tissue papillae, plus the prominent, dilated, and thin capillaries in them, accounts for the color. In whites the lips vary from pink to red, whereas in blacks the melanin pigment may cause a purple to brown color range.

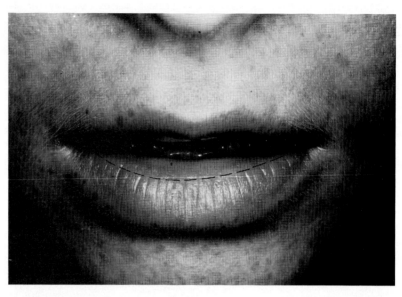

Fig. 16-6. Wet line of lower lip, which separates vermilion border from labial mucosa.

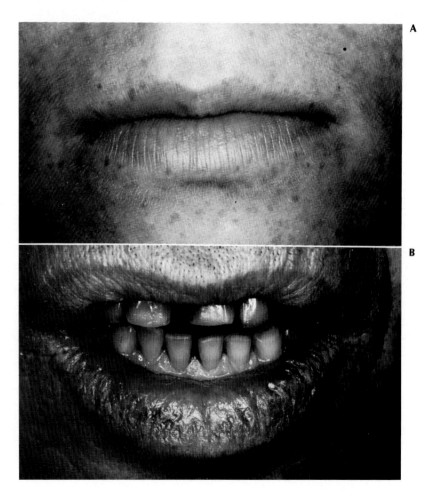

A

B

Fig. 16-7. A, Normal smooth texture of lips of young adult. **B,** Roughened texture in older patient or one exposed to elements.

232

Examination

To perform an adequate examination of any of the oral soft tissues, a good light source, mouth mirrors, and gauze sponges are essential. The mouth mirror serves as a retractor and allows the reflection of light to less accessible areas of the mouth. The gauze sponges may aid in the retraction of moist surfaces and the drying of excessively moist surfaces. In many instances it is advisable to lightly wipe the soft tissue with a gauze sponge to remove any materia alba (soft, white deposits consisting of epithelial cells, leukocytes, and bacteria) or food particles, which may simulate disease changes.

The lips should be carefully inspected for evaluation of any functional or structural changes. Observable functional changes are evidenced by abnormal motor function or glandular activity. Structural changes may appear as abnormal changes in form, texture, or color.

Bidigital palpation of the lips (Fig. 16-8) is essential and requires only a few moments to accomplish. Palpation can assist in the detection of textural change, consistency of the tissues, submucosal nodules or masses, and tenderness.

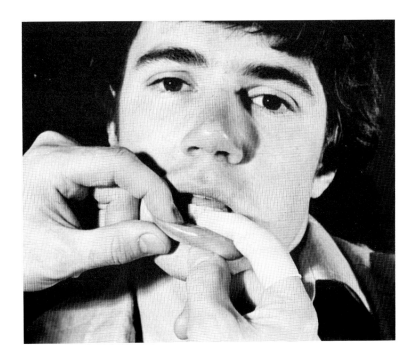

Fig. 16-8. Bidigital palpation of lips.

Abnormalities

The more common functional abnormalities of the lip are usually related to seventh cranial nerve disturbances, which were discussed in Chapter 14. The major developmental abnormality of the upper lip is clefting. This was discussed in Chapter 8. Small developmental pits may be found involving the lower vermilion zone (lip pits) (Fig. 16-9) and the corners of the mouth (commissural pits, Fig. 16-10). The small (1 to 2 mm) depressed lesions may be blind-end defects, or they may have minor accessory glands associated with them, in which case they will secrete a variable mucous flow. These pits are usually normal pink in color.

One of the more common changes noted on the lips is an alteration in texture. This change may indicate a spectrum ranging from chapped lips to an early stage of cancer. An excessive dryness of the lips may cause a fissuring and crusting surface change. This in turn usually results in an abnormal white color change. However, if the condition persists for an extended period, the fissuring may be accompanied by a serous exudate that results in a yellow to brown crusting. This was discussed in Chapter 6.

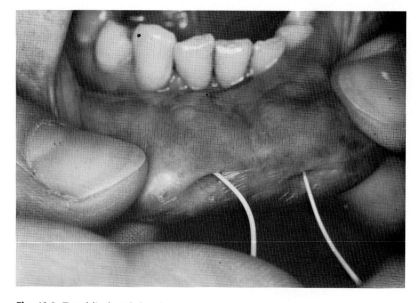

Fig. 16-9. Two blind-end developmental lip pits.

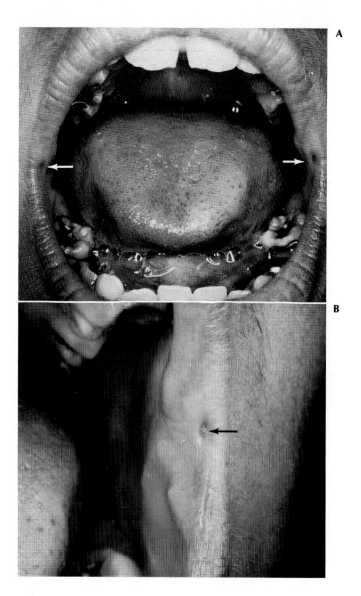

Fig. 16-10. A, Bilateral commissural pits. **B,** Close-up view of typical commissure pit.

Chapping and drying of the lips may result from weather changes or exposure to a cold, windy environment. It can also be associated with habits of sucking, biting, or excessive licking of the lips. Mouth breathing may cause a similar change, usually to a milder degree.

Prolonged exposure to the elements either from occupations such as farming and sailing or from living in a warm climate may induce lip changes referred to as actinic cheilitis (Fig. 16-11) and actinic keratosis (Fig. 16-12).

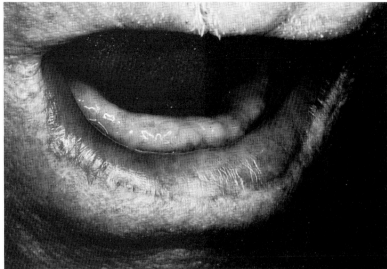

Fig. 16-11. Early textural and color change in sun-damaged lip. Diagnosis: Actinic cheilitis.

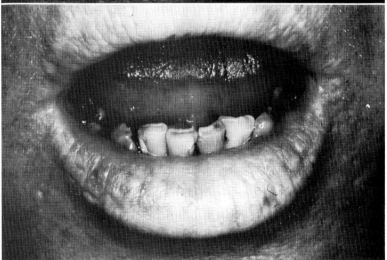

Fig. 16-12. More severely damaged lip resulting in hyperkeratosis. Diagnosis: Actinic keratosis.

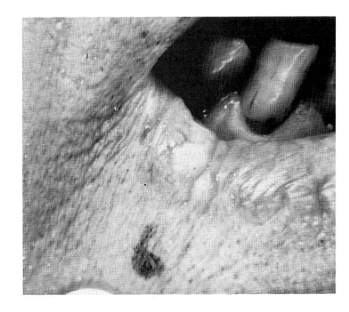

With actinic cheilitis there is marked individual variation in susceptibility to ultraviolet rays, either as natural sunlight or as artificial irradiation. In general, individuals with fair skin and light hair, particularly those with blue eyes, react quickest and exhibit the most pronounced effects. Repeated overexposure for months and years, particularly in those susceptible individuals, may finally result in permanent damage. Chronic actinic cheilitis is common on the lower lip, especially in seamen and in agricultural workers. It first develops after many years of exposure as dryness and fine scaling. The epithelium initially becomes thinned. Later the epithelium becomes visibly and palpably thickened with small grayish white plaques. Vertical fissuring and crusting may occur. The underlying dermis changes also, undergoing a basophilic degeneration and solar elastosis. Actinic cheilitis may develop into actinic keratosis.

Actinic keratosis (leukokeratosis of the lips) is a dermatosis commonly limited to sun-exposed areas, occurring after middle age and appearing as plaque-like areas of adherent hyperkeratosis. It is the result of changes in the epidermal cells, which may later progress to squamous cell carcinoma. The first evidence of actinic keratosis is usually a dry, rough, adherent, dirty brown-colored scale. This can be picked off only with difficulty, and a hyperemic base with bleeding points is revealed. At times the scale will spontaneously disappear, only to reoccur at a later date. The vermilion border of the lower lip is most frequently involved, usually the lateral portions. The upper lip is seldom involved, probably because its anatomic position protects it from the sun. Actinic keratoses are potentially malignant. The transition to malignancy may be subtle and is suggested by the induration at the base of the keratosis. Only about 25% of keratoses become malignant, and the latent period is at least 10 years.

Occasionally, nonspecific hyperkeratosis may be found on the lips, appearing as white, slightly elevated plaques. These should be managed in the same manner as hyperkeratosis or leukoplakia occurring in any oral site. A histologic examination is essential to evaluate the cellular changes occurring in such lesions.

Angular cheilitis (Fig. 16-13) is another common condition involving the corners or commissures of the mouth. This also appears as a fissuring change that is usually inflamed, thereby causing a red color. In longstanding chronic angular cheilitis, secondary infection by *Candida albicans* is frequently a factor and can result in a red and white lesion. Other etiologic factors that must be considered for angular cheilitis are a closed vertical dimension, which creates a natural fissure, providing an ideal environment for ulceration and chronic inflammation. Habits similar to those causing chapped lips, iron deficiency anemia, and avitaminosis (B complex) are other factors that may play a role in angular cheilitis.

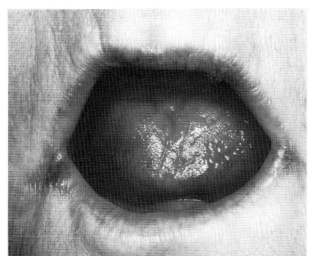

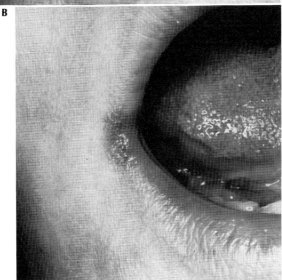

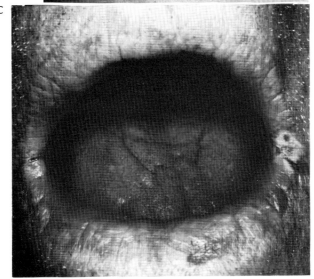

Fig. 16-13. A, Bilateral involvement of commissures in denture-wearing patient. Diagnosis: Angular cheilitis. **B,** Similar condition in patient with natural dentition. Cytologic findings of lesion were positive for *Candida albicans.* **C,** Bilateral angular cheilitis with white changes. Chronic problem that was also positive for *Candida albicans.* Note other changes on lower lip.

Color changes alone, without textural change, of the vermilion zones of the lips can indicate systemic disease. This site is unique for more obvious color changes because of the thin epithelial surface combined with the rich underlying capillary beds. Diseases that affect the numbers of red blood cells or the relative quantities of reduced hemoglobin and oxyhemoglobin in the red cells can alter the color. The change may be an increased whiteness (pallor), an increased redness, or a bluish color (cyanosis). For example, anemias may cause an abnormal pallor, polycythemia may cause increased redness, and cardiac failure and emphysema may induce varying degrees of cyanosis.

Several significant abnormalities that may be manifested on the lips appear as focal areas of color change or pigmentation. Peutz-Jeghers syndrome (hereditary intestinal polyposis) may cause multiple small (1 to 5 mm) brown to black macules on the vermilion zones and skin of the lips (Fig. 16-14). These macules result from melanin depositions and may be present from birth. Nevi may appear as solitary brown to black macules on the lips.

Patients with hereditary hemorrhagic telangiectasia may have multiple red, macular-papular lesions involving the lips (Fig. 16-15). These may be slightly elevated lesions, since they represent multiple telangiectatic or dilated capillaries.

Fordyce's granules, which are ectopic sebaceous glands, may be found in various oral sites in varying degrees of concentration (Fig. 16-16, A). When they involve the lips in great numbers, they can appear as multiple small papules having a slightly yellow color. The upper lip is more commonly involved. A dense concentration of these glands can cause a plaque formation (Fig. 16-16, B).

Fig. 16-14. Multiple melanotic macules. Diagnosis: Peutz-Jeghers syndrome.

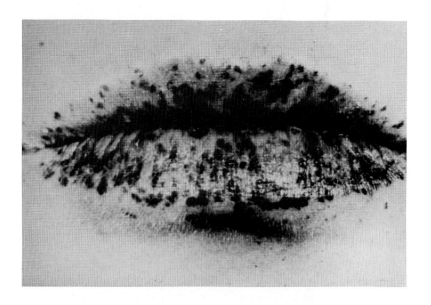

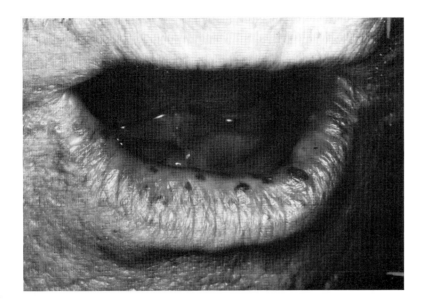

Fig. 16-15. Multiple red, maculopapular lesions involving vermilion border and labial mucosa of patient with hereditary hemorrhagic telangiectasia.

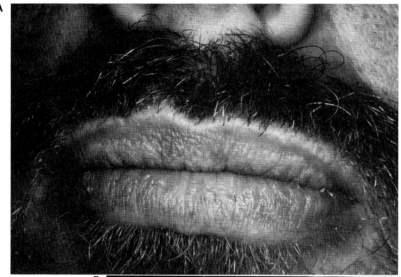

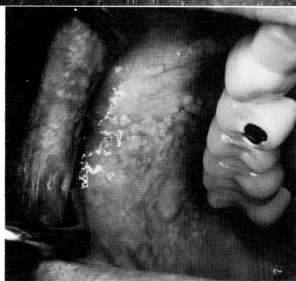

Fig. 16-16. A, Plaquelike lesions of upper vermilion border. Diagnosis: Fordyce's granules. **B,** Multiple yellow papules on buccal mucosa. Diagnosis: Fordyce's granules.

Most other diseases or disorders of the lips cause more obvious structural alterations and can be included in the basic morphologic categories of elevated or depressed lesions.

Angioedema often affects the lips and may occur in the dental office (Fig. 16-17). This usually allergic type of reaction causes a generalized edematous swelling of one or both lips. The swelling is usually very rapid in onset and may appear as normal tissue color or may have varying degrees of redness. The upper lip is more commonly involved, and other sites, such as the eyelids, may be affected.

Other generalized enlargement of the lips would most likely indicate a neoplasm. Hemangiomas, though not necessarily considered true neoplasms, may be large elevated tumescences that vary considerably in size and extent of tissue involvement. These usually show a blue color change because of their blood-filled spaces, and they may blanch on diascopic examination (Fig. 16-18).

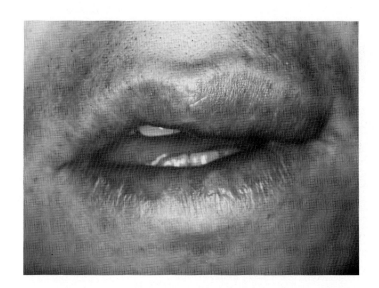

Fig. 16-17. Sudden spontaneous onset of generalized swelling of upper lip. Diagnosis: Angioedema.

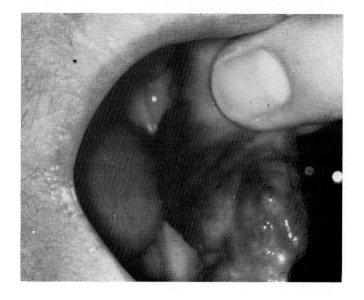

Fig. 16-18. Blue, blood-filled tumescence involving the lip and buccal mucosa, present since birth. Diagnosis: Hemangioma.

Herpes simplex commonly involves the lips in both the primary and recurrent infections. The initial or primary lesions for both primary and recurrent herpes infection are vesicles that arise in clusters. In the oral region most vesicles rupture soon after development, which results in ulcer formation. The primary infection is usually diffuse, involving multiple sites with extensive ulcerations. The recurrent infection is unique in that fewer vesicles are present, and they are either limited to the lips, where they involve the junction of the skin and the vermilion zone as recurrent herpes labialis, or also involve the hard palate or gingiva as recurrent intraoral herpes simplex (Figs. 16-19 and 16-20).

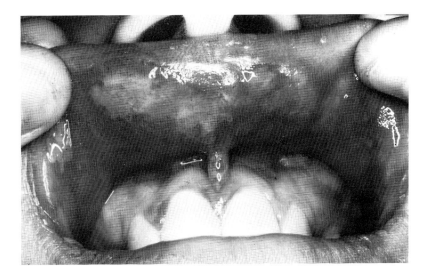

Fig. 16-19. Diffuse ulceration of upper labial mucosa. Note gingival involvement. Diagnosis: Primary herpes simplex.

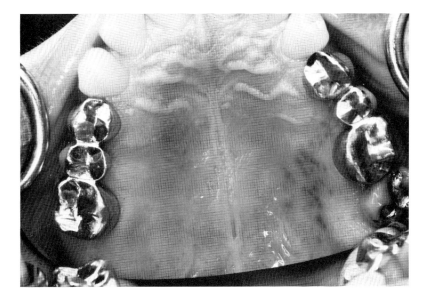

Fig. 16-20. Cluster of coalescing, punctate ulcers typical of recurrent herpes simplex.

Erythema multiforme, also discussed in Chapter 10, is another vesiculoerosive disease that quite characteristically involves the lips in a high percentage of cases. The lip lesions have a rapid onset and arise as vesicles or bullae that ruputre very rapidly, leaving diffuse ulcerations whose exudate on the lips tends to dry and form crusts, which may cause adherence of the upper and lower lips during sleep (Fig. 16-21).

A significant number of patients with oral lesions of lupus erythematosus will have lesions involving the skin or vermilion zones of the lips. These changes may be very subtle and appear as scaly, erythematous plaques or as superficial ulcerations (Fig. 16-22).

Fig. 16-21. Crusting ulcerative lesions of lips characteristic of erythema multiforme.

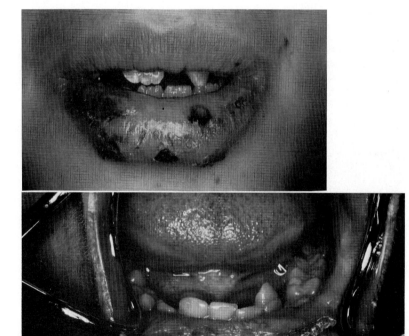

Fig. 16-22. Scaly, erosive lesions of lip in patient with chronic discoid lupus erythematosus. Note similar lesion on skin beneath lip.

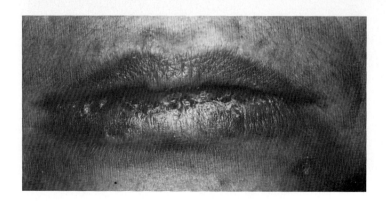

A common dermatologic disease with oral mucosa involvement is lichen planus (see Chapter 10). The disease may be manifested on the lips in two forms. Bullous lichen planus (Fig. 16-23) may appear as vesicles or bullae on the lips or labial mucosa. The most characteristic mucosal lesions of lichen planus are multiple co-alescing papules that form various patterns, such as linear, reticular, or annular, and are referred to as Wickham's striae (Fig. 16-24).*

_____

*Wickham's original description referred to striae on the papules and plaques of skin lesions. ·

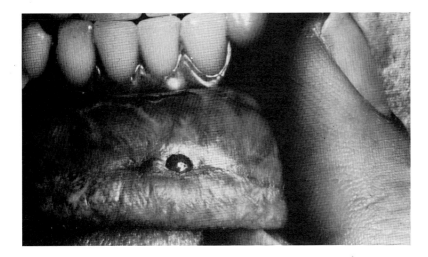

Fig. 16-23. Bulla and striae. Diagnosis: Bullous lichen planus.

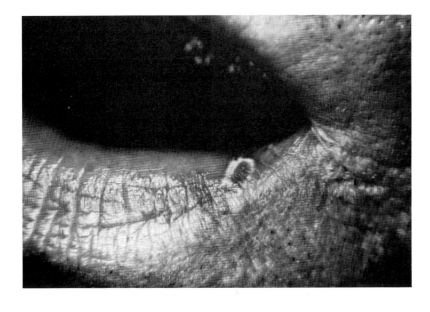

Fig. 16-24. Red and white annular lesion of lichen planus on lower lip.

Fig. 16-25. Chronic ulcer of lower lip. Diagnosis: Well-differentiated squamous carcinoma.

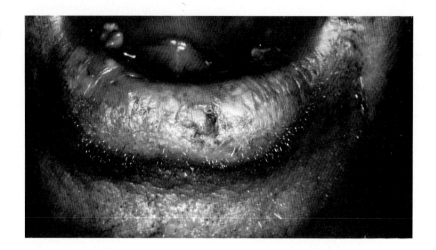

Fig. 16-26. Large chronic ulcer with rolled, indurated margins. Diagnosis: Well-differentiated squamous carcinoma.

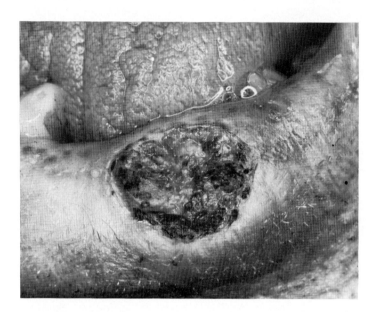

Fig. 16-27. Chancre. Diagnosis: Primary syphilis.

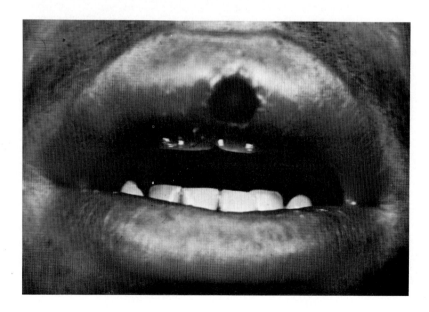

There are several diseases that cause discrete ulcers of the lips of varying size. The occurence of epidermoid carcinoma in conjunction with actinic and nonspecific keratoses was discussed in Chapter 10. A characteristic appearance of lip cancer is a chronic nonhealing, indurated ulcer that may vary in size from 2 or 3 mm to several centimeters (Figs. 16-25 and 16-26).

The chancre of primary syphilis may appear as a lesion identical to carcinoma (Fig. 16-27). The primary difference between carcinoma and a syphilitic chancre is that the latter usually heals spontaneously after a few weeks.

LABIAL MUCOSA
Anatomy

Retraction of the lips away from the teeth and gingiva exposes the labial mucosa. The labial mucosae are the rectangular areas between imaginary lines drawn from the commissures to the distal surfaces of the maxillary and mandibular cuspids, extending from the vermilion border into the vestibule (Fig. 16-28). In the midline of the upper and lower vestibule, a fold of mucosa extends from the mucosal surface to the alveolar mucosa. These are the labial frenula (Fig. 16-28).

The texture of the labial mucosa is normally smooth, soft, and elastic, with the mucosa fixed to the underlying muscle fascia. Stretching of the mucosa will reveal varying degrees of prominent vessels and ductal orifices of the minor salivary glands. These glands can sometimes cause the surface of the labial mucosa to be nodular or granular.

The color of the labial mucosa is normally pink to purple depending on the racial pigment. The area is rich in vascularity and minor salivary glands.

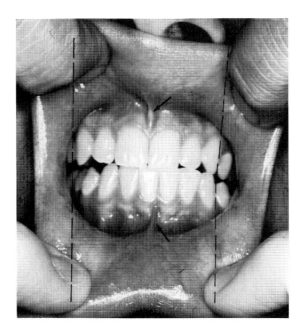

Fig. 16-28. Approximate outline of upper and lower labial mucosa. Arrows indicate labial frenula.

Examination

The labial mucosa can be easily inspected by reflection of the lips (Fig. 16-29). Palpation of the area is accomplished when the lips are examined. Bidigital palpation should extend from commissure to commissure with extension into the vestibular sulcus to detect any submucosal changes.

Abnormalities

A developmental anomaly that may cause some cosmetic problem occurs on the labial mucosa in the form of a secondary fold of tissue. This has been called a double lip and may be more obvious when the lips are slightly pursed (Fig. 16-30).

The labial mucosae are common locations for various traumatic lesions, particularly those associated with habits such as lip biting and lip chewing (moriscatio labiorum). The lesions that result from these various habits show a broad spectrum of textural change and can be diagnostic problems without a cooperative history from the patient (Figs. 16-31 and 16-32). Prolonged chronic irritation from any source is likely to induce a hyperkeratosis in addition to the roughened texture.

Fig. 16-29. Reflection of lower labial mucosa showing slightly granular texture because of the numerous superficial minor salivary glands. These should not be confused with Fordyce's granules.

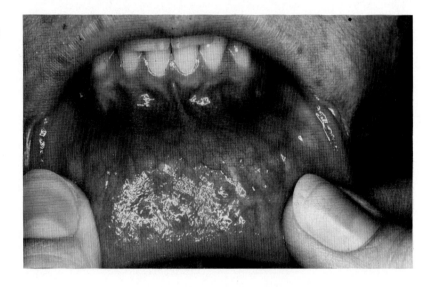

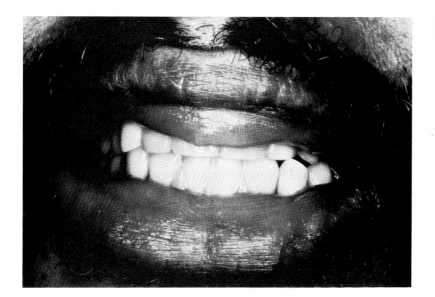

Fig. 16-30. Redundant tissue of upper labial mucosa or double lip.

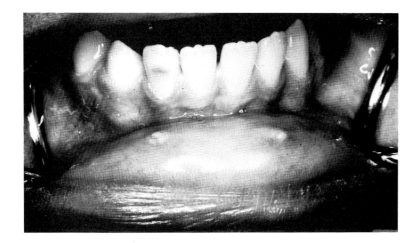

Fig. 16-31. Two white papular lesions on lower labial mucosa from chronic lip-biting habit.

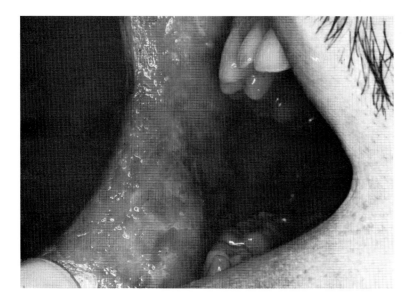

Fig. 16-32. Chronic "nibbler" of labial mucosa and commissure.

Trauma is considered to be the major etiologic factor causing mucoceles (mucous retention phenomenon). Mucoceles commonly occur on the lower labial mucosa as sessile or pedunculated blisterform lesions (Fig. 16-33). If the lesions persist untreated, some of them will undergo fibrosis and remain as fibroepithelial polyps (Fig. 16-34). Occasionally, irritation fibromas may develop from chronic trauma. The inner aspects of the commissures are common locations for these lesions (Fig. 16-35). Fibromas may be sessile or pedunculated lesions having a normal intact epithelial surface and color. The consistency of fibromas on palpation can vary considerably from very soft to firm lesions.

Pigmented macules, other than the purple to brown racial pigmentation, may be seen from amalgam or other foreign body tattoos. The color of such tattoos varies from blue to black, depending on the foreign substance and the depth of the material in the tissues (Fig. 16-36).

The lower labial mucosa is a common site for varices. These are dilated veins that usually appear as small blue to purple elevated, sessile lesions. A varix may or may not blanch on diascopic examination, depending on the presence of a thrombus or the ease with which the blood may be forced through the emptying venule (Fig. 16-37).

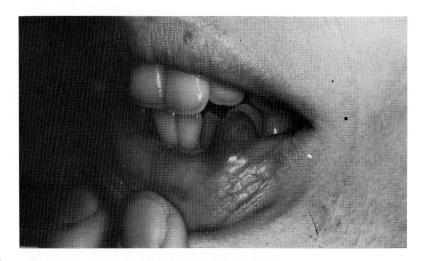

Fig. 16-33. Sessile, mucus-filled lesion of lower labial mucosa. Diagnosis: Mucocele.

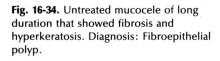

Fig. 16-34. Untreated mucocele of long duration that showed fibrosis and hyperkeratosis. Diagnosis: Fibroepithelial polyp.

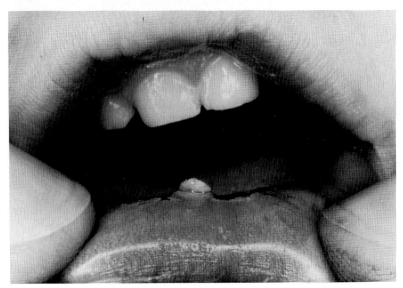

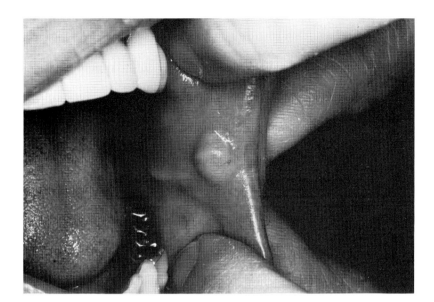

Fig. 16-35. Soft pink nodule near commissure. Diagnosis: Fibroma.

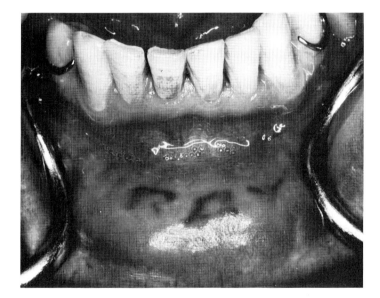

Fig. 16-36. Unique tattoo.

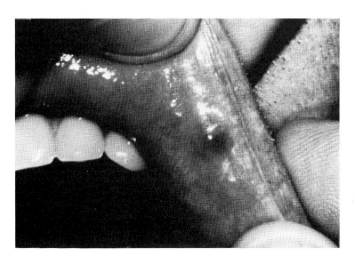

Fig. 16-37. Small blue blood-filled lesion. Diagnosis: Varix.

One of the most common oral ulcer problems that the dentist encounters is recurrent aphthous ulcers (RAU). The upper and lower labial mucosae are two of the most frequent sites for these lesions. They typically appear in the minor form as 2 to 4 mm superficial ulcers that are regular in outline with smooth margins, a necrotic central portion, and a red periphery (Fig. 16-38). A major form of RAU can cause extremely large, deep ulcers (Fig. 16-39). This is one of the few oral lesions that may heal with scarring. Major RAU is also referred to as Sutton's disease and periadenitis mucosa necrotica recurrens (PMNR).

Fig. 16-38. Single superficial ulcer with regular outline, smooth margins, necrotic yellow center, and red periphery. Diagnosis: Recurrent aphthous ulcer (RAU).

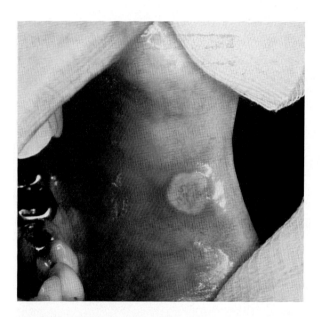

Fig. 16-39. Single deep ulcer with irregular outline, raised margins, and necrotic white center. Diagnosis: Periadenitis mucosa necrotica recurrens (major RAU).

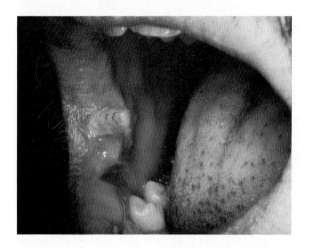

BUCCAL MUCOSA AND VESTIBULAR SULCUS
Anatomy

The buccal mucosa is bounded superiorly and inferiorly by the reflection of the mucous membrane onto the alveolar process. The buccal mucosa is the entire lining mucosa of the cheeks that is confluent anteriorly with the labial mucosa and commissure and extends posteriorly to a fold, the pterygomandibular raphe (Fig. 16-40). The pterygomandibular raphe is a tendinous strip that attaches to the hamulus process above and the retromolar triangle below.

The buccal mucosa has one important landmark, the parotid papilla, which varies considerably from one person to another. In some people it may have a prominent elevation, but in others it may be just a slight indentation. This represents the orifice of Stensen's duct (Fig. 16-40). Approximately at the middle of the buccal mucosa in most individuals there is a longitudinal fold of tissue extending from a point near the commissure posteriorly to a point close to the pterygomandibular raphe. This is known as the linea alba buccalis, or occlusal line (Fig. 16-41).

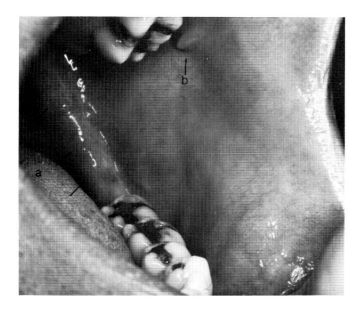

Fig. 16-40. *a,* Normal buccal mucosa extending to pterygomandibular raphe *(arrows on left).* *b,* Prominent parotid papilla (Stensen's duct) *(arrow on right).* Palpation of parotid gland will activate secretion at this point.

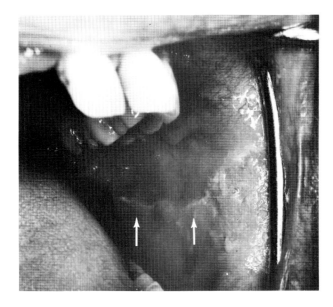

Fig. 16-41. Occlusal line or linea alba buccalis will vary considerably in prominence. Cheek-biting habits will accentuate prominence. There is evidence of cheek biting on anterior portion and commissure.

The buccal mucosa contains primarily the buccinator and masseter muscles. Posteriorly, it contains the parotid gland and varying amounts of fat, which form the buccal fat pad. Scattered throughout the buccal mucosa are numerous minor salivary glands; it may also contain sebaceous glands (Fig. 16-42).

The texture of the buccal mucosa is very similar to that of the labial mucosa. The mucous membrane is soft and fixed to the inner fascia of the buccinator muscle. In some people the numerous mucous and mixed glands in the submucous tissue will result in a nodular texture. There are frequently prominent sebaceous glands, or Fordyce's granules, adjacent to the commissures and extending to the molar region. These may feel granular to the touch (see Fig. 16-16). The buccal fat pad can vary considerably in its degree of prominence. It usually decreases in prominence from childhood into adulthood. More easily palpated than viewed, it lies beneath and distal to the parotid papilla.

The color of the buccal mucosa is normally pink in whites but bluish or bluish gray in blacks. This bluish color in blacks may have a patchy distribution and may contain brown to black areas of pigmentation.

Although the vestibular sulcus, or fornix, and buccal mucosa are confluent, the vestibular sulcus is the horseshoe-shaped furrow formed by the reflection of the superior and inferior borders of the buccal mucosa and labial mucosa. This area is sometimes referred to as the mucobuccal fold, the buccal gutter, or the vestibule, among other terms (Fig. 16-43). The vestibular sulcus may have several folds of tissue traversing the alveolar mucosa and buccal mucosa. These are the lateral frenula or buccal frenula, usually present in the area of the cuspids or bicuspids in both the maxilla and mandible (Fig. 16-43).

The mucous membrane of the vestibular sulcus is thin, and the many small blood vessels present are easily seen. The submucous tissue attaching the mucous membrane to muscles and bone is very loose in texture, allowing for the marked mobility of the lips and buccal mucosa. This mobility decreases in the molar region, as does the amount of this loose connective tissue.

Fig. 16-42. Anatomic structures in buccal mucosa.

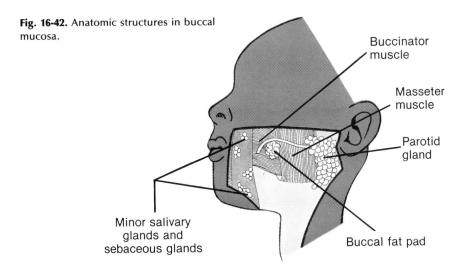

Buccinator muscle

Masseter muscle

Parotid gland

Buccal fat pad

Minor salivary glands and sebaceous glands

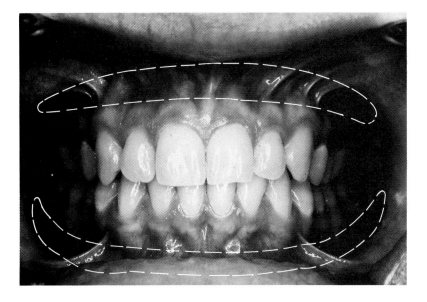

Fig. 16-43. Outline of vestibular sulcus with prominent lateral (buccal) frenula.

Examination

The examination of the buccal mucosa and vestibular sulcus requires good lighting to view the boundaries and to detect any subtle textural or color changes. Reflection and rolling of the buccal mucosa over the fingertips (Fig. 16-44) will enhance the visual inspection and allow palpation of the tissues at the same time.

Bidigital or bimanual palpation (Fig. 16-45) is extremely important for this area. Submucosal lesions associated with the lymphatic system, salivary glands, muscle, fat, or connective tissue may occur and not be obvious to inspection for many months. During the palpation of the parotid gland area, the examiner should observe the orifice of Stensen's duct for normal flow and consistency of secretion. A small quantity of clear, serous fluid should be expressed by this manipulation.

Fig. 16-44. Rolling buccal and labial mucosa over fingertips allows examiner to inspect and palpate area simultaneously.

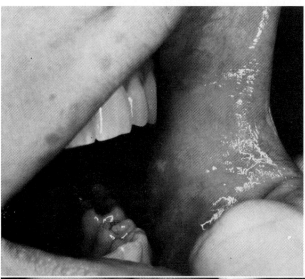
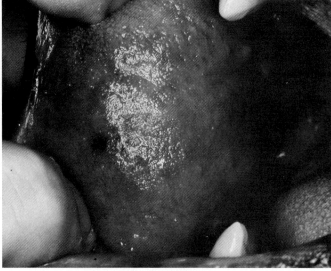

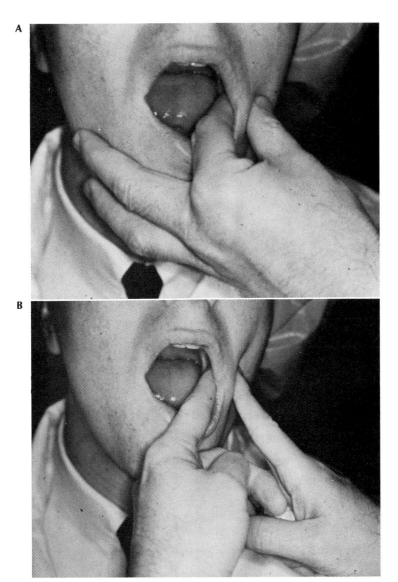

Fig. 16-45. A, Bidigital palpation of buccal mucosa. **B,** Bimanual palpation of buccal mucosa.

Abnormalities

There are several conditions affecting the buccal mucosa that can be considered as variations of normal but that at first glance may appear grossly abnormal. The number and concentration of sebaceous glands (Fordyce's granules) can vary considerably, thereby altering both the texture and color from a smooth, soft, pink surface to a granular, yellowish mucosa (Fig. 16-46).

Leukoedema is another variation seen quite prominently, involving most of the buccal mucosa. This change is caused by an abnormal intracellular fluid accumulation in the epithelial cells that causes the tissues to be abnormally white with a milky appearance (Fig. 16-47). This color alteration is reversible to a normal pink color by stretching the mucosa over the fingers. The condition is reported to occur in approximately 40% of white and 85% of black adults.

Two hereditary diseases, white sponge nevus and hereditary benign intraepithelial dyskeratosis (HBID), affect the buccal mucosa, causing a similar but more extensive white change. There is usually a marked thickening of the mucosa that results in a very irregular surface (Fig. 16-48).

Fig. 16-46. Variation of normal buccal mucosa, having numerous Fordyce's granules.

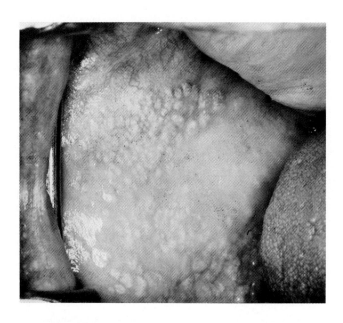

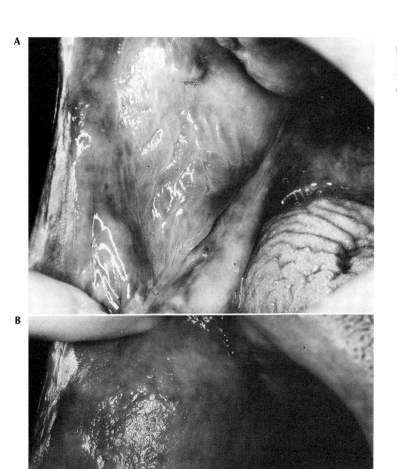

Fig. 16-47. A, White appearance seen in leukoedema. B, Stretching mucosa over fingertips results in temporary reversal of color change.

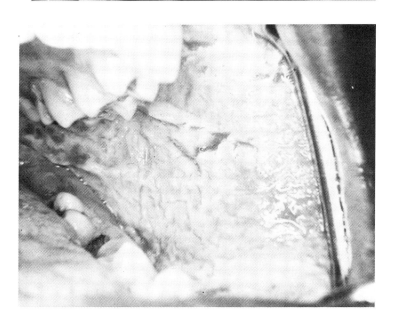

Fig. 16-48. White sponge nevus.

The prominence of the linea alba buccalis (occlusal line) is another highly variable feature of the buccal mucosa. This longitudinal fold may be accentuated by a number of factors, such as muscle pressure against the teeth or habits of sucking or biting the cheeks. The same irregular roughened textural changes and frictional keratoses as described for the labial mucosa may be seen even more frequently on the buccal mucosa (Fig. 16-49). Fibromas frequently arise along the occlusal line (Fig. 16-50).

The lower half of the buccal mucosa and mandibular vestibular sulcus, in addition to being a natural pooling area for secretions, foods, and beverages, is also a favorite site for dissolving lozenges and medications, and for holding various tobacco products. Consequently, this is not an unusual site for a varying range of leukoplakia and erythroplasia changes. Because of the significant premalignant changes that a certain percentage of such lesions may show, careful evaluation is essential (Fig. 16-51).

The dissolving of aspirin tablets in the vestibular sulcus is a popular home remedy treatment for various dental and periodontal pain problems. Aspirin acts as a mild chemical cautery agent to the epithelial cells and results in white lesions that may be plaque-like and vary greatly in extent. Necrosis of the epithelium results in sloughing that in turn can lead to ulceration (Fig. 16-52).

Fig. 16-49. Typical roughened textural change from chronic cheek biting.

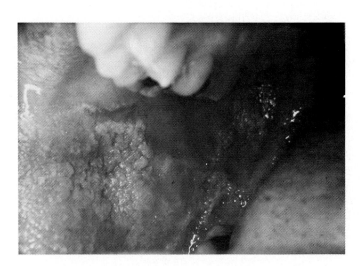

Fig. 16-50. Soft pedunculated nodule arising on occlusal line of buccal mucosa from repeated irritation. Diagnosis: Fibroma.

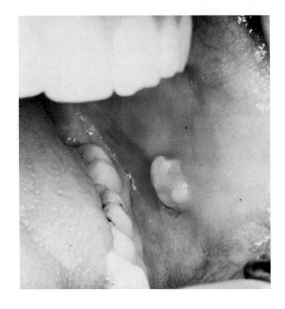

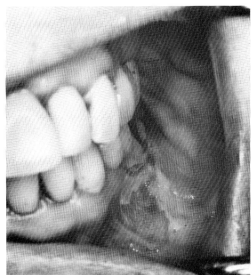

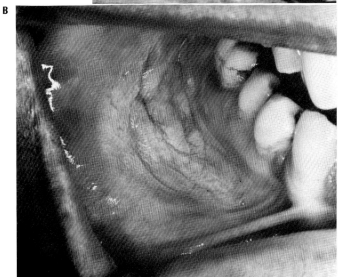

Fig. 16-51. A, White plaque in vestibular sulcus extending onto buccal mucosa. **B,** Roughened white textural change with increased firmness and thickness to mucosa. Associated with use of snuff. Diagnosis (**A** and **B**): Keratosis without atypia.

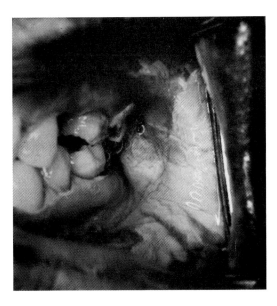

Fig. 16-52. Extensive white change indicating superficial necrosis of epithelium. Diagnosis: Aspirin burn.

Abnormal pigmentation involving the buccal mucosa may be an early manifestation of a diverse group of disturbances. Perhaps the most common pigmentation other than normal racial pigmentation is amalgam tattoos, which may be found in most any intraoral site. These are usually small discrete macules ranging in color from blue to black (Fig. 16-53). Other focal areas of pigmentation may indicate nevi. More diffuse areas of abnormal melanin pigmentation may be seen in patients with Addison's disease and occasionally in patients with an internal malignancy. The history of duration and increasing pigmentation is usually significant.

The buccal mucosa and vestibular sulcus are common sites for lichen planus. Various patterns of striae may be seen (Fig. 16-54).

Fig. 16-53. Bluish black macules. Diagnosis: Amalgam tattoo.

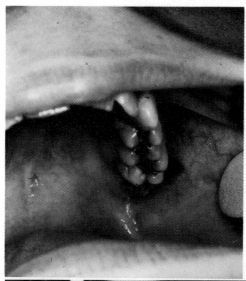
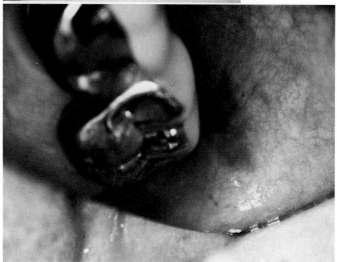

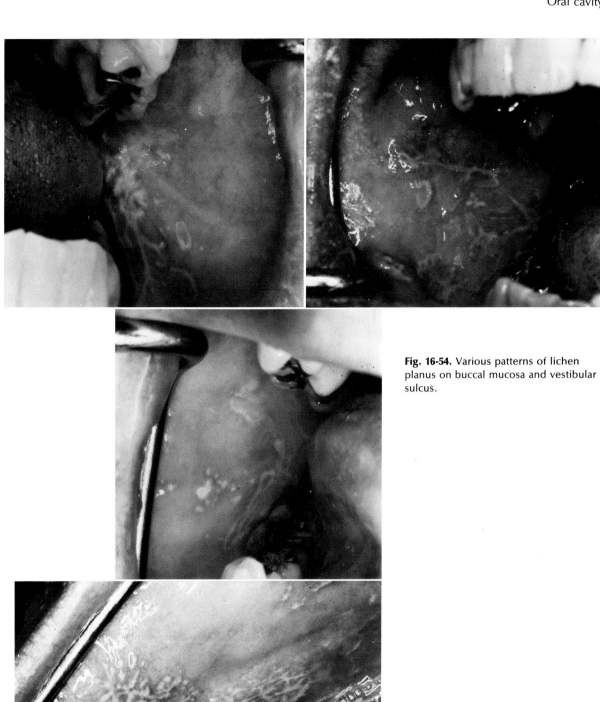

Fig. 16-54. Various patterns of lichen planus on buccal mucosa and vestibular sulcus.

Traumatic ulcers, recurrent aphthous ulcers, and ulcerations associated with bullous lichen planus and lupus erythematosus, erythema multiforme, or pemphigus may all be seen involving the buccal mucosa and vestibular sulcus (Fig. 16-55).

Fig. 16-55. A and **B,** Factitial traumatic ulcers.

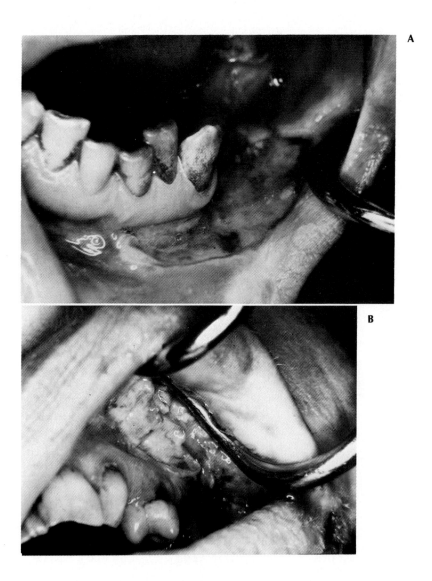

A

B

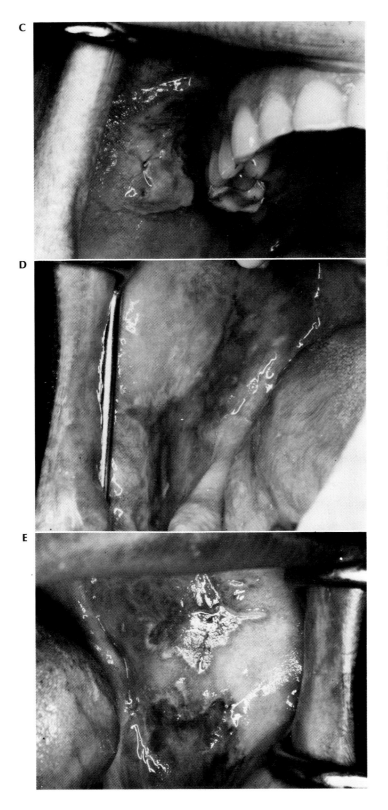

Fig. 16-55, cont'd. C, Iatrogenic traumatic ulcer from possible combination of topical anesthetic, cotton roll burn, superficial anesthetic injection, repeated impressions, and eugenol burn from temporary crown. **D,** Ulcerations from erosive lichen planus. **E,** Ulcerations from oral lupus erythematosus.

GINGIVA AND ALVEOLAR MUCOSA
Anatomy

From the vestibular sulcus the mucous membrane continues over the tooth-supporting bone to the cervical areas of the teeth. This area may be subdivided into two zones: the zone adjacent to the vestibule is the alveolar mucosa; the zone adjacent to the teeth is the gingiva (Fig. 16-56). In the anterior zone the alveolar mucosa and gingiva are separated from each other by a sharp scalloped line that parallels the free margin of the gingiva, the mucogingival junction (Fig. 16-57).

The gingiva is subdivided into the attached and the free gingiva. The free gingiva extends into the interdental spaces, such as the gingival papilla, and ends in a knife-like edge closely adapted to the teeth circumferentially. The gingival sulcus is the crevice between the free marginal gingiva and the point of attachment to the teeth at or near the cementoenamel junction (Fig. 16-58).

Fig. 16-56. Imaginary line dividing alveolar mucosa and gingiva.

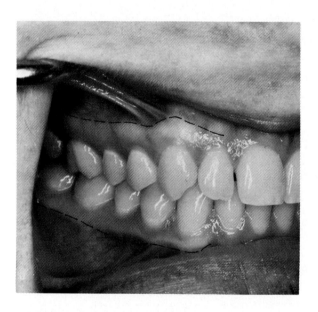

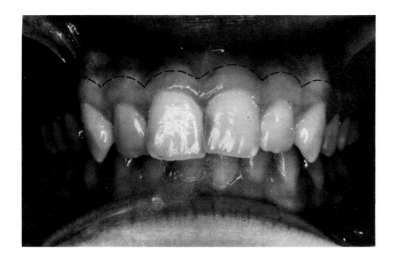

Fig. 16-57. Scalloped dividing line on anterior gingiva resulting from difference in color of tissue.

A

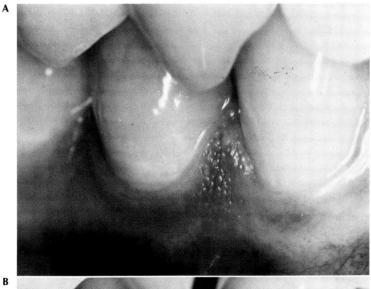

B

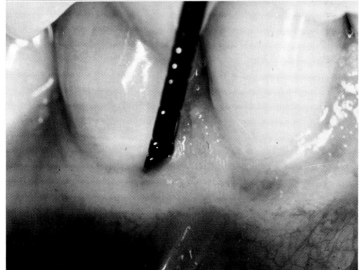

Fig. 16-58. A, Normal gingiva with interdental papilla. **B,** Periodontal probe in gingival sulcus.

The surface of the attached gingiva and the interdental papilla is generally stippled. There is considerable variation in the degree of stippling, even in healthy gingiva. The texture may vary from a light stippling similar to velvet to heavier stippling similar to the surface of an orange. The free gingival margin and borders of the interdental papillae are smooth (Fig. 16-59, *A*). The alveolar mucosa is characterized by a more delicate texture, greater mobility, and a darker red color than the gingiva. This darker color is caused by the larger number of blood vessels, plus a nonkeratinized epithelium. The alveolar mucosa is smooth, without stippling.

The normal color of the attached and the free gingivae is a pale pink in whites, but in black and other dark-skinned races varying amounts of melanin pigment may be scattered in irregular patterns (Fig. 16-59, *B* and *C*). The normal color varies from one individual to another. The vascularity, hemoglobin content, and reduced hemoglobin in the blood, as well as the density of connective tissue, width of epithelium, and degree of keratinization, have an effect on the color, shade, and intensity.

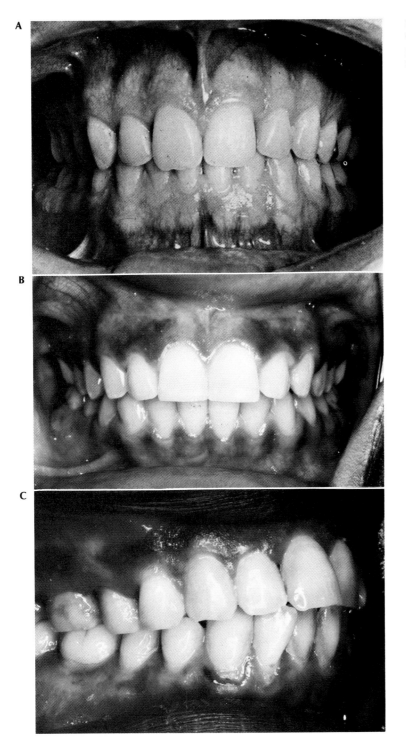

Fig. 16-59. A, Normal gingiva. **B** and **C,** Varying patterns of racial melanin pigment involving gingiva and alveolar mucosa.

Examination

Careful visual inspection of the gingiva is the primary means of evaluating early and subtle changes. Textural change that usually involves the stippling character of the gingiva may be one of the earliest changes from normal health. The overall contours and form of the tissues are also important considerations. Alterations in form or contour may result from developmental factors, disease, or previous treatment of gingival or bony disease. The change may indicate atrophy, recession, loss of tissue, hypertrophy, or enlargement (Fig. 16-60). The consistency of the tissues can best be determined by palpation with the index finger. When obvious enlargement of the gingiva is noted, either focal or generalized, it is important to determine by palpation if the enlargement indicates edema, or fibrous or bony change. Normally, because of the relative thin nature of the gingiva and the fact that all but the marginal gingiva is firmly bound down, the consistency is firm and resilient, with the contours of the supporting bone being readily palpated. During palpation, the examiner should look carefully at the marginal gingiva for the presence of any exudate.

The level of attachment of the gingiva, the depth of the gingival crevice, and consequently the amount and form of marginal unattached gingiva should be noted carefully. A more detailed discussion of pocket depth is discussed in the section on the periodontium.

Evaluation of the color of the gingiva is an extremely important phase of the examination. Because of the variation of physiologic pigmentation, there is a great range in the normal color of the gingiva from one individual to another. In the same individual normal color can change with age and with stages of the dentition. Color changes frequently accompany textural changes (Fig. 16-61). These changes may involve either the marginal or attached gingiva or both. The pigmentation may be focal or diffuse in distribution.

The interdental papillae contour, texture, and color should also be carefully noted, since some diseases characteristically begin with involvement of the papillae.

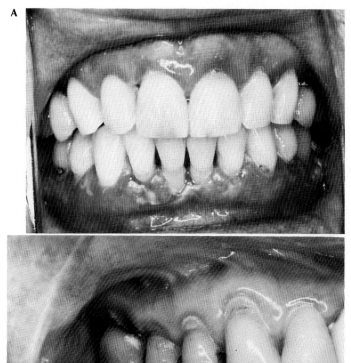
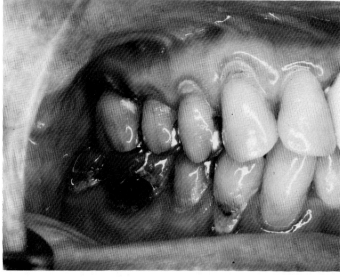

Fig. 16-60. A, Maxillary gingiva showing increased redness of marginal gingiva and change of contour indicating early periodontal disease. Mandibular gingiva shows gingival recession with loss of interdental papillae and cleft formation labial to central incisor. **B,** Extensive gingival recession and dental abrasion of cervical areas.

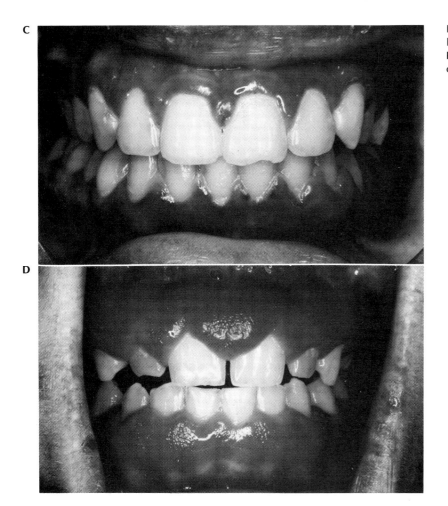

Fig. 16-60, cont'd. C, Gingival hypertrophy and marginal gingivitis. **D,** More severe gingival hypertrophy and diffuse erythematous change.

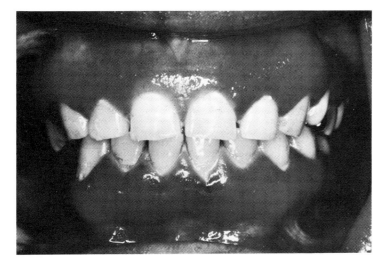

Fig. 16-61. Severe erythema with loss of normal stippling. Diagnosis: Atypical gingivitis associated with chewing gum allergy.

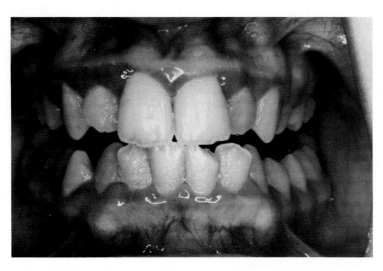

Fig. 16-62. Marginal gingivitis with sharply demarcated red color change.

Abnormalities

The most common abnormalities involving the gingiva are gingivitis and periodontitis. It is rare to find a patient without some degree of marginal gingivitis (Fig. 16-62). This may appear as an increased redness of the free gingiva around one or many of the teeth, and the gingiva may or may not be enlarged. The condition is usually an inflammatory response to local irritating factors that range from collections of soft debris to large deposits of calculus.

Pericoronitis is a localized but more acute form of gingivitis that is common in teenage and young adult patients with partially erupting third molars. This usually indicates a bacterial infection between the crown of a tooth and a flap of overlying gingival mucosa before the crown is fully erupted and a normal gingival sulcus is present.

Fig. 16-63. Typical parulis associated with fistula from necrotic dental pulps.

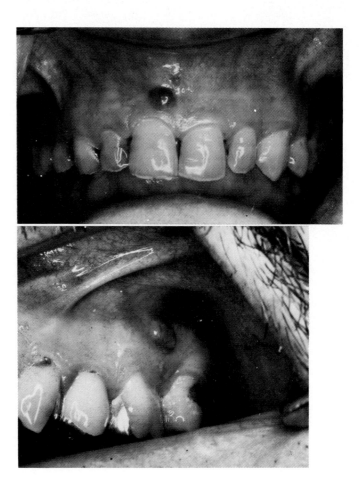

There are two abscess conditions that may appear as gingival lesions. The periapical abscess that stems from a nonvital dental pulp is seen in all age groups. The gingival lesion resulting from a periapical abscess most frequently appears as a parulis (gum boil), which indicates the drainage point of a fistula from the apex of a tooth root (Fig. 16-63). A parulis may appear as a red papule, nodule, or pustule of varying size. This elevated lesion is usually a mass of granulation tissue attempting to heal the fistula. This condition generally is associated with a subacute to chronic periapical abscess. In some acute abscess conditions the gingival lesion may be a more generalized red, painful enlargement (Fig. 16-64).

The pyogenic granuloma is a pseudotumor mass that most commonly occurs on the gingiva as a pedunculated nodule, usually arising from the interdental papilla. It is usually soft to palpation and may vary in color from pink to red. A pyogenic granuloma may range in size from a few millimeters to several centimeters. When it occurs during pregnancy, it is referred to as a granuloma gravidarum (Fig. 16-65).

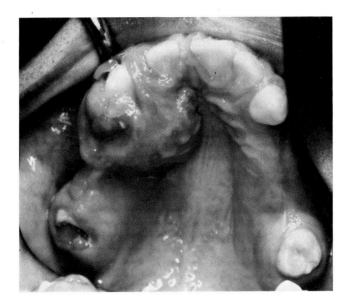

Fig. 16-64. Acute periapical abscess.

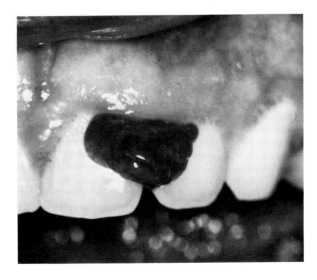

Fig. 16-65. Pyogenic granuloma.

Exostoses are common elevated lesions that occur on the attached gingiva. They are frequently multiple lesions, bony hard to palpation, and appear as sessile or pedunculated nodules. They occur on the mandible or maxilla (Fig. 16-66). The most common foci of exostoses are the palatal torus (torus palatinus) and the lingual mandibular torus (torus mandibularis) (Fig. 16-67).

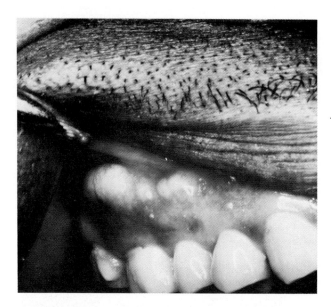

Fig. 16-66. Multiple exostoses of maxilla.

Fig. 16-67. A, Large torus palatinus. **B,** Torus mandibularis.

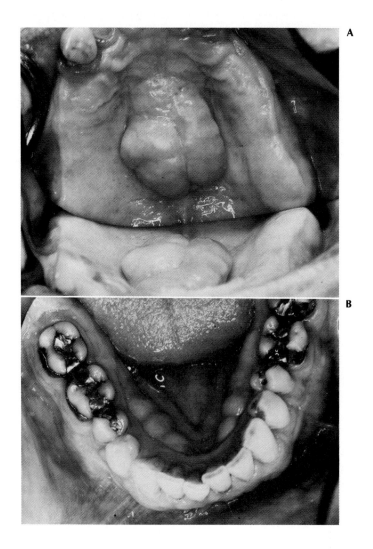

A

B

A more generalized enlargement of the gingiva may be seen as idiopathic fibromatosis or phenytoin (Dilantin) hyperplasia (Fig. 16-68). On inspection, gingival hyperplasia may be difficult to distinguish from bony enlargement, such as occurs in Paget's disease or other fibroosseous diseases. However, the consistency and resiliency on palpation should assist the examiner in distinguishing these similar-appearing clinical conditions. Of course, the radiographic examination should readily separate fibroosseous conditions from soft tissue hyperplasia.

Dentigerous cysts, tumors, and various fibroosseous lesions may cause localized expansion of the jaws that can appear clinically as a large sessile nodule or tumescent enlargement of the gingiva (Fig. 16-69). Palpation of such lesions may assist the examiner in distinguishing cystic lesions by their rebound sensation.

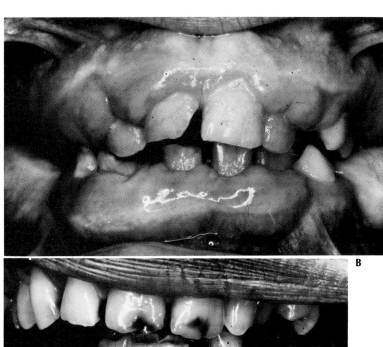

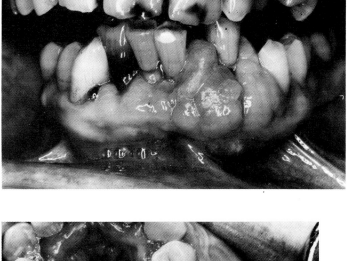

Fig. 16-68. A, Idiopathic gingival hyperplasia (fibromatosis). **B,** phenytoin (Dilantin)-associated hyperplasia.

Fig. 16-69. Expansion of maxillary alveolar process, bony hard to palpation. Diagnosis: Fibrous dysplasia.

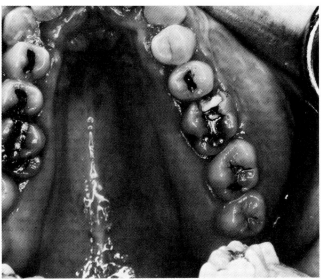

The peripheral giant cell granuloma is a unique lesion that occurs exclusively on the gingiva, usually as a pedunculated nodule or tumor. The purple color that is characteristic of most of these lesions helps distinguish them from the fibromas and pyogenic granulomas (Fig. 16-70).

Some other specific conditions that affect the gingiva are Vincent's disease, desquamative gingivitis, and allergic reactions. Vincent's disease, or acute necrotizing ulcerative gingivitis, is characterized by the early necrotic involvement of the interdental papillae. This necrosis results in a gray membrane covering, and eventually the interdental papilla is sloughed, leaving punched-out craterform areas between the teeth (Fig. 16-71).

Desquamative gingivitis or gingivosis usually appears as a nonspecific erythematous and atrophic lesion of the gingiva (Fig. 16-72). The desquamation or peeling of the epithelium may not be obvious either to inspection or to palpation; hence the gingiva may have a bright red color simply from the increased vascularity and atrophy of the epithelium. The condition is extremely painful, and minimal stimulation or irritation causes bleeding. Both these symptoms discourage good oral hygiene habits. This condition may indicate a localized early manifestation of benign mucous membrane pemphigoid; special immunofluorescent studies are indicated to make this diagnosis.

Fig. 16-70. Purple tumescence arising from alveolar mucosa. Diagnosis: Giant cell tumor.

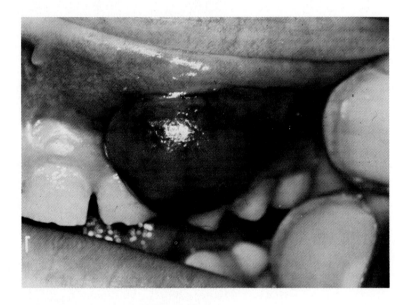

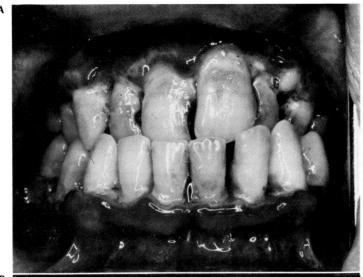

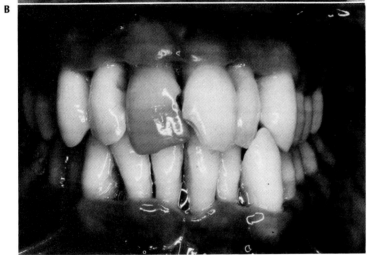

Fig. 16-71. A, Acute necrotizing ulcerative gingivitis before treatment. **B,** A similar case after conservative treatment, showing loss of interdental papillae.

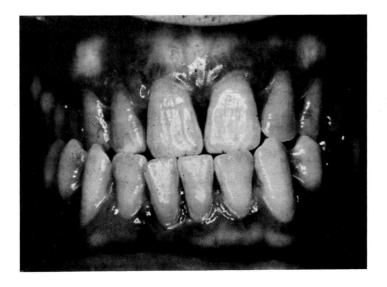

Fig. 16-72. Desquamative gingivitis.

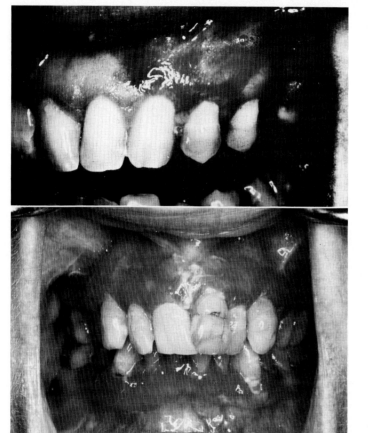

Erosive lichen planus can also simulate gingivosis, especially if no Wickham's striae are present and only the gingivae are involved (Fig. 16-73). Biopsy may help distinguish between the two conditions. Other oral sites, as well as the skin and genital areas, should be inspected for more characteristic lesions of lichen planus.

In recent years a unique form of allergic gingivitis, referred to as atypical gingivitis or plasma cell gingivitis, has been noted, which also causes a bright red color change similar to gingivosis but without obvious desquamation (Fig. 16-74). The cause in many of these cases was an allergic response to chewing gum.

Fig. 16-73. Erosive lichen planus.

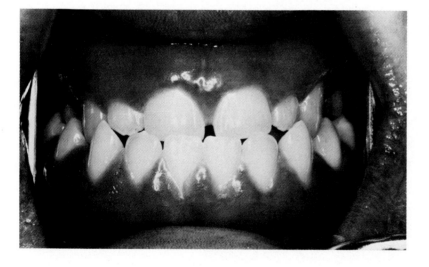

Fig. 16-74. Atypical or plasma cell gingivitis.

Several gingival conditions are characterized by inflammatory hyperplasia, particularly involving the interdental papillae and marginal gingiva. Localized involvement may simply indicate a response to local irritants, such as plaque, calculus, teeth with sharp margins, or sharp restoration margins (Fig. 16-75). More generalized involvement is seen with pubertal and pregnancy gingivitis (Fig. 16-76). In addition to the local factors, there appears to be a hormonal influence as well. Leukemic gingivitis is also characterized by marked enlargement (Fig. 16-77). The local factors may be minimal in this condition. The enlargement is caused by infiltration of the gingiva with neoplastic white blood cells. In all these conditions the enlarged gingiva is spongy and bleeds readily. With leukemia and other blood dyscrasias, the gingiva may show spontaneous hemorrhage.

Inflammatory gingival hyperplasia that persists and is untreated may tend to undergo fibrosis. Phenytoin (Dilantin) hyperplasia appears to be an example of such an exaggerated gingival hyperplasia in patients undergoing long-term phenytoin therapy (Fig. 16-68, B).

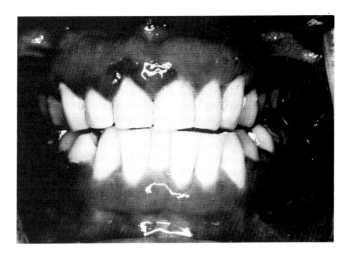

Fig. 16-75. Inflammatory gingival hyperplasia.

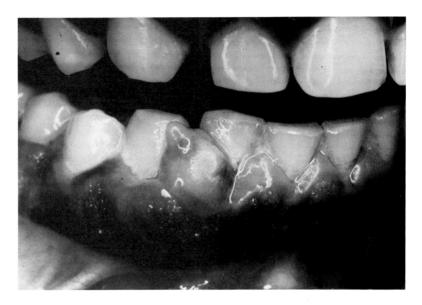

Fig. 16-76. Gingival hyperplasia during pregnancy.

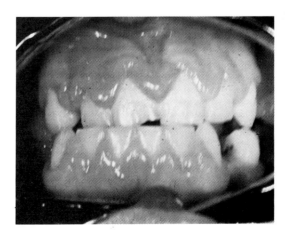

Fig. 16-77. Gingival hyperplasia in patient with leukemia.

It was mentioned previously that recurrent herpes simplex has an affinity for gingival and palatal tissue. The lesions are characteristically clusters of small coalescing vesicles that rapidly result in punctate ulcers (Fig. 16-78; see also Fig. 16-20). Cytologic tests can often be helpful in confirming the diagnosis because of the unique cytopathogenic effect of the virus in the epithelial cells. Other discrete ulcers that may be found on the gingivae are most likely traumatic in origin. Occasionally recurrent aphthous ulcers may involve the frenula or the more loose alveolar mucosa near the vestibular sulcus (Fig. 16-79).

Pigmented macules indicating amalgam tattoos are the most common pigmented lesions of the gingiva. These are usually blue to bluish black macules varying in size from a few millimeters to a centimeter or more (Fig. 16-80). There may or may not be radiographic evidence of amalgam particles in the area; however, there is usually evidence of large restorations in present or previously extracted teeth. Large, diffuse areas of pigmentation may result in areas where endodontic retrograde amalgams have been placed. This can be cosmetically disturbing to some patients, particularly when the anterior region is involved. There is usually evidence of the surgical scar, which can assist in the diagnosis of such pigmentation.

Heavy metal poisoning, which may result from therapy with arsenic, mercury, silver, and bismuth preparations, can also cause a unique pigmentation of the gingiva that usually appears as a narrow band of blue to black pigmentation in the marginal gingiva.

Fig. 16-78. Coalescing punctate ulcers. Diagnosis: Recurrent herpes simplex.

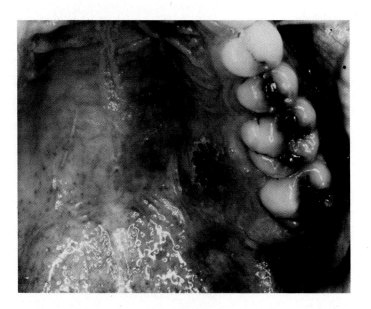

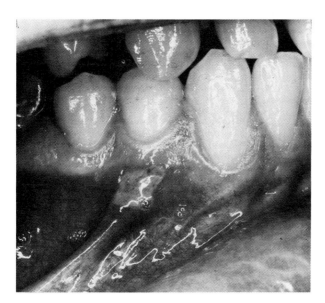

Fig. 16-79. RAU involving buccal frenulum.

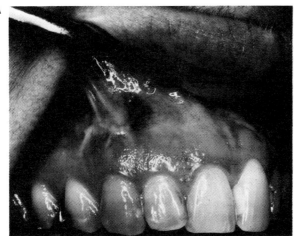

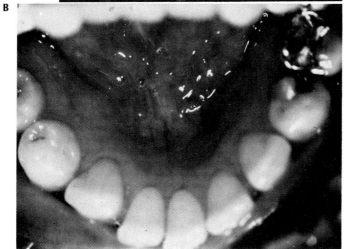

Fig. 16-80. A, Amalgam tattoo following retrograde amalgam endodontic treatment. Surgical scar is evident and would be helpful in suggesting this diagnosis. **B,** Small amalgam tattoo remote from restored teeth indicating probable implantation from high-speed cutting of tooth having an amalgam restoration.

279

PALATE
Anatomy

The roof of the oral cavity proper is formed by the *hard palate* anteriorly and the *soft palate* posteriorly. The hard palate extends peripherally to become the palatal gingiva. At the posterior end of the hard palate, there are frequently two small depressions, the *fovea palatinae*. The hard palate terminates at an imaginary line running through or close to the fovea palatinae. In the midline there is a narrow elevated ridge, the *palatine raphe*. It extends from a small projection, the *incisive papilla,* posteriorly over the entire length of the hard palate. On the anterior hard palate, radiating from the incisive papilla and anterior portions of the palatine raphe, are irregular branching ridges termed the *palatine rugae.* The mucous membrane covering the anterior hard palate is keratinized and firmly attached to the underlying bone and therefore is not movable. The peripheral zone is firm but more resilient toward the gingiva (Fig. 16-81).

On the posterior hard palate, the lateral portions between the palatine raphe and the gingiva contain numerous mucous glands, nerves, and blood vessels in the submucosa. This area may be soft to palpation because of the fat and mucous glands. Posterior to the last molar, the hard palate mucosa fuses peripherally with the vestibular gingiva and posteriorly with the pterygomandibular raphe. This prominent ridge is the *alveolar tuberosity.* The concavity distal to the tuberosity is the *hamular notch.*

The hard palate is normally pale pink in color in whites and blacks. However, a bluish gray hue may be normal.

The soft palate begins posteriorly to the imaginary line running laterally near the fovea palatinae. It is a thick fold of mucous membrane that extends posteriorly and downward to end as the *uvula.* This fold of mucous membrane provides an important boundary between the *oral cavity,* the *nasal cavity,* and the *oral pharynx.* Laterally, the soft palate extends downward to fuse with the *pillars of the fauces* (Fig. 16-82).

The soft palate mucosa is thin and nonkeratinized. The prominent vascularity may give a slightly darker red color than the hard palate. Sometimes the prominent fat tissue or lipids in the area may cause the soft palate to be more pale yellow in color. The smooth texture may be interspersed with prominent ductal orifices from the mucous glands.

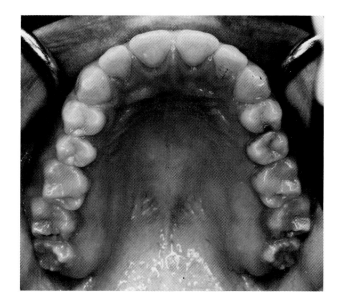

Fig. 16-81. Normal hard palate.

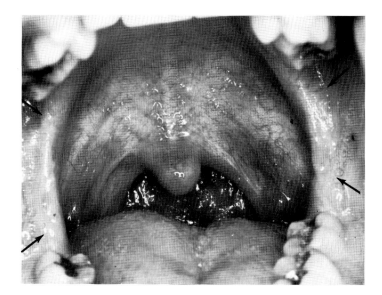

Fig. 16-82. Normal soft palate showing slight erythematous change in faucial pillar area. Also shows good example of prominent pterygomandibular raphe *(arrows)*.

EXAMINATION

The palate should be inspected carefully for any abnormal developmental anomalies, such as clefts, prominent palatine rugae, or raphes. Since the hard palate mucosa is bound tightly to the underlying bone, any abnormality in form or texture should be readily apparent. Today most patients with clefts have had surgical repair during infancy. The surgery may still leave varying abnormal defects in form to the palate.

Palpation of the posterior hard palate and soft palate should be a routine examination procedure. There is a wide range of normal variation in these areas because of the quantity of fat and minor accessory glands in the submucosa. Palpation may detect early submucosal changes, such as salivary gland tumors.

Subtle color changes, particularly erythematous change, should be carefully noted in the mucosa of these posterior palatal sites. The variation in the vascularity and thickness of the mucosa in the soft palate causes a marked degree of color variation from one individual to another.

Abnormalities

Since the periphery of the hard palate represents the palatal gingiva, it is susceptible to the various abnormalities discussed in the section on the gingiva. The periapical abscess, particularly from the molars, may be found extending well onto the hard palate (Fig. 16-83).

The torus palatinus is a fairly common finding (approximately 20% of the population) on the hard palate. These exostoses appear in varying sizes and shapes (Fig. 16-84). The palatal torus arises along the palatine raphe and is very hard to palpation. The color is usually pale pink because of the thin, tightly bound surfacing mucosa. The lesions are not neoplasms but usually develop gradually over a period of years. Many patients are unaware of its presence or consider it to be normal for everyone. Other patients may suddenly discover the mass and become alarmed that it may indicate a neoplasm. Tori are significant only when they interfere with the adaptation and wearing of a dental prosthesis.

On the anterior hard palate, in the area of the incisive papilla, the incisive canal cyst may appear as a sessile nodule with a normal pink color (Fig. 16-85). If secondary infection has occurred, then the color may be red, and a draining fistulous tract may be present. Another developmental or inclusion-type cyst, the median palatal cyst, may occur in the midline, more posteriorly. The softness of these lesions on palpation readily distinguishes these swellings from a bony torus or exostosis.

Fig. 16-83. Palatal-oriented abscess of pulpal and periapical origin.

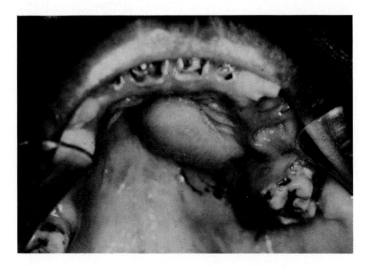

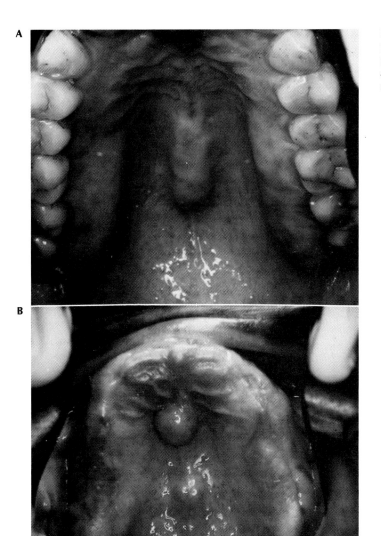

Fig. 16-84. A, Typical elongated torus palatinus. **B,** Two tori are present: round pedunculated nodule slightly off midline and smaller sessile nodule in posterior midline.

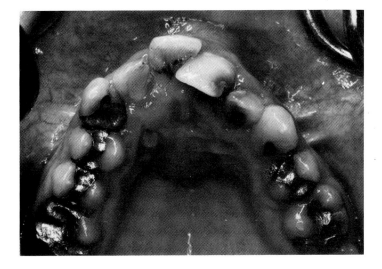

Fig. 16-85. Palatal swelling involving incisive papilla. Diagnosis: Nasopalatine duct cyst.

Salivary gland tumors arising in the minor accessory glands usually appear as sessile or pedunculated nodules or tumors on the posterior aspect of the hard palate. A tumor is more firm to palpation than the cystic lesions just described, and it is unusual for a salivary gland tumor to arise symmetrically in the midline (Fig. 16-86).

One of the most common conditions involving the hard palate is papillary hyperplasia. It appears as multiple small papules, most frequently under denture bases. Most of the area involved is very red and may form an outline of the prosthesis (Fig. 16-87).

Candidiasis may be associated with some cases of papillary hyperplasia. However, candidiasis frequently appears as an erythematous change involving large areas of the hard palate without any papular hyperplasia and may be seen in nondenture wearers as well as in the denture-wearing patient (Fig. 16-88). Severe cases of candidiasis may show collections of soft white plaques in addition to the erythematous change.

Fig. 16-86. Pedunculated nodule on hard palate that would be rubbery on palpation, in contrast to bony hard sensation of torus. Diagnosis: Pleomorphic adenoma (mixed salivary gland tumor).

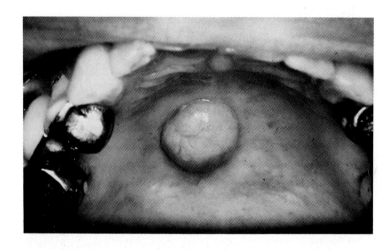

Fig. 16-87. Multiple coalescing red papules on hard palate of denture wearer. Diagnosis: Papillary hyperplasia.

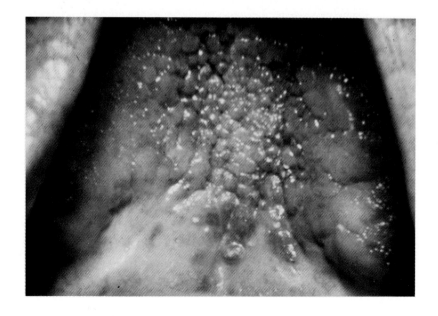

Nicotine stomatitis is a unique condition found on the palates of heavy smokers. It occurs on the hard palate and may extend onto the soft palate. The condition is characterized by an inflammatory change in the ducts of the minor mucous glands that causes discrete red macules or papules approximately 1 mm in diameter. The epithelium of the mucosa is usually hyperkeratotic, causing a white change with the overall texture of the mucosa and showing a rough surface containing fissures and cracks (Fig. 16-89).

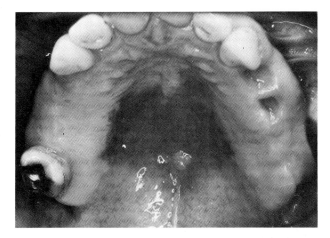

Fig. 16-88. Erythematous change in palatal mucosa. Diagnosis: Candidiasis.

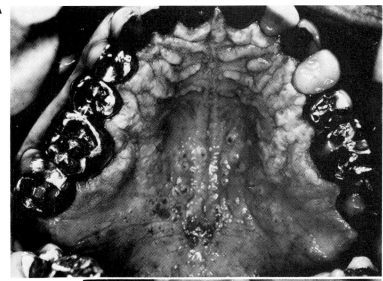

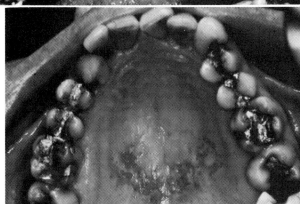

Fig. 16-89. A, Severe case of nicotine stomatitis in patient with long history of pipe smoking. B, Less severe case of nicotine stomatitis.

285

Intraoral recurrent herpes simplex infections characteristically involve the hard palate. These lesions arise as clusters of small discrete vesicles that rupture and leave punctate red ulcers that may coalesce (Fig. 16-78).

The palate also lends itself to traumatic ulcers from various causes. Once the cause is determined and removed, the lesions usually heal in a few days. Traumatic ulcers that occur on a palatal torus, however, may be slow to heal because of the thin and rather avascular surfacing mucosa (Fig. 16-90).

The soft palate is one of the more common sites for papillomas. These usually occur as pedunculated lesions, varying in size from a few millimeters to a centimeter or more (Fig. 16-91). Papillomas can usually be distinguished clinically from fibromas because of the numerous fronds that project from the lesion, giving it a pebbled, rough texture. The color varies from pink to red or white.

Petechiae of the soft palate may be a prodromal sign of infectious mononucleosis, various blood dyscrasias, or habits that cause a vacuum-like pressure to the area (Fig. 16-92). These may appear as diffuse ecchymosis.

Fig. 16-90. Palatal torus with traumatic ulcer.

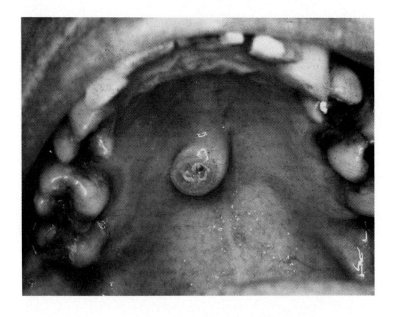

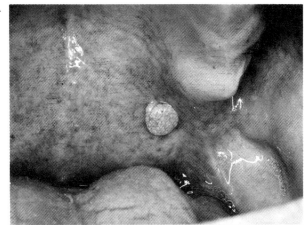

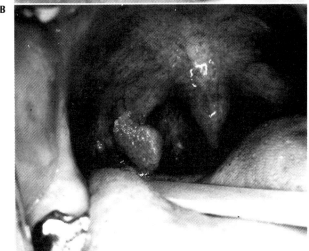

Fig. 16-91. A, Soft pedunculated papule with cauliflower-like texture. Diagnosis: Papilloma. **B,** Pedunculated tumor with similar roughened texture. Diagnosis: Papilloma.

Fig. 16-92. Petechiae and areas of ecchymosis from contact allergy.

Ulcers of the soft palate may be associated with RAU. RAU lesions of this site may be larger and more persistent in relation to other intraoral sites (Fig. 16-93).

The uvula is a highly variable structure that may show numerous developmental anomalies (Fig. 16-94).

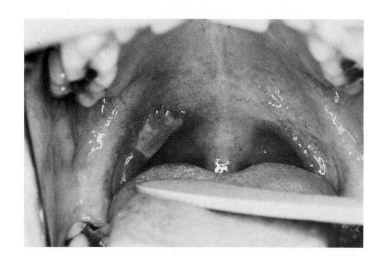

Fig. 16-93. RAU.

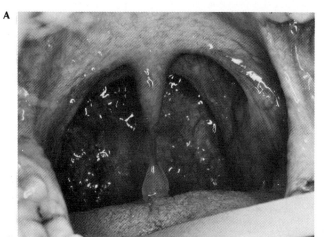

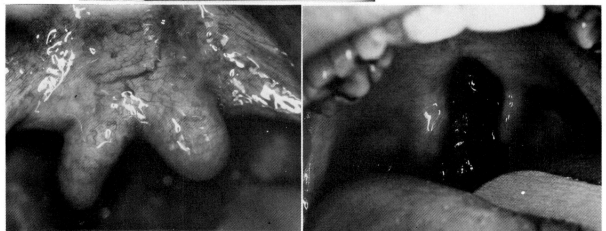

Fig. 16-94. A, Elongated malformed uvula. **B,** Bifid uvula. **C,** Bifid uvula and soft tissue cleft.

288

FAUCES AND PHARYNX
Anatomy

The junction between the mouth and the oropharynx is a narrow passageway (isthmus faucium) bounded superiorly by the soft palate, laterally by the anterior and posterior pillars of the fauces, and inferiorly by the tongue (Fig. 16-95). This circular area contains several clusters of lymphoid tissue and is referred to as Waldeyer's ring. It is composed of adenoids (nasopharyngeal tonsil), lateral pharyngeal bands, palatine tonsils, and lingual tonsils.

The pillars of the fauces are two vertically directed projections that descend from the soft palate. The anterior pillar is the *glossopalatine arch*, and the posterior pillar is the *pharyngopalatine arch*. These arches form a somewhat triangular space between them called the *tonsillar niche*, which contains the *palatine tonsils*. The anterior pillar ends at the lateral part of the base of the tongue, and contains the palatoglossal muscle. The posterior pillar gradually flattens out on the lateral wall of the pharynx and contains the palatopharyngeal muscle.

The *pharynx* is a mucous membrane–lined tubular space subdivided for descriptive purposes into three parts. From above downward, these are the *nasopharynx*, the *oropharynx*, and the *laryngopharynx* (Fig. 16-96). The pharynx consists of a posterior wall and two lateral walls, all of which are continuous and fuse anteriorly on each side with the posterior pillars of the fauces.

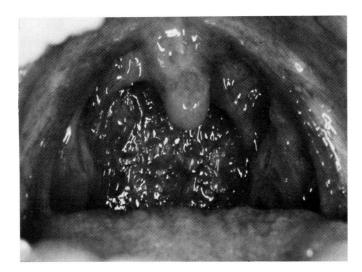

Fig. 16-95. Normal oropharynx with prominent palatine tonsils.

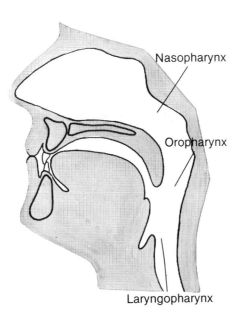

Nasopharynx

Oropharynx

Laryngopharynx

Fig. 16-96. Major divisions of pharynx.

The fauces and oropharynx show marked variation in form and size. The quantity and size of the lymphoid tissue in Waldeyer's ring vary greatly from one individual to another and from time to time in the same individual. Generally there is a physiologic enlargement in children that gradually decreases in adult life. Of course, lymphoid tissue enlarges dramatically in response to infections and other immunologic stress or stimulation.

The palatine tonsils usually form the major aggregate of lymphoid tissue in the oropharynx. Normally the tonsils do not protrude much beyond the limits of the tonsillar pillars. The palatine tonsils are present at birth and gradually increase in size until approximately the age of 12 years. Subsequently, they slowly atrophy. At times they become so small that it appears as if they have been removed. After a tonsillectomy remnants of tissue frequently persist in the tonsillar niche and are referred to as tonsillar tags.

The palatine tonsils are covered by a nonkeratotic stratified squamous epithelium that invaginates, forming deep crypts. These crypts may become filled with desquamated cells, lymphocytes, bacteria, other cellular detritus, and food particles. This material may appear as white or yellow spots on the tonsils and usually has a cheesy consistency. The covering mucosa of the tonsils is the same color as the other mucous membranes.

Soft palate function is intimately coordinated with the pharynx in a constrictor mechanism functioning as the velopharyngeal valve. The actions of this mechanism are essential for normal swallowing and speech.

The mucosal surface of the fauces and oropharynx is normally moist. The soft, smooth surface mucosa may show small elevated aggregates of lymphoid tissue (subepithelial lymphoid tissue) scattered randomly over the oropharynx (Fig. 16-97).

The vascularity may be very prominent, and vascular dilation can influence the degree of redness of this area. The color is normally a bright pink.

Fig. 16-97. Several prominent aggregates of lymphoid tissue on posterior pharyngeal wall.

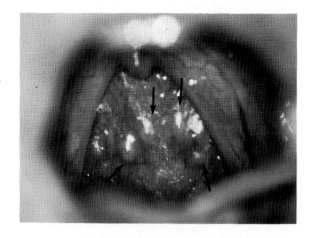

Examination

The oropharynx may be a difficult site to examine in some patients because of the relative small size of the fauces plus the obstruction from a large and difficult-to-control tongue. For inspection it is essential to depress the tongue with the aid of a tongue blade and to have an adequate light source that can be readily focused to cover the area from various angles.

It is extremely important for the examiner and patient to be at ease before this portion of the examination. The patient should be sitting erect and well back in the chair with the head projected slightly forward. The patient should open the mouth without protruding the tongue. The examiner should have a firm grasp on a tongue blade or mouth mirror and press its free end firmly down on the midpoint of the arched tongue, exerting a downward and forward pressure (Fig. 16-98).

The posterior placement of the tongue blade or mirror is critical. If it is too far posterior it may cause gagging, as well as press the tongue farther back. If the blade is placed anteriorly, it may cause posterior bulging of the tongue, which obstructs the view. Securing optimal inspection of the oropharynx usually requires several lateral placements of the tongue blade. The patient should be instructed to say "Ah," which will test the ninth and tenth cranial nerves by raising the soft palate. The uvula will be drawn upward in the midline.

Further inspection of the soft palate, together with the anterior and posterior pillars, tonsils, and posterior pharynx should be done, noting the color, symmetry, and evidence of exudate, edema, ulceration, or tonsillar enlargement. Palpation of this area is usually difficult without the aid of topical anesthetics. However, the gag reflex is a highly variable reflex from one patient to another. Each patient must be evaluated independently according to any positive findings from the inspection.

On the posterior pharyngeal wall the prominent vascularity, together with the small aggregates of lymphoid tissue, may cause the beginning student to suspect inflammatory changes. The color of these small aggregates can vary from pink to red to yellow. Behind the posterior pillars one may find the lateral pharyngeal bands that extend from the nasopharynx downward toward the base of the tongue. These bands are also composed of lymphoid tissue.

Any positive or suspected findings from the dentist's examination of the oropharynx should demand referral to the patient's physician or to an otolaryngologist for consultation, diagnosis, and treatment.

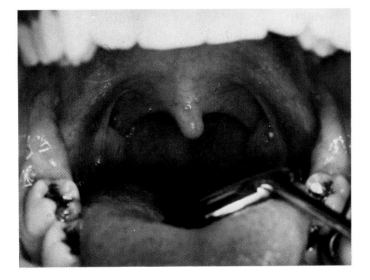

Fig. 16-98. Proper placement of mouth mirror on tongue to gain maximal view of oropharynx.

Abnormalities

Perhaps the most common abnormal finding of the oropharynx is inflammatory disease of bacterial or viral origin. This is usually characterized by erythema, edema, ulceration, and purulent exudate. The tonsillar crypts serve as a natural harbor for bacterial infections. Distinguishing between bacterial and viral pharyngitis may be difficult or impossible without the aid of laboratory cultures. Viral pharyngitis usually causes a generalized, dull, increased redness and enlargement of the lymphoid tissues without generalized edema or purulent exudates. Bacterial pharyngitis often has a more rapid onset, severe sore throat, high temperature, and bright red and edematous mucosa with obvious small tonsillar abscess formation. Cervical lymph nodes are commonly tender and enlarged.

Streptococcal pharyngitis is characterized by a brilliant red mucosa that ends abruptly near the back of the soft palate as if painted on. Abscess formation is not as prevalent as with staphylococcal infections.

Tonsils may be enlarged or hypertrophied without being infected. Acute tonsillitis is usually easy to recognize because of the pain, color change, abscess formation, and associated lymphadenopathy. Chronically enlarged tonsils from any source may interfere with respiration and swallowing and thereby be of concern to the dentist because of mouth breathing, tongue thrusting, and other muscular reflex habits affecting the dentition and oral health. Benign and malignant neoplasms can also arise from the tonsils and pharyngeal mucosa. Consequently, areas of erythroplasia or hyperkeratosis should be considered to have the same malignant potential as discussed for other oral sites. Generally, the more posterior the squamous carcinoma is located, the higher the grade and the poorer the prognosis.

Ulcers of the oropharynx may represent a wide range of entities, such as traumatic ulcers, RAU, or secondary lesions of vesiculoerosive diseases. Herpangina (apthous pharyngitis) is characterized by small vesicles that rupture to leave small aphthous-like ulcers that are usually limited in distribution to Waldeyer's ring.

Oral lesions of pemphigus often have a history of arising in the pharynx as bullae that rapidly rupture and result in areas of ulceration. Sore throat may be the first clinical symptom before more obvious oral lesions develop.

TONGUE
Anatomy

The tongue is a mobile muscular organ attached with its base and central part of its body to the floor of the mouth. The *body* of the tongue makes up the horizontal anterior two thirds of the organ. It has two surfaces: the *dorsal* (superior) surface (or dorsum) and the *ventral* (inferior) surface (Fig. 16-99). The base and body are separated by a shallow V-shaped groove, the *terminal sulcus,* which varies in prominence among individuals.

The dorsum is sometimes marked by a slight midline groove, the *median sulcus.* This runs from the anterior end to a depression near the apex of the terminal sulcus, the *foramen cecum* (Fig. 16-100). The mucosa of the dorsum forms numerous small elevations called papillae, giving the tongue a very characteristic roughened surface.

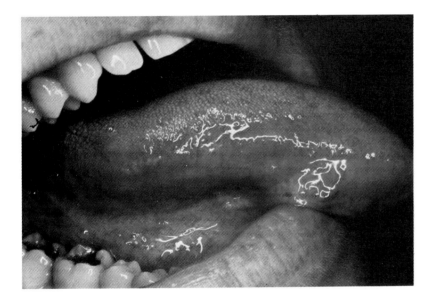

Fig. 16-99. Lateral view of body of tongue.

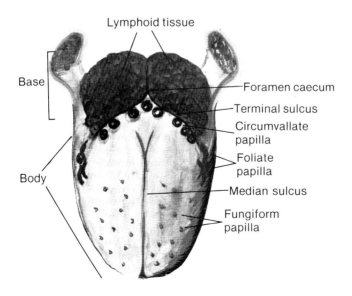

Fig. 16-100. Anatomic features of tongue.

Lymphoid tissue

Base

Body

Foramen caecum

Terminal sulcus

Circumvallate papilla

Foliate papilla

Median sulcus

Fungiform papilla

293

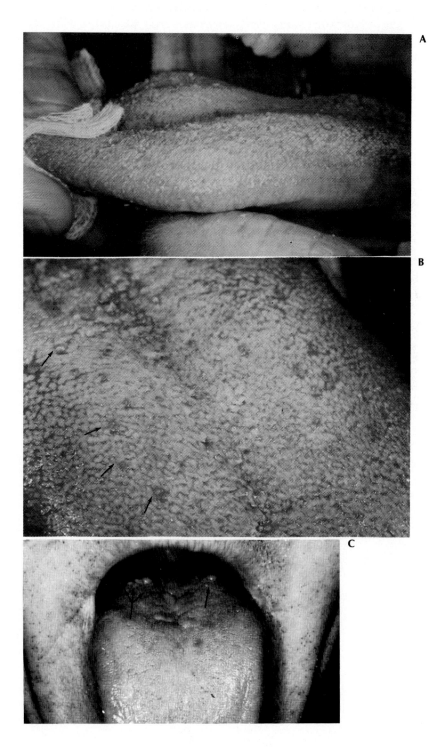

Fig. 16-101. A, Most numerous papillae are filiform. **B,** Scattered among filiform papillae are numerous fungiform papillae. **C,** Prominent circumvallate papillae.

There are three major types of papillae (Fig. 16-101): the filiform, the fungiform, and the circumvallate papillae. The *filiform papillae,* the most numerous, are slender, conical, pink structures that cover the dorsal surface. The degree of keratinization of the many filiform papillae and the presence of chromogenic bacteria are the major causes of color variation on the dorsal surface. The *fungiform papillae* are less numerous but are scattered widely along the sides and at the apex of the tongue. They are shaped like small mushrooms, with a rounded surface and deeper red color than the filiform papillae. The *circumvallate papillae* are the largest, but fewest in number, and are prominent because of

their deep red color. They form a V-shaped line just anterior and parallel to the terminal sulcus. They may be interpreted as pathologic.

The dorsal surface is fairly uniform in appearance, soft to palpation, and grayish pink with no or minimal racial variation.

The *base* or root of the tongue makes up the posterior one third and is the more fixed, vertical part of the organ. It is more closely associated with the oropharynx than with the oral cavity proper. The mucous membrane covering the base is thick and presents an irregular rough surface because of underlying prominences of lymphoid tissue, the lingual tonsils (Fig. 16-102; see also Fig. 16-100).

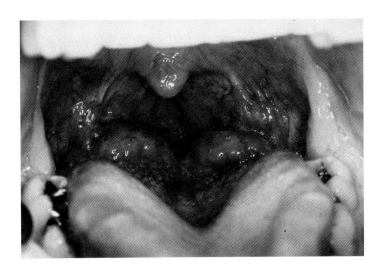

Fig. 16-102. Extremely large lingual tonsils projecting from posterior third of tongue.

The ventral surface is smooth with a thin mucous membrane, tightly adherent to the tongue musculature. The mucosal surface reflects onto the floor of the mouth. In the midline there is a distinct, elevated mucosal fold called the *lingual frenulum,* which attaches the free portion of the tongue to the floor of the mouth. The normal color varies from pink to red. There may be large prominent veins on this surface, which will cause a bluish color (Fig. 16-103).

The lateral border of the tongue usually shows a sharp contrast in texture and color where the dorsum and ventral surfaces merge. There is a deeper red color as the dorsal papillae end and the smooth ventral surface begins.

At the posterior part of the lateral border there may be irregular, vertically elevated folds of mucosa, the *foliate papillae.* The prominence of these structures exhibits a wide range of variation from one individual to another (Fig. 16-104), but they are usually bilaterally symmetrical.

Fig. 16-103. Normal ventral surface of tongue with prominent lingual frenulum and lingual veins.

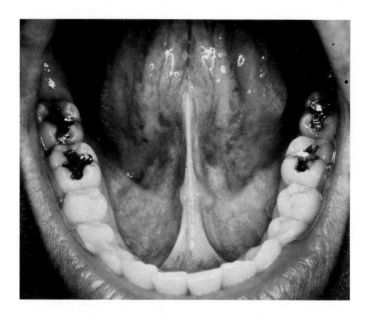

A

B

C

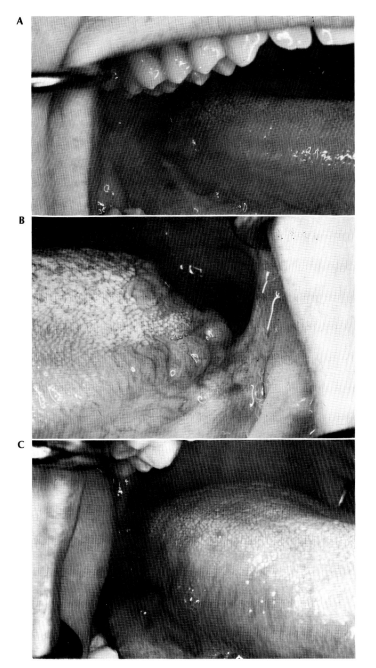

Fig. 16-104. A and **B,** Several variations in size of foliate papillae. **C,** Absence of foliate papillae.

Examination

Thorough examination of the tongue requires both careful visual inspection and palpation. The tongue should be inspected in its normal resting position and then in a protruded position. The ability to protrude the tongue varies considerably from one patient to another, and it is rare that a patient can voluntarily protrude the tongue adequately for thorough examination. The examiner should grasp the end of the tongue with a gauze sponge in order to gently retract and manipulate the full length of the tongue while inspecting and palpating with the index finger of the other hand (Fig. 16-105). The tongue is primarily muscle and should have the same consistency throughout on palpation. The posterior lateral margins are an extremely important area to view and palpate, since the presence of prominent foliate papillae causes the surface to be very irregular. Oral cancer may arise in this area as a rather subtle textural or color change. Superficial erosions or ulceration of this area should be palpated carefully for any signs of induration.

Fig. 16-105. Retraction of tongue for inspection and palpation.

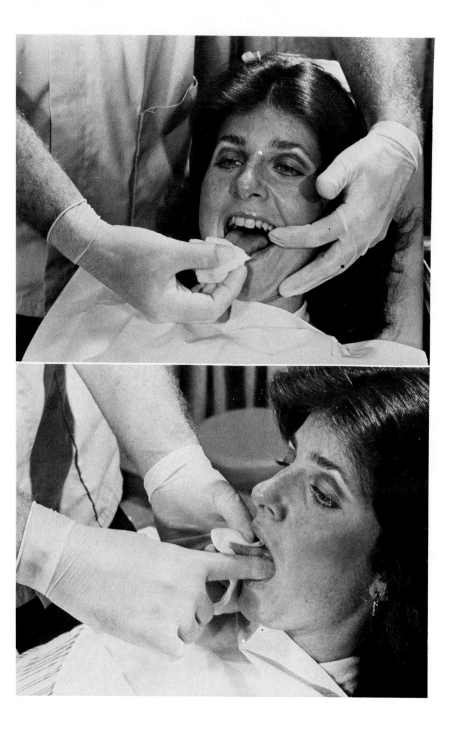

The dorsal surface textural features, specifically referred to as the coating of the tongue, has received a lot of emphasis in the past as an indicator of various systemic health problems. Actually, the coating, which indicates varying degrees of keratinization of the filiform papillae, varies rather markedly among individuals. Generally, excessive keratinization of the papillae is of little significance other than the possible cosmetic appearance of a heavily coated tongue. Hairy tongue (Fig. 16-106) represents an extreme keratinization that usually becomes secondarily stained by tobacco, food dyes, and chromogenic bacteria, resulting in an unsightly coating that varies in color from black to brown to gray.

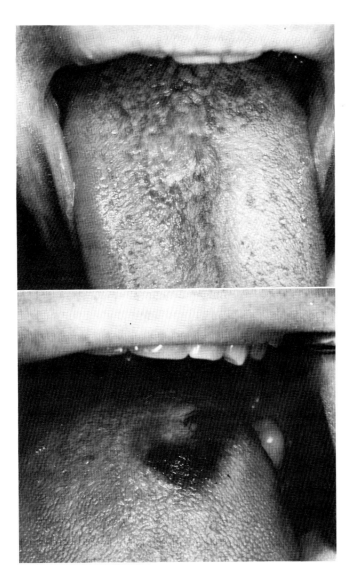

Fig. 16-106. Two examples of hairy tongue.

Less dramatic color changes may be associated with the use of lozenges and medications containing bismuth (Fig. 16-107).

The loss or absence of papillae on the dorsum is also highly variable among individuals. This may be a significant finding in some patients.

Evaluation of the mobility of the tongue is an important part of the examination. In children an abnormal lingual frenulum can restrict the mobility of the tongue, resulting in swallowing and speech abnormalities. An extremely short frenulum, which markedly limits tongue movement, is referred to as ankyloglossia (Fig. 16-108).

Limited mobility, deviation on protrusion, or atrophy, in the absence of any specific disease or lesion of the tongue, may indicate a disturbance of the hypoglossal (twelfth) nerve.

Fig. 16-107. Black discoloration of dorsum of tongue following use of antacid preparation containing bismuth.

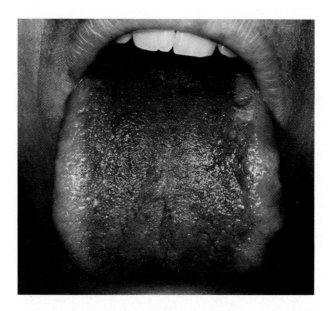

Fig. 16-108. Ankyloglossia.

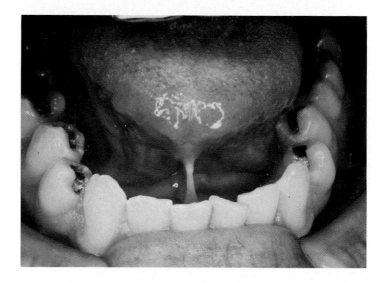

Abnormalities

Macroglossia is a generalized symmetrical enlargement of the tongue that may be a developmental abnormality or may be associated with conditions such as cretinism, mongolism, myxedema, acromegaly, and amyloidosis. A clinical sign often associated with macroglossia is crenation, or scalloping of the borders, caused by pressure of the enlarged tongue against the teeth. This may in turn cause diastema between the teeth (Fig. 16-109). Asymmetric macroglossia may result from hemangioma, lymphangioma, or neurofibroma involvement (Fig. 16-110). Some instances of macroglossia may be transient changes, as occur in angioedema, hematoma, or drug reactions.

Fissured or scrotal tongue (Fig. 16-109) is the presence of numerous grooves or crevices in the dorsal surface and lateral margins. These may tend to increase with age and, other than the problem of entrapment of food and bacteria, are seldom significant.

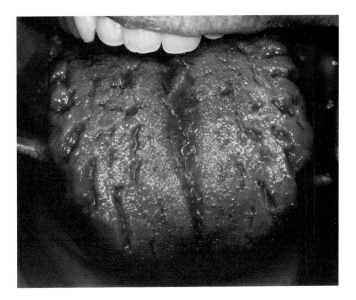

Fig. 16-109. Macroglossia with deep fissures (fissured tongue) and crenated lateral margins.

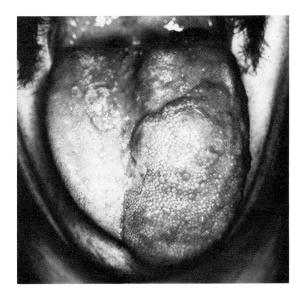

Fig. 16-110. Macroglossia of half of tongue because of hemangioma.

Two conditions of the tongue are characterized by the partial loss of normal papillae. Median rhomboid glossitis may occur as a flat lesion on the posterior dorsum of the tongue, involving the midline, usually in the area of the foramen cecum. The area is devoid of normal papillae and may have various outline patterns. Occasionally the condition may appear as an elevated, nodular, or mammillated change but again without the normal surface papillae (Fig. 16-111). Median rhomboid glossitis has been considered a developmental disturbance. However, recent studies indicate that it may be a transitory condition caused by candidiasis.

Migratory glossitis or geographic tongue is a common condition (Fig. 16-112). The typical lesions of migratory glossitis are circinate red areas with white borders. On the dorsum of the tongue the red areas result from the loss of filiform papillae, and the white borders are due to hyperkeratosis of filiform papillae just before exfoliation. The name refers to the periodic changes in the outline of the lesions, the condition tending to be chronic with periods of complete spontaneous remission. Histological-ly, the changes are similar to those seen in psoriasis of the skin. In recent years similar lesions to those seen on the lateral borders and ventral surface of the tongue have been reported occurring on the floor of the mouth, buccal mucosa, and vestibular sulcus. This has been called benign migratory stomatitis, stomatitis areata migrans, and erythema migrans oralis.

Fig. 16-111. Median rhomboid glossitis.

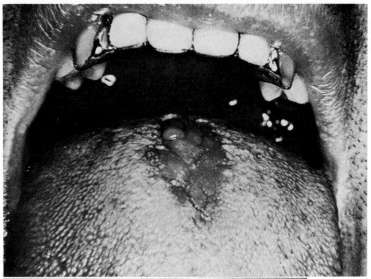

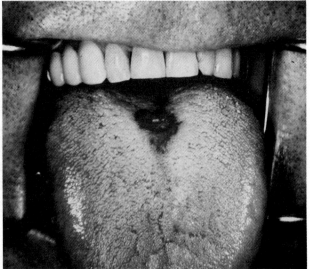

A diffuse or focal loss or atrophy of tongue papillae results in a bald, smooth, slick textural appearance. This change may be associated with nutritional deficiencies, especially vitamin B deficiency, iron deficiency anemia, and pernicious anemia; it may also result from physical, thermal, or chemical injuries or drug reactions.

The complaint of painful tongue (glossodynia) or burning tongue (glossopyrosis) may accompany the loss of papillae in the conditions listed above. Many times the complaint of painful or burning tongue is not accompanied by any textural or color change, and the possibility of a psychosomatic cause must be considered.

Fibromas are localized elevated lesions that frequently occur on the lateral margins of the tongue (Fig. 16-113). There is often an association with trauma. These may be pedunculated or sessile but usually have an intact normal mucosal surface.

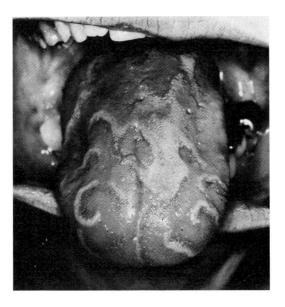

Fig. 16-112. Migratory glossitis (geographic tongue).

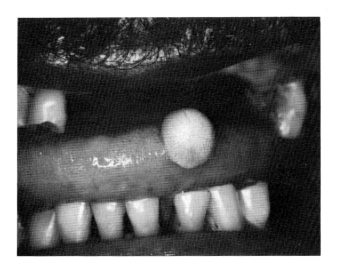

Fig. 16-113. Irritation fibroma.

Hemangiomas and lymphangiomas can vary considerably in their size, from extensive lesions to well-circumscribed lesions (Figs. 16-110 and 16-114). The blue to purple color change is usually helpful in suspecting a vascular lesion. It is compressible and may blanch.

Varices are much smaller, localized elevated lesions that may occur on the lateral borders or ventral surface of the tongue. These also have a blue to purple color and are usually sessile lesions (Fig. 16-115). Lingual varicosities are fairly common on the ventral surface of the tongue, particularly in older individuals, but are usually not significant changes (Fig. 16-116).

In addition to the prominent lingual tonsils that are present on the dorsal surface of the tongue posterior to the terminal sulcus, lymphoid aggregates can be seen along the lateral borders in addition to the foliate papillae. These may appear as pink or yellow, single or multiple, usually pedunculated papules or nodules (Fig. 16-117).

Fig. 16-114. Hemangioma.

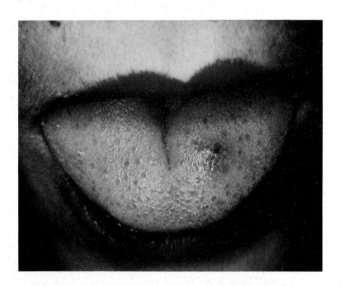

Fig. 16-115. Varix on lateral margin of tongue.

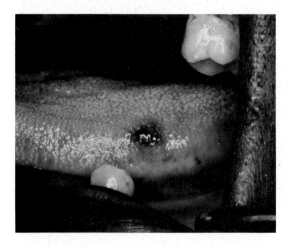

Occasionally, in the midline of the dorsal surface near the foramen cecum, a sessile nodule indicating lingual thyroid may be found. Since this may represent the only thyroid tissue present in the body, radioisotope studies are indicated before biopsy or excision of the mass (Fig. 16-118).

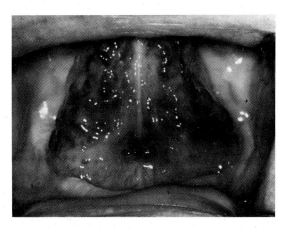

Fig. 16-116. Varicosities of sublingual veins, also referred to as phlebectasia linguae or caviar spots

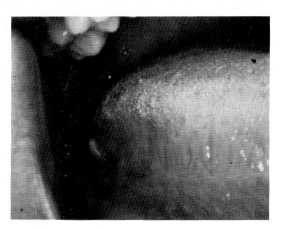

Fig. 16-117. Pedunculated yellow papule on lateral border of tongue. Diagnosis: Lymphoid tissue.

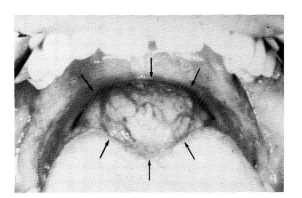

Fig. 16-118. Lingual thyroid mass on dorsum of tongue.

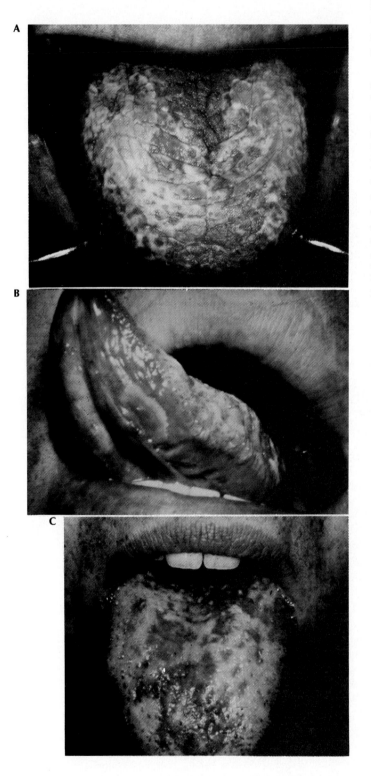

White plaques of the tongue may indicate lichen planus, candidiasis, hyperkeratosis, or mucous patches of secondary syphilis or other diseases (Fig. 16-119). Careful examination and evaluation are necessary to make a definitive diagnosis.

Ulcers of the tongue can also indicate a diverse spectrum of disease. Traumatic ulcers, minor and major aphthous stomatitis, primary herpetic stomatitis, erosive lichen planus, erythema multiforme, syphilis, tuberculosis, and mycotic diseases are some of the diseases that may appear as ulceration of the tongue. Aphthous ulcers are commonly found involving the lateral borders and ventral surface. These are usually quite painful and have the same morphologic characteristics as those described on the labial mucosa (Fig. 16-120).

Fig. 16-119. A, Lichen planus. **B,** Mucous patch of syphilis. **C,** Allergy to antibiotics.

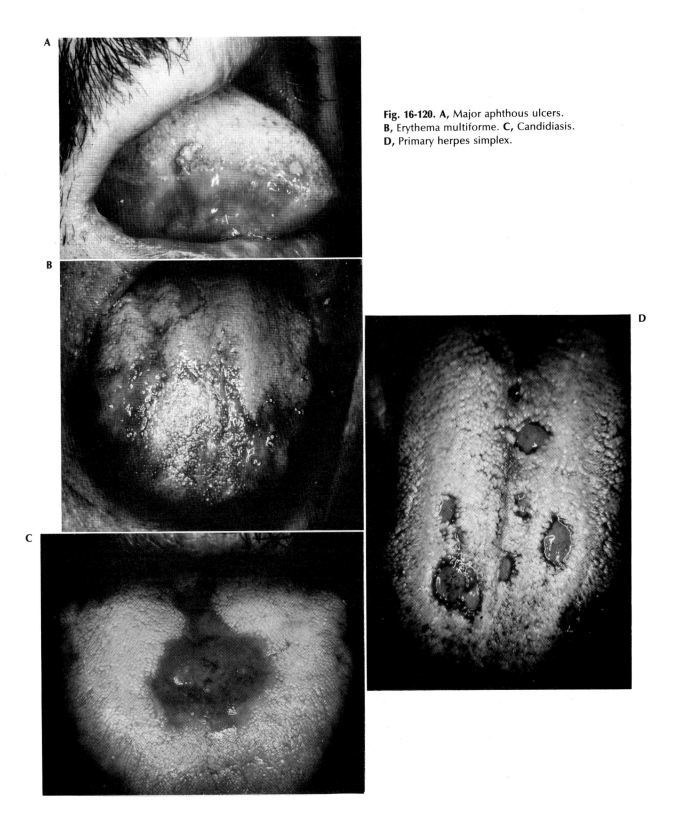

Fig. 16-120. A, Major aphthous ulcers.
B, Erythema multiforme. **C,** Candidiasis.
D, Primary herpes simplex.

Erosive lichen planus is usually seen as a superficial ulceration that may arise as bullae. These ulcerations vary greatly in size and shape. Usually, there are typical papular lesions of the reticular type of lichen planus involving either the tongue or other sites (Fig. 16-121).

Traumatic ulcers vary considerably in size and depth (Fig. 16-122). Some traumatic ulcers of the tongue can be chronic and resistant to therapy and may simulate carcinoma.

Major aphthae (periadenitis mucosa necrotica recurrens), primary syphilis (chancre), tuberculosis, and mycotic ulcers are frequently deep and irregular ulcers that involve the tongue.

As was mentioned previously carcinoma of the tongue may vary from a white plaque to a superficial erosion of various size, shape, and depth of ulceration. Induration of the borders is characteristic of carcinoma, but other deep ulcers, particularly on the tongue, may also have this feature.

Fig. 16-121. Erosive lichen planus.

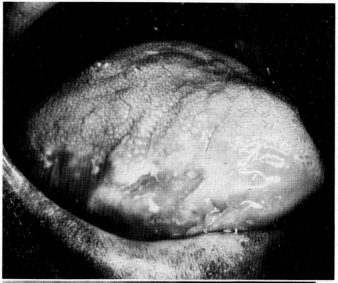

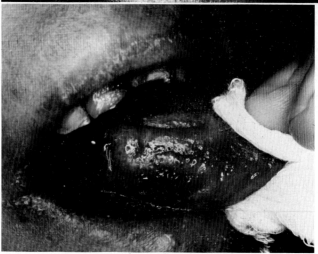

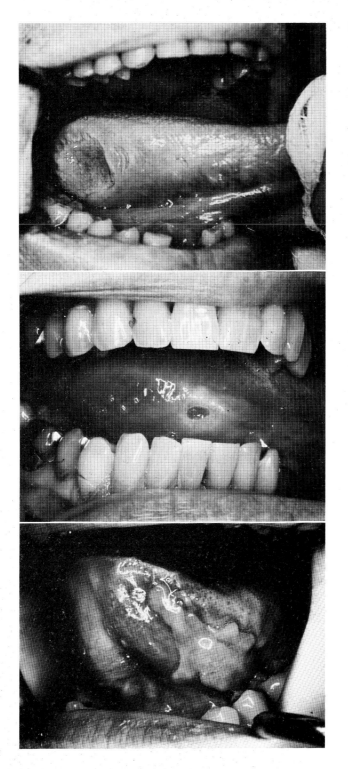

Fig. 16-122. Traumatic ulcers.

FLOOR OF MOUTH
Anatomy

The inferior boundary of the oral cavity proper is the floor of the mouth. When the tongue is elevated, there is a horseshoe-shaped space that extends laterally and anteriorly from the tongue to the alveolar mucosa of the mandible. This is the floor of the mouth. The mucosa is nonkeratinized, soft, and smooth except for the sub-lingual ridges (Fig. 16-123). A number of important anatomic structures are located beneath the surface in the lateral spaces formed by the lingual frenulum. Each of these lateral spaces contains the *genioglossus* and *genio-hyoid muscles,* the *sublingual gland,* and its ducts (Fig. 16-124). These lateral spaces also contain the upper portion of the *submandibular glands* and their ducts, nerves, lymph nodes, and

Fig. 16-123. Normal floor of mouth.

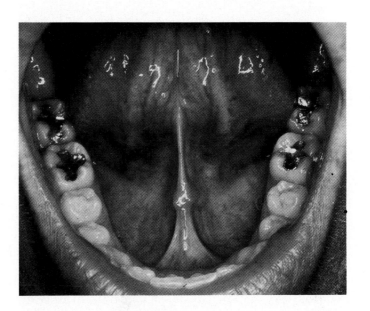

Fig. 16-124. Cross-section illustration of anatomic structures in floor of mouth.

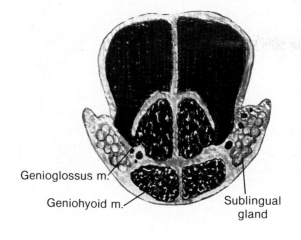

Genioglossus m.

Geniohyoid m.

Sublingual gland

abundant fat tissue (Fig. 16-125). The underlying important structures influence the surface features of the floor mucosa. The sublingual glands and the ducts of the submandibular glands cause bilateral elevations close to the lingual frenulum that are called the *sublingual folds* or ridges. Each sublingual fold ends anteriorly in a small round papilla called the *sublingual caruncle* (Fig. 16-126). These carun- cles contain openings for the flow of secretions of the submandibular and sublingual glands. Minor sublingual ducts open along the crest of the sublingual fold. The color of the floor mucosa is pink, with minimal or no racial difference. The vascular network may vary in prominence.

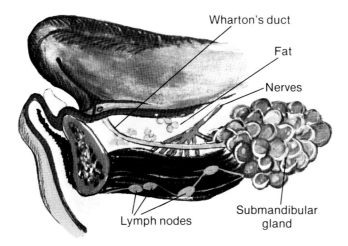

Fig. 16-125. Lateral view of floor of mouth.

Wharton's duct

Fat

Nerves

Submandibular gland

Lymph nodes

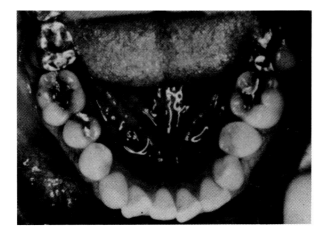

Fig. 16-126. Sublingual folds and caruncles.

Examination

Inspection of the floor of the mouth can begin by having the patient open the mouth and touch the tip of the tongue against the anterior hard palate. The examiner can readily evaluate the lingual frenulum for its length and position of attachment, as well as inspect the surface mucosa, sublingual folds, and caruncles. It is important to reflect the light with the mouth mirror to adequately inspect the mucosa at the anterior aspect of the floor and lingual gingiva (Fig. 16-127).

To inspect the distal aspects of the floor, the examiner should carefully retract the tongue (Fig. 16-128) away from the mandible with the aid of a mouth mirror. Adequate lighting is essential to carefully evaluate the mucosa for the most subtle textural or color change. As was mentioned for the posterior lateral aspects of the tongue, carcinoma arising in the floor of the mouth can cause a minimal surface change in the early stages of the disease (Fig. 16-129).

Fig. 16-127. Using mouth mirror to reflect light to most anterior portion of floor of mouth.

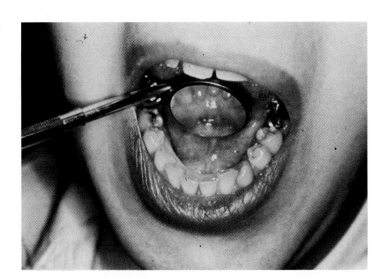

Fig. 16-128. Using mouth mirror to retract tongue for better view of posterior floor of mouth. Arrows indicate a subtle textural change, which was carcinoma.

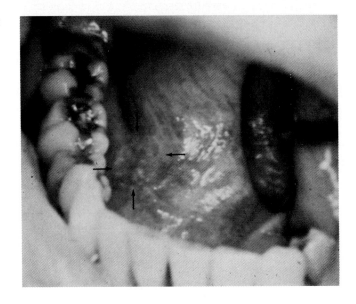

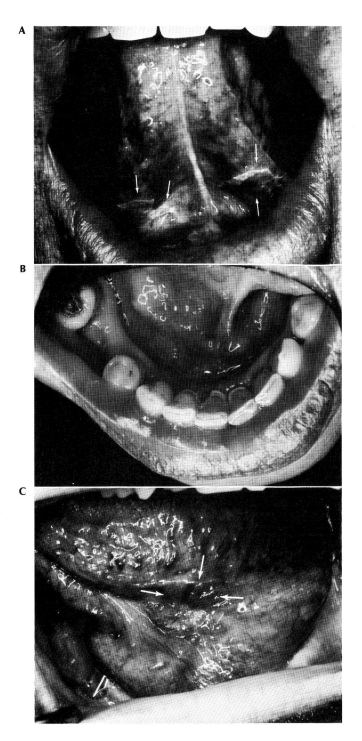

Fig. 16-129. A, Subtle white change. Diagnosis: Carcinoma in situ. **B,** Erythematous change. Diagnosis: Carcinoma. **C,** Superficial ulcer. Diagnosis: Carcinoma.

The examination of the floor is not complete without careful palpation of the entire sublingual and submandibular fossa areas. This is best accomplished by bimanual palpation (Fig. 16-130). It is important that the patient be relaxed as much as possible with the head in an upright position. Using the index finger of one hand, the examiner palpates against the supporting fingers of the opposite hand. Alternating the hands between the left and right sides allows an easier and more complete examination with minimal discomfort to the patient.

With experience, the examiner will become familiar with the normal consistency of the sublingual tissues, including the sublingual glands, the submandibular ducts and glands, the geniomuscles, and the varying amount of fat that may be found in the floor. Any abnormal consistency of these tissues, swellings, or submucosal masses should be further evaluated to rule out a disease.

In some edentulous patients who have had marked resorption of the alveolar process, the geniomuscle group can be extremely prominent, and extended calcification of the geniotubercles may cause a hard, slightly elevated mass to be palpable in the anterior floor of the mouth.

The periphery of the horseshoe-shaped floor of the mouth becomes confluent with the lingual alveolar mucosa, and this area is conveniently inspected and palpated at the same time as the floor.

Fig. 16-130. Bimanual palpation of floor of mouth.

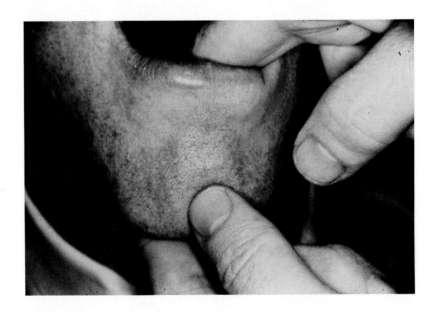

Abnormalities

Sialadenitis is inflammation of the salivary glands. This more commonly affects the submandibular gland, and the gland may be tender to palpation and enlarged. The patient may complain of increased swelling at mealtime or during salivary flow stimulation. Blockage of the duct with mucous plugs or various-sized sialoliths may be the cause. The stones may be palpated or seen on occlusal radiographs. Inflammation of the duct, referred to as sialodochitis, usually results from blockage or retrograde infections (Fig. 16-131). Two common abnormalities seen in the floor of the mouth are the mucous retention phenomenon (mucocele) and the mucous retention cyst (Fig. 16-132). Hippocrates used the Greek word *ranula,* meaning "little frog," to describe this lesion because it looks like a frog's belly. It usually appears as a soft, sessile, blisterform lesion varying in size from one to several centimeters. It may be pink or bluish in color with a translucent character caused by the mucous content.

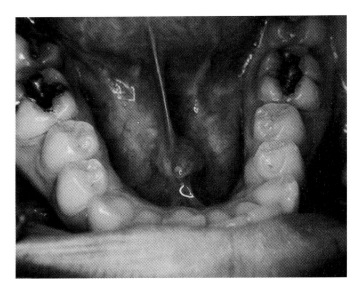

Fig. 16-131. Blockage and inflammation of Wharton's duct associated with small sialolith.

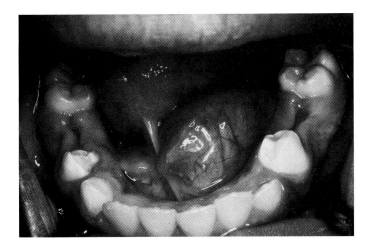

Fig. 16-132. Mucous retention cyst.

Occasionally, dermoid cysts may involve the floor. They also appear as a sessile, fluid-filled mass, but they are usually more opaque, firmer in consistency, and less likely to fluctuate in size than the mucocele (Fig. 16-133).

Neoplasms arising from the salivary glands or connective tissue may also appear as sessile lesions but are usually much more firm to palpation. These would likely interfere with normal tongue mobility or with the swallowing reflex.

Of course, cellulitis from the mandibular teeth may spread into the spaces of the floor of the mouth and can vary in consistency, but usually the classic signs of acute inflammation are present.

A unique lesion, a small lymphoepithelial cyst, occurs in the floor of the mouth as a yellow submucosal nodule. It seldom exceeds 2 cm in overall diameter.

Most of the other significant changes that occur in the floor of the mouth relate to possible carcinoma. Because of the possible rapid metastasis via the lymphatics, which may be ipsilateral, contralateral, or bilateral, early detection of carcinoma in this site as well as in the posterior tongue cannot be overemphasized.

Color changes, particularly red or white, that cannot be readily explained as inflammatory or traumatic should be evaluated carefully. White plaques or red and white plaques should usually be biopsied without delay.

Ulcers that cannot be explained as inflammatory or traumatic should also be biopsied for definitive diagnosis.

BIBLIOGRAPHY

Degowin, E.L., and Degowin, R.L.: Diagnostic examination, ed. 3, New York, 1976, Macmillan, Inc.

Prior, J.A., Silberstein, J.S., and Stang, J.: Physical diagnosis: the history and examination of the patient, ed. 6, St. Louis, 1981, The C.V. Mosby Co.

DuBrul, E.L.: Sicher's oral anatomy, ed. 7, St. Louis, 1980, The C.V. Mosby Co.

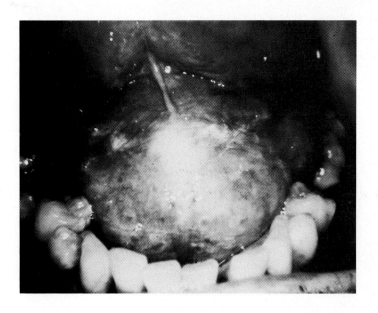

Fig. 16-133. Dermoid cyst.

17 Periodontium, dentition, and occlusion

PERIODONTIUM
Anatomy

The supporting tissues of the teeth are referred to collectively as the periodontium (from the Greek words *peri,* around; *odontos,* tooth). These tissues consist of the gingiva, periodontal ligament, cementum, alveolus, and supporting bone.

The functions of the periodontium are to:

1. Attach the tooth to the bony housing.
2. Resist and resolve forces of mastication, speech, and deglutition.
3. Maintain the integrity of the body surface by separating the external and internal environments.
4. Adjust for structural changes associated with wear and aging through continuous remodeling and regeneration.
5. Defend against the noxious external environmental influences that are present in the oral cavity.

Since the gingiva has been discussed previously, the following discussion focuses primarily on the other components of the periodontium. The free marginal gingiva and the interdental gingiva are usually the initial sites of gingival and periodontal disease. The free marginal gingiva and the coronal portion of the interdental gingiva are not attached to bone, but they are united organically through the junctional epithelium to the tooth surface. This union of the gingival soft tissue with the tooth has been a controversial issue for many years, but with the aid of electron microscopy the union of functional epithelial cells to the tooth surface by hemidesmosomes and a basal lamina has been established and demonstrated.

The attached gingiva is bound firmly by the periosteum to the alveolar bone and by the gingival collagen fibers to the cementum, resulting in its characteristic immobility.

Beneath the gingival attachment to the tooth, a complex network of gingival collagen fibers serves to suspend and attach the teeth in their alveolar root sockets. These fibers are organized into groups of fiber bundles. These bundles have been described classically on the basis of their location, origin, and insertion as the dentogingival, dentoperiosteal, alveologingival, circular, and transseptal fiber groups (Fig. 17-1).

The dentogingival fibers originate from the root cementum near the cementoeneamel junction, splay out into the gingiva in a coronal direction, and laterally terminate near the basal lamina of the free gingival margin. The dentoperiosteal fibers have the same origin, but they bend apically over the alveolar crest and insert into the buccal and lingual periosteum.

The alveolar gingival fibers originate from the crest of the alveolar bone and extend coronally, terminating in the free marginal gingiva. The circular fiber group passes circumferentially around the cervical region of the tooth into the free gingiva. The transseptal fibers originate from the cementum of one tooth, traverse the interdental bone, and insert into the cementum of the adjacent tooth. The transseptal fibers collectively form an interdental ligament connecting all the teeth of the arch. These fibers appear to be extremely important in maintaining the integrity of the dental arch. They rapidly reform after excision, but following inflammatory disease they usually re-form at a more apical level.

Beneath the fiber system, the periodontal ligament envelops the roots of the teeth (Fig. 17-1). The periodontal ligament is differentiated from the loose connective tissues investing the tooth bud, the dental follicle. It forms as the tooth develops, erupts into the oral cavity, and completes its final form on the tooth reaching occlusion. The mature periodontal ligament is organized into the principal and secondary fiber bundles. The principal bundles traverse the periodontal space obliquely and insert into the cementum and alveolar bone as Sharpey's fibers. The secondary bundles are randomly oriented between the principal bundles.

The periodontal ligament and space contain a rich network of blood vessels, lymphatics, and nerves.

Cementum forms the interface between root dentin and the connective tissue fibers of the periodontal ligament. It is a specialized calcified tissue that has many similarities to bone from a structural standpoint but differs in several functional aspects. There is normally a primary layer of cementum enveloping the entire root surface that is cell free. Cementum deposition, like bone, does not cease after tooth development and eruption but continues intermittently throughout life. After tooth eruption, secondary cementum is deposited in response to functional demands. Secondary cementum may entrap cells and is usually less uniform than primary cementum.

Cementum may be fibrillar or afibrillar. Fibrillar cementum usually has a dual collagen fiber system laid down by cementoblasts and oriented randomly or parallel to the root surface. These fibers, which form the intrinsic fiber system, are interwoven with the principal fibers of the periodontal ligament (Sharpey's fibers) as the tooth erupts and reaches functional occlusion. Sharpey's fibers then form an extrinsic fiber system, which is produced by fibroblasts.

The remaining structure of the periodontium is the alveolar bone (Fig. 17-1). The alveolar processes are the thin bony plates surrounding the roots that hold the roots; they are tooth-dependent structures. They develop as the teeth develop and are absorbed to a great extent following the loss of the teeth. The overall structure of the alveolar processes depends on tooth form and position. The alveolar bone, together with the fiber systems, has to withstand the forces of occlusion, mastication, deglutition, and phonation. The maintenance of heavy alveolar bone is the primary goal of preventive periodontics and periodontal therapy.

The alveolar bone begins formation by the deposition of calcium salts in localized areas of connective tissue matrix near the developing tooth buds. These foci continue to develop, enlarge, fuse, and remodel by a constant metabolism of osteoblastic and osteoclastic activity. This bone growth and remodeling continues at the demands of the developing and erupting teeth until the bone finally becomes a mature structure characterized by a buccal and lingual cortical plate, which encloses a delicate, interconnecting network of trabeculae and marrow-containing spaces. The thickness of the cortical plates varies considerably from one individual to another, as do the size, shape, and thickness of the trabeculae.

As the teeth erupt and the roots form, another cortical plate much thinner and more delicate than the buccal and lingual cortices is formed adjacent to the periodontal space, which is known as the lamina dura (Fig. 17-1). The multiple small openings scattered over the lamina dura create a sievelike structure. The openings, which come from the marrow spaces to communicate with those of the periodontal ligament, serve as foramina for the delicate vascular network.

The remaining bone of the mandible and maxilla, composed of the same buccal and lingual cortical plates and cancellous bone, is referred to as the alveolar supporting bone.

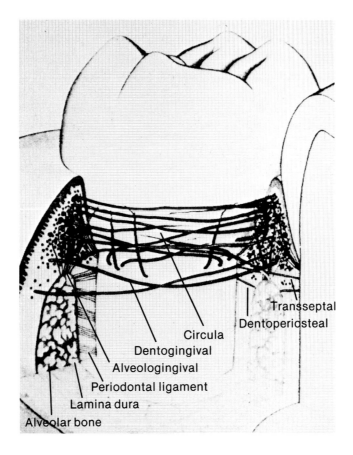

Fig. 17-1. Periodontal fiber system and alveolar bone.

Transseptal
Dentoperiosteal
Circula
Dentogingival
Alveologingival
Periodontal ligament
Lamina dura
Alveolar bone

Examination

Early recognition is, as in all preventive procedures, critical to diagnosis and optimal therapy of gingival and periodontal diseases. The examination of the periodontium requires not only inspection and palpation but also a very careful, systematic probing examination of the gingival sulcus around every tooth. In addition, a review of an adequate radiographic survey is essential to properly evaluate the continuity of the lamina dura, the periodontal ligament space, the height of the alveolar crest, and the surrounding character of bony trabeculation and marrow spaces.

In addition to the examination procedures described for the gingiva, particular care must be taken to evaluate the interproximal papillae for color, shape, and attachement. Normally the interdental papillae assume a pyramidal or conical shape in the anterior region but become more blunt and assume the shape of a col in the premolar and molar regions. The size and shape of the interdental space change with age and normal wear of the teeth; consequently the form of the papillae is altered to coincide with these changes.

Some type of periodontal chart is invaluable for recording the level of the gingiva, the depth of the surrounding gingival sulcus, and the level of the alveolar bone. Other findings that are pertinent to the evaluation of the periodontium are a measure of plaque and calculus deposits, mobility of the teeth, malposition of the teeth, and, of course, the absence of teeth and furcation involvement. Such a chart establishes the periodontal history at the time of examination. This becomes a baseline from which future examinations reveal the status of health, the process of disease, or the effects of treatment.

The periodontal probe is probably the most significant diagnostic "tool" in the evaluation of the periodontium (Fig. 17-2). The visual examination and the radiographic examination have various limitations that may become very obvious on the simple but direct procedure of probing for periodontal pockets. The probe should be small and calibrated so that millimeter measurement of pocket depth can be done. Most periodontal charts have horizontal lines of 1 mm gradations. The gingival margin should be outlined in its relationship to the cementoenamel junction. As a systematic continuous circumferential probing of each tooth is performed, a second line would indicate the pocket depth. This procedure must be done carefully with minimal discomfort to the patient to gain the maximal information. It is preferable to probe as nearly parallel to the long axis of the tooth as possible. If it is readily apparent that this is impossible as the contact area is approached, angulation of the probe is essential to evaluate these interradicular areas (Fig. 17-3). Another critical point in the probing examination is determining furcation involvement and extent of involvement. This may require a special instrument, such as a "cowhorn" explorer (Fig. 17-4).

The shape of the crown and roots, the position of the teeth in the dental arch, overhanging restorations, and developmental anomalies all serve to make the probing examination more difficult. The examiner must use sound judgment to compensate for these irregularities. The correlation of radiographic findings with the probing examination is vital to obtaining the most comprehensive periodontal evaluation.

The mobility of all teeth should be tested and a numerical reference used to indicate the degree of mobility. Teeth with a healthy periodontium will show normal physiologic mobility. Incisors tend to be more mobile than cuspids, premolars, and molars, indicating that the total surface of root attachment is important. Normal mobility of the teeth is greatest when one arises after sleep and decreases progressively during waking hours. A significant decrease in normal mobility is noted after chewing.

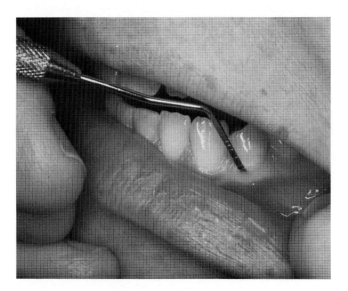

Fig. 17-2. Examination with periodontal probe.

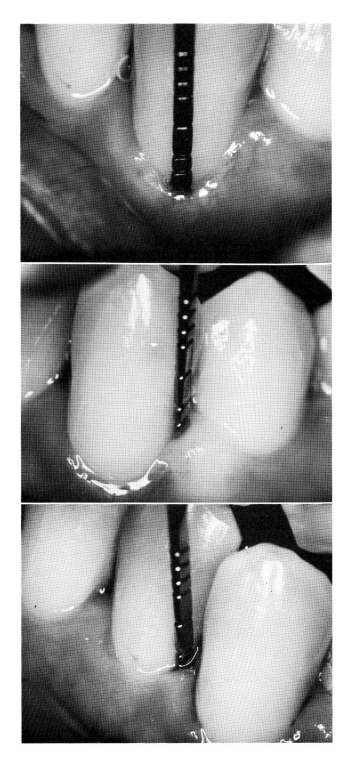

Fig. 17-3. Probing parallel to long axis of tooth in circumferential manner.

The most common approach to testing tooth mobility is to hold the crown of the tooth from the lingual surface with an instrument handle or finger and press on the facial surface with a second instrument handle (Fig. 17-5). The degree of mobility is scored on either a 1 to 4 or I to III scale, with the higher number indicating the greater movement both buccolingually and apically. Abnormal mobility findings must be carefully evaluated on an individual basis. Ex-cessive tooth mobility is generally an alarming sign of a disturbed attachment apparatus, most often related to alveolar bone loss, alteration in width of the periodontal ligament, or a combination of these factors. With the inexperienced examiner, the degree of mobility is often much less than would be expected from the initial cursory clinical and radiographic impressions.

Fig. 17-4. Using cowhorn-type explorer to determine furcation involvement.

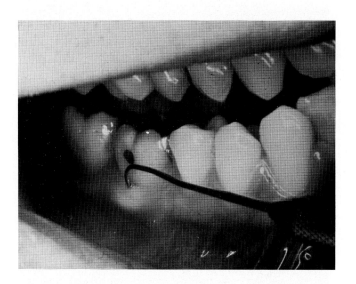

Fig. 17-5. Testing mobility of teeth using handles of two dental instruments.

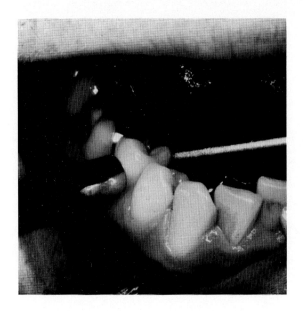

Abnormalities

The more common gingival abnormalities have been discussed. The range of clinical expression, the rate of progress of periodontal disease, and the interreaction of local and systemic factors constitute an extremely complex subject. Although much progress has been made in both prevention and treatment, the essential pathogenesis of periodontal disease is still not completely understood. It is now recognized that periodontal disease is not limited to middle-aged and older patients; thus, all practitioners of dentistry must be alert to early diagnosis and management.

There is much confusion in terminology and classification as a result of the relatively poor understanding of the causes and pathogenesis of the numerous diseases of the periodontium. For the most part, even in cases in which discrete clinical entities can be described, multiple causes may be at work. What may appear to be multiple distinct diseases may in fact be only stages of the same disease modified in expression by time and individual response.

To resolve the nomenclature and classification problems, the American Academy of Periodontolgy formed a Committee on Nomenclature. The efforts of this committee have resulted in clarification of many aspects of the nomenclature problem.[3]

A classification of periodontal diseases based on the clinical manifestations, pathologic alterations, and causes was devised (Table 5). The diseases were designated as inflammatory, degenerative, atrophic, hyperplastic, and traumatic. Two inflammatory lesions were acknowledged. Gingivitis was defined as the inflammatory lesion confined to the tissues of the marginal gingiva, and periodontitis was the term accepted to describe the inflammatory lesion extending into the deeper tissues.

Gingivitis was subclassified on the basis of its presumed causes into local and systemic forms. Locally caused forms of gingivitis included those resulting from food impaction, calculus, irritating restorations, and drug reactions. Gingivitis with systemic causes included lesions seen in pregnant women and in individuals with various systemic diseases, such as diabetes, endocrine dysfunctions, tuberculosis, syphilis, and leukemia. Additional systemic causes included drug reactions, allergies, and hereditary predisposition. Cases that could not be resolved etiologically were classified as idiopathic. In general, this approach to classifying the various forms of gingivitis continues to be used.

Subdivision of periodontitis into simplex and complex forms as originally suggested by Box was accepted. *Periodontitis simplex* was defined as the lesion evolving from gingivitis and resulting principally from local factors. It progresses relatively slowly, exhibiting shallow wide-mouthed pockets distributed throughout the mouth, with generalized bone loss. The pockets are generally filled with plaque and debris, and there is an acute inflammatory reaction in the gingiva. The inflammatory reaction is most apparent in the perivascular areas, and it progresses into the alveolar bone and eventually into the periodontal membrane through the perivascular tissues. Periodontitis complex was considered to be caused predominantly by systemic disease or to be a periodontitis of local origin superimposed on a base of periodontosis. When the cause is apparent, the disease is named accordingly as tubercular, diabetic, leukemic, or syphilitic. When the cause is inapparent or not known, the disease is classified as idiopathic. The lesion can be further subclassified as acute, chronic, ulcerative, purulent, or suppurative.

Table 5. Periodontal disturbances

Type	Disturbance
Inflammatory	Gingivitis (local origin, systemic origin)
	Periodontitis (simplex, complex)
Degenerative	Periodontosis (systemic, hereditary, idiopathic)
Atrophic	Periodontal atrophy (traumatic, presenile, senile, caused by disuse, idiopathic, inflammatory)
Hypertrophic	Gingival hyperplasia (chronic irritational, drug-induced, genetic, idiopathic)
Traumatic	Periodontal traumatism

Periodontosis was accepted as a general term and defined to include degenerative noninflammatory destruction of any one or more of the tissues of the periodontium. The characteristics of periodontosis include (1) loosensing and migration of the teeth in the presence or absence of secondary epithelial proliferation and (2) pocket formation or secondary gingival disease. The disease was considered to have three pathologic stages: (1) the connective tissue fibers degenerate, and the ligament space widens; (2) the epithelium near the sulcus proliferates and migrates apically to deepen the sulcus and convert it into a pocket; and (3) the attachment completely separates from the tooth, leaving a deep pocket.

Periodontal atrophy was accepted as an entity separate from periodontitis and defined as a decrease in the size of an organ or part by virtue of the loss of its cellular elements after it has attained mature size. Two forms of atrophy were distinguished. *Gingival recession* is the most commonly observed form of periodontal atrophy. In this condition there is a noninflammatory loss of periodontal tissue, with concurrent apical movement of the soft tissue attachment to the tooth without pocket formation. The causes may include trauma (for example, from the vigorous long-term use of a hard-bristled toothbrush), excessive occlusal forces, and aging. A second form is *atrophy of disuse,* in which the functional forces have been removed from the tooth and in which there is a loss of alveolar bone and the principal fibers of the periodontal ligament without gingival recession; the alveolar bone proper persists, but the supporting bone trabeculae become thin and finally disappear as the marrow spaces increase in size. The ligament space becomes narrowed, and new cementum is deposited.

Periodontal traumatism was defined as a form of pressure necrosis characterized by thrombosis, hemorrhage and resorption of the bone and cementum, resulting from mechanical trauma. The affected teeth may loosen, become sensitive to percussion, and contact prematurely in centric and excentric functional movements of the mandible. The term *primary occlusal traumatism* has been used when the affected teeth are otherwise healthy, the periodontium normal, and the force excessive; *secondary occlusal traumatism* is the term used for teeth around which the periodontium has been pathologically altered to the extent that otherwise normal occlusal forces cannot be tolerated.

Since publication of the intial recommendations of the American Academy of Periodontology, the accepted nomenclature and classification of the various periodontal diseases have undergone considerable change. In general, the changes have resulted from attempts to avoid vagueness in terminology and to attain simplification in classification.

The term *gingivitis* continues to be used to designate inflammatory lesions that are confined to the marginal gingiva, regardless of the cause. The types most frequently encountered are plaque-associated gingivitis, acute necrotizing ulcerative gingivitis, hormonal gingivitis, and drug-induced gingivitis. There is a consensus that periodontitis begins as gingivitis, although transient forms of gingivitis that may not progress to periodontitis appear to occur.

Although most investigators and clinicians agree that marginal periodontitis is not a homogeneous entity, it is no longer subclassified as periodontitis simplex and periodontitis complex. In spite of intensive efforts extending over several decades to refine the criteria, it has never been possible to definitively diagnose most cases of periodontitis as being one type or the other. This is not to deny that cases differ greatly with regard to the extent and distribution of lesions, the amount of associated plaque and calculus, the rate of progression, the age of the individuals affected, and the characteristic bone and soft tissue alterations. In addition, it is clear that while most cases respond well to therapeutic measures, such as improved oral hygiene, root planing, and pocket elimination, directed toward control of the growth and accumulation of plaque, significant numbers of cases do not respond to therapy, regardless of the aggressiveness with which it is applied. In spite of these differences, subclassification either according to local versus systemic etiologic factors or according to the superimposition of an inflammatory lesion on previously existent degenerative lesion does not appear to be justified. The data now available appear to support subclassification of marginal periodontitis into juvenile and adult types.

The meaning and usage of the term periodontosis remain controversial. The disease was considered to be a primary lesion of alveolar bone, to be noninflammatory in character except in the advanced stages, and to result from systemic or constitutional causes.

Periodontosis, as described by Gottlieb and subsequently by others, was considered to be noninflammatory degenerative lesion of the periodontium, occurring generally in the absence of debris or deposits on the teeth, and leading to migration, loosensing, and exfoliation of the teeth. It was generally conceived that in advanced stages the lesion could become complicated by the presence of inflammation. Gottlieb considered the lesion to result from a pathologic alteration in cementum, although other investigators believed that it could start as a noninflammatory degeneration of the principal fibers of the periodontal ligament. Systemic factors were considered to be the principal cause of the disease.

The general conclusion is that periodontosis, as it is usually defined, does not exist as a specific disease, but there seems little doubt that a form of periodontitis exhibiting features permitting definitive differentiation from the usual form does exist. The disease occurs principally in young people, especially adolescent girls, who are otherwise normal and healthy in all respects and who exhibit clean teeth; it appears to have a hereditary component. It has a predilection for the central incisors and first molars, but it is not confined to these teeth. The lesions, which may also affect the primary dentition, exhibit blatant inflammation; rapid progress; formation of isolated, deep, tortuous pockets; drifting and mobility of the teeth; and lack of response to standard therapeutic measures.

Several investigators have suggested classification of the disease as juvenile periodontitis in contrast to adult periodontitis. This subclassification of periodontitis appears to have a firm scientific basis. In addition to the distinctive clinicopathologic manifestations noted, the immune response of persons exhibiting the juvenile lesion appears to differ both from that of normal persons and from that of persons with the adult form of the disease.

There are many other osseous diseases that may affect the periodontium. These are considered to be beyond the realm of this book.

DENTITION
Anatomy

The dental anlagen develop at approximately 6 weeks of intrauterine life. The tooth germs or buds arise from the dental lamina, which consists of a U-shaped band in the maxilla and mandible of proliferating oral epithelium, extending into the underlying mesenchyme. Fig. 17-6 is a diagrammatic illustration of the series of subsequent events in the life cycle of a tooth. The normal primary dentition comprises 20 teeth, and the permanent dentition contains 32. Generally, the first primary teeth begin eruption into the oral cavity at 6 months of age, and by the age of 2 or 2½ years, the child has a full complement of 20 primary teeth. They function in the chewing apparatus for the greater part of 4 years and then are gradually resorbed and replaced by the permanent dentition.

As illustrated in Fig. 17-6, the dentition represents a continuous dynamic cycle involving multiple tissues. The developmental stages are dominated by dentogenesis (formation of dentin), amelogenesis (formation of enamel), and cementogenesis (formation of cementum). These processes represent the mineralized tissues of the dentition that enclose a soft tissue component (the dental pulp), which represents a highly vascularized and innervated connective tissue organ, rich in cells that have a pleuripotential capability. With eruption, function, and age the overall pulp size is gradually decreased, and the mineralized surfaces are subject to wear.

The general architecture of the teeth can be described as a structure consisting predominantly of dentin that has an enamel-covered crown portion with its coronal pulp chamber in the center and a cementum-covered root portion containing a central pulp canal. The pulp canal communicates with the periodontium at the apical foramen, which many times actually consists of multiple accessory foramina, as opposed to one central opening. At a slight constriction between the crown and root is the cervical line, or the cementoenamel junction. On the proximal surfaces of the teeth, the cementoenamel junction is convex in a coronal direction, thereby increasing the area of attachment of supporting fibers of the periodontium.

A distinction should be made between the terms *anatomic crown* and *clinical crown*. That part of the tooth that is exposed to the oral cavity at a given time is the clincial crown. In young patients not all the anatomic crown may be exposed because of the gradual eruption process. Normally the anatomic root is completely embedded and in organic connection with the periodontium, but in fact after early periodontal disease a portion of the root may be exposed to the oral cavity, together with the anatomic crown.

The color of the crown depends on the color and translucency of the enamel. Normally, enamel is a light yellow because the underlying dentin's yellow color is seen through the translucent enamel. The thickness and overall structure of the enamel can vary considerably, and consequently various shades of yellow to white will be seen in dentitions.

The dentition is divided into the anterior teeth, consisting of the central incisors, lateral incisors, and canines; and the posterior teeth, comprising the premolars and molars.

The terms used to designate the surfaces of teeth are essentially universally accepted. The surfaces of teeth are named according to the anatomic structures opposite them. These surface designations are: *labial* (next to or toward the lips; *buccal* (next to or toward the cheek); *lingual* (next to or toward the tongue); *proximal* (adjacent to another tooth in the same arch); *mesial* (proximal surface toward the median line); *distal* (proximal surface away from the median line); *incisal* (cutting edge of anterior teeth); and *occlusal* (biting surface of posterior teeth, made up of a variable number of elevations called *cusps*). The term *facial* is used as a collective term for both labial and buccal. It is preferred by some, since it avoids concern of whether it is applied to an anterior or posterior tooth.

Several different systems are used throughout the world for designating individual teeth. The three systems that have gained the most popularity are the Universal system, which was officially adopted by the ADA in 1968, the Palmer/Zsigmondy system, and the Federation Dentaire International (FDI) system.

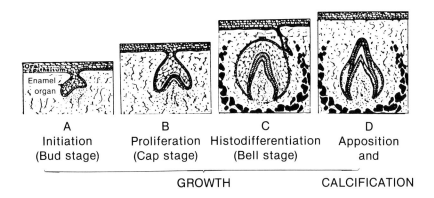

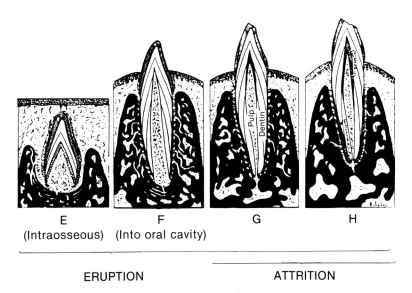

Fig. 17-6. Diagrammatic illustration of life cycle of tooth. Stage *C* shows active morphodifferentiation as well as histodifferentiation. (Modified from Schour and Massler.)

The Universal system is used by a number of dental schools, the federal services, and most insurance companies. In this system, each tooth in the permanent dentition is given a number from 1 to 32. The mandibular right third molar, for example, is number 32 (Fig. 17-7). The primary teeth are indicated in the same sequence, using capital letters A through T.

The Palmer/Zsigmondy system was taught by many dental schools in the past and is therefore still in common use throughout the world. This system uses a grid based on the quadrant in which the tooth is found. The teeth in each quadrant are numbered, with 1 being the central incisor and 8 being the third molar. The grid symbols are right angles derived from a standard quadrant diagram (Fig. 17-8). The number for the specific tooth is placed inside the grid symbol. The primary dentition is designated by using capital letters in place of numbers, with A being the central incisor and E the second molar.

The FDI system is more recent, and it combines the Palmer system with numbers used to designate the various quadrants. This results in a two digit code for each tooth, with the first digit representing the quadrant and the second representing the tooth. The permanent dentition has the quadrants numbered from 1 to 4, and the teeth in each quadrant are numbered 1 to 8 as in the Palmer system (Fig. 17-9). The primary dentition numbers the quadrants 5 through 8, and the teeth in each quadrant are numbered 1 to 5 instead of A through E.

A nomenclature of classification of cavity preparation was developed by Dr. J.V. Black and is now used to describe the tooth surfaces involved with caries; it also applies to dental restoration as follows:

Class I: Pit and fissure cavities on the occlusal surface of premolars and molars and lingual surfaces of maxillary incisors.

Class II: Cavities on the proximal surfaces of the premolars and molars.

Class III: Cavities on the proximal surfaces of incisors and canines that do not involve the incisal angle.

Class IV: Cavities on the proximal surfaces of incisors and canines that involve the incisal edge.

Class V: Cavities on the gingival third of the facial or lingual surfaces of all teeth.

Class VI: Cavities on the incisal edge of anterior teeth or on the occlusal cusp heights of posterior teeth.

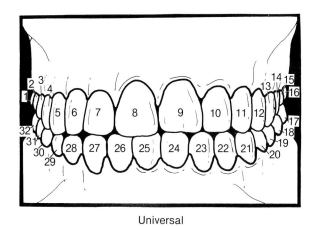

Fig. 17-7. Universal system.

Universal

Fig. 17-8. Palmer/Zsigmondy system.

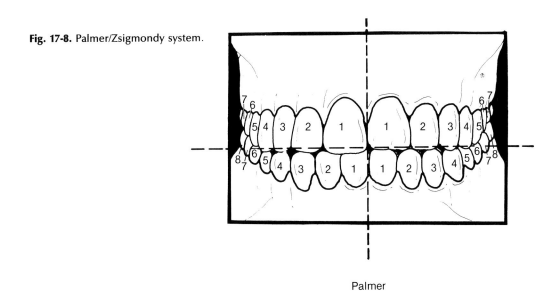

Palmer

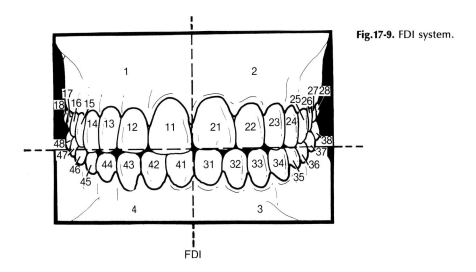

Fig.17-9. FDI system.

FDI

Examination

When the dentition is examined, the following factors should receive careful attention: number of teeth present, both erupted and unerupted; size, form, and structure of both crowns and roots; color of the crowns; contact relationship; and vitality. The examination of teeth can be separated into three different procedures according to the specific area that is being examined. When the examination procedures are divided into those that involve the (1) surface of the tooth, (2) pulp, and (3) periapex, it becomes apparent that somewhat different techniques are used, though at times they may overlap. It should also be apparent that different diseases can involve these different areas, though usually they are interrelated and result from the extension of a common disease process—dental caries.

Before the *surfaces of the teeth* are examined, it is essential that the teeth be thoroughly cleaned so that all the plaque, stain, debris, and calculus are removed. This is obviously important if all the tooth surfaces are to be adequately inspected. The following equipment is necessary to conduct a thorough clinical examination:

1. Bright artificial light
2. Sharp, fine explorers
3. Mouth mirror
4. Compressed air (air-water syringe)
5. Dental floss

The mouth mirror facilitates visual observation by providing reflected light and allowing the examiner to see areas that otherwise could not be directly observed. The explorer serves as an extension of the examiner's fingers, allowing him or her to perceive (palpate) the character of the tooth surface being examined. Also, the relative hardness of the tooth surface can be determined.

The teeth must be examined in a systematic fashion to avoid overlooking lesions. Generally it is best to begin in the maxillary right quadrant and move to the left. Then one should proceed to the mandibular quadrant and move from the lower left to the right. Individual teeth should be examined in the following order:

1. Occlusal-incisal surface.
2. Facial surface extending from the mesial to the distal embrasure.
3. Lingual surface extending from the mesial to the distal embrasure.

The interproximal surfaces of teeth usually cannot be examined adequately by either an explorer or direct vision. The detection of early carious lesions is difficult, especially in posterior teeth. In this situation other techniques, such as bite-wing radiography or transillumination, are useful in demonstrating demineralization of the surface enamel. Bite-wing radiographs are most useful in the posterior teeth, as opposed to transillumination, which is most effective when used on the anterior teeth.

Transillumination has become a more useful technique in recent years because of the availability of a high-intensity light source that can be concentrated on a small area. When the anterior teeth are examined, the light source should be placed on the facial surface of the proximal areas. The examiner should view the teeth from the lingual aspect with a mirror, looking for dark areas. Demineralized enamel has a lower index of light transmission than sound enamel and appears as a dark area.

Dental floss can be extremely helpful in evaluating interproximal surfaces, contact areas, recurrent interproximal caries, and faulty restoration margins. Thin, round, unwaxed floss should be used, and careful insertion and removal are essential to gain optimal value from this part of the examination.

The techniques for determining *pulp vitality* are relatively poor and unreliable. The techniques that are available include thermal (hot and cold), electric, and test cavity. They basically reflect gross changes; a tooth may have only a segment of viable pulp tissue and still give a normal response. Conversely, a normal pulp may not respond at all. Radiographic evidence of changes in the size or shape of a pulp chamber or root canal may be of value in assessing the status of the pulp. In spite of the shortcomings associated with pulp vitality examination, every effort should be made to ascertain the vitality of pulps whenever there may be a question from the examiner's findings or from the patient's signs or symptoms. It is usually preferable to delay a permanent cast type of restoration on a questionable tooth until the pulpal health status is established.

Irreversible pulp disease will eventually involve the *apical tissues* of the tooth. Depending on the nature of the response, the signs and symptoms will be variable. Apical disease may be totally asymptomatic and demonstrated only by radiographic examination; this occurs in chronic conditions. When problems are acute or subacute, percussion and palpation will reveal notable changes. The tooth will almost invariably be tender to percussion, and the transmission of force to an edematous apical area will result in increased pressure and pain. Frequently, the apical region of a tooth will be tender to palpation and may in fact be slightly enlarged. The enlargement is usually a firm, discrete swelling of the alveolar process.

It should be obvious from the preceding discussion that examination of the dentition requires careful correlation between visual inspection findings and radiographic findings. It is seldom that either is independently sufficient. The particular format that one follows is not important, but a routine should be established that will ensure correlation of both aspects of the examination. The examiner should be ever aware of the deficiencies and possible pitfalls related to radiographic angulations and other technique limitations. Every surface, together with all pits, grooves, and fissures, must be examined with care. The tooth surfaces beneath the gingival margins, whether they be enamel or cementum, must be carefully explored. Areas of radiographic cervical burnout can be very difficult to interpret without careful clinical correlation.

Most of the dentition examination findings lend themselves to diagrammatic charting. There are numerous approaches to dental charting, and various types of printed forms with varying anatomic tooth charts and individual symbols are used with no universally accepted standardization. Some charts combine periodontal findings with those of the dentition.

Regardless of the particular format adopted, there are certain requirements for a good charting system. Charts are a vital part of any dental health record, and the same considerations apply to them as were outlined in Chapter 4. Charts, in addition to their serving as an important medicolegal document in case of malpractice proceedings, also serve as a convenient and quick reference for patient treatment plans and progress of treatment. The role of dental charts as a forensic dentistry mechanism for identification was also discussed in Chapter 4. The initial charting for a new dental patient should provide an accurate record of missing teeth and existing restorations. It is usually wise to keep this chart in its original, permanent form; other charts can be used to identify existing pathosis. Existing pathosis should include all carious lesions, including recurrent caries and other defective restorations, residual tooth fragments, fractured teeth, impactions, and other radiographic findings, such as periapical diseases, retained roots, and cysts. The other important purpose of charting is to record restorative treatment as it progresses. The symbols used should distinguish between the basic types of restorative materials and between individual cast restorations and bridges and removable prostheses. Symbols are frequently used to indicate the following: teeth to be extracted, impacted teeth versus unerupted teeth, retained primary teeth, open contacts, poor contacts, food impaction, drifted teeth, rotated teeth, intruded and extruded teeth, overhangs, plunging cusps, bifurcation involvement, periodontal pocket depth, frenum attachment, loss of papillae, and others.

Study casts can be an important examination aid as well as a treatment planning aid. Minor dentition defects may be enhanced on study casts, and the overall arch relationship and occlusion can be evaluated in more depth.

Abnormalities

The major disease that involves the dentition is, of course, dental caries. The criteria for the diagnosis of caries and particularly for deciding on which lesions should be restored vary considerably and are unfortunately highly subjective. The following discussion is a condensation of some of the latest suggestions from the literature in an attempt to standardize the evaluation of dental caries. The diagnostic criteria were adopted by the Caries Measurement Task Group of the American Dental Association in 1968.[1]

The process of dental caries can be influenced by many different factors, and as a consequence, it can present a range of clinical changes. This range is in part exemplified by the various classifications of caries that have been proposed.

CLASSIFICATION OF CARIES
1. Tissue involved
   a. Enamel
   b. Dentin
   c. Cementum
2. Anatomic location
   a. Pit and fissure
   b. Smooth surface
   c. Cusp tip
   d. Root
3. Stage in natural history of the disease (degree of tissue destruction)
   a. Preclinical
   b. Incipient ("white spot")
   c. Cavitation
   d. Gross destruction
4. Rate of disease progression
   a. Acute (rapid, rampant)
   b. Chronic (slowly progressive)
   c. Arrested
5. Prior history of disease
   a. Primary (virgin) attack
   b. Secondary (recurrent) caries

Each of the above classifications is valid and useful, though none is complete or embodies all the information. As can be seen, many if not all of the classifications can be applied to one carious lesion. The classification that is probably used most often relates to the rate of progression of the lesions: acute, chronic, or arrested.

The initial clinical lesion seen in smooth surface enamel caries is a "chalky" white spot that is hard and shows no cavitation. This change is caused by initial surface demineralization of the enamel, followed by subsurface demineralization. This results in an increased porosity of the tissue that leads to color change. The initial white lesion becomes stained, progressing to a light brown and then to a darker brown. With the progressive color change, there is also a partial softening and roughing of the enamel surface. There is usually no evidence of cavitation at this time. As the lesion progresses to dark brown and black it becomes softer, and cavitation is readily apparent. The color change results from either a change in the amino acid composition of the matrix or the accumulation of stains from foods, products of bacterial metabolism, and tobacco.

Dentinal caries has been classified into three groups: active, chronic, and arrested:

Active
   Color—pale yellow
   Consistency—soft and cheesy
   Pain—painful with sweets and
      probing with explorer
Chronic
   Color—dark center (brown to
      black) with pale periphery
   Consistency—leathery center
      and soft edges
   Pain—usually no pain
Arrested
   Color—dark brown or black
   Consistency—hard
   Pain—none

CRITERIA FOR DIAGNOSIS OF DENTAL CARIES

I. Frank lesions: The detection of these lesions on the basis of gross cavitation usually does not present a problem in diagnosis. When cavitation is present, the diagnosis is positive.
   A. Cavitation in this context may be defined as a discontinuity of the enamel surface caused by loss of tooth substance.
   B. Cavitation that is the result of the caries process must be distinguished from fractures and smooth lesions of erosion and abrasion.

II. Lesions not showing frank cavitation: The most difficult part of the examiner's task is the detection of lesions where there is not frank cavitation. These are the lesions that are close to the decision point between carious and sound. The criteria for detection of these lesions are summarized in three categories, each presenting its special problems.
   A. Detection of pit and fissure lesions of the occlusal, facial, and lingual surfaces.
      1. Area is carious when the explorer "catches" or resists removal after the insertion into a pit or fissure with moderate to firm pressure and when this is accompanied by one or more of the following signs of caries.
         a. Softness at the base of the area.
         b. Opacity adjacent to the pit or fissure as evidence of undermining or demineralization.
         c. Softened enamel adjacent to the pit or fissure that may be scraped away with the explorer.

      2. Area is carious if there is loss of the normal translucency of the enamel, adjacent to a pit, which is in contrast to the surrounding tooth structure. This condition is considered to be reliable evidence of undermining. In some of these cases, the explorer may not catch or penetrate the pit.
   B. Detection of lesions on smooth area of facial and lingual surfaces.
      1. Area is carious if surface is etched or if there is a white spot as evidence of subsurface demineralization and if the area is found to be soft by one of the following.
         a. Penetration with explorer.
         b. Scraping away enamel with explorer.

C. Detection of lesions on proximal surfaces. It is not possible to attain agreement on a single set of criteria, since procedures used for diagnosis of proximal surfaces vary considerably. Some examiners depend largely on visual-tactile methods, some depend largely on radiographs and transillumination, and others use combinations of these procedures. The following is intended to be a composite of the best elements from all procedures.

1. Areas exposed to direct visual and tactile examination are diagnosed as under II B for smooth areas.
2. Hidden areas not exposed to direct visual-tactile examination.
   a. Visual examination: If the marginal ridge shows an opacity as evidence of undermined enamel, the proximal surface is carious.
   b. Tactile examination: Any discontinuity of the enamel in which an explorer will enter is carious if it also shows other evidence of decay, such as softness, shadow by transillumination, or loss of translucency.
   c. Radiography: Any definite radiolucency indicating a break in the continuity of the enamel surface is evidence of caries.
   d. Transillumination (used mostly for anterior teeth): A loss of translucency producing a characteristic shadow in a calculus-free and stain-free proximal surface is adequate evidence of caries.

Stain and pigmentation should not be regarded as evidence of caries, since they occur on sound teeth. In borderline conditions a decision of sound or carious must be made. It was concluded that the generally accepted procedure for classifying conditions about which the examiner is doubtful should be: "When in doubt, call it sound."

The criteria that are used for the radiographic diagnosis of caries are somewhat rigid in that any break in the continuity of enamel is labeled caries. This is somewhat in contrast to the criteria that are used for other smooth surfaces. It is well known from experience that proximal lesions seen on radiographs do not always show cavitation or in fact are soft. The presence of softness or cavitation is usually related to the depth of the enamel lesion. It is difficult to assess the clinical stage of these interproximal lesions, since direct visual observation is usually awkward or impossible unless the adjacent tooth is missing.

A recent study[1] correlating the radiographic depth of proximal carious lesions with their clinical appearance noted that approximately 30% of the teeth that have radiographic lesions limited to the outer half of enamel have cavitation. Since the lesion extends to the dentinoenamel junction, it follows that 61% have cavitation.

It must be emphasized that this information correlates only two observations: (1) radiographic evidence of the depth of the carious lesion (demineralization) and (2) whether the surface enamel shows cavitation. Numerous studies have demonstrated that carious lesions are much deeper, as demonstrated by histologic techniques and mineral content, than the changes on radiographs appear to indicate. The process of dental caries can range from clinically imperceptible surface demineralization to frank destruction of enamel and dentin. This correlation of information can be useful when enamel lesions are present and a decision must be made as to whether the tooth should be restored or observed for evidence of progression of caries at subsequent examinations.

Clinical studies have shown that the progression of proximal lesions, as demonstrated by radiographs, may be very slow. One study[1] reports that 50% of the lesions on proximal surfaces did not progress during an interval of 4 years. As the study continued, only 33% of the proximal lesions did not progress in 6 years and 26% in 8 years.

Studies have also shown that intact enamel surfaces that are demineralized can be remineralized under certain conditions. In theory, early enamel caries may be reversible if the surface remains intact. At times caries may be reversible or "arrested" even when there is cavitation. This is most dramatically demonstrated by "eburnated" caries or eburnation of dentin. It must be noted that the remineralized enamel is not normal in structure or hardness, but for clinical purposes it is "healed." The most effective method to promote remineralization is the topical use of fluoride. Laboratory studies suggest that the sequential and dual application of acidulated phosphate fluoride and stannous fluoride is the most effective technique.

333

Fig. 17-10. A, Attrition: Normal physiologic wear particularly noticeable on first molars. **B** and **C,** Radiographs of same patient showing attrition.

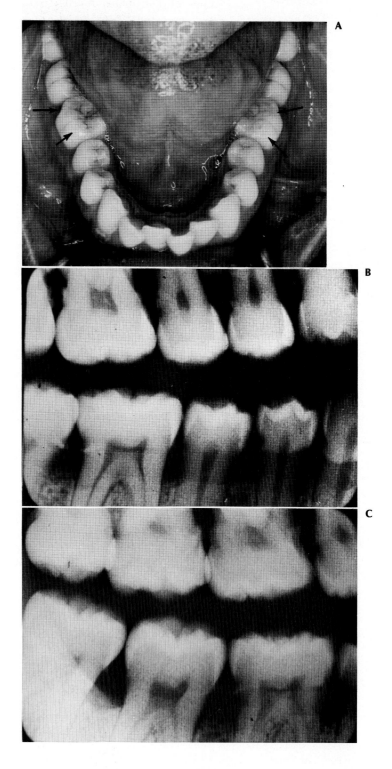

A note of caution is important in regard to informing the patient of the total number of carious lesions that may be present in his or her mouth. At times patients are apprised only of the teeth that will be restored, and enamel lesions are not mentioned. This in part leads to the disparity in the number of "cavities" that different dentists may find in the same patient. If the same diagnostic criteria are used, there should be few if any differences in the number of carious lesions that are diagnosed. A disparity, if it exists, would be in the number that are designated for restoration, since this is a value judgment based on primarily subjective criteria.

In patients with or without dental caries, the dentition is subject to wear after the teeth erupt into occlusion. *Attrition* is the correct term to refer to physiologic wear, and this accounts for the normal wear facets that are found on any tooth surfaces that contact other teeth (Fig. 17-10). When wear becomes excessive, then the term *abrasion* is used to indicate pathologic wear (Fig. 17-11). Generally, abrasion results from a mechanical wearing by some physical agent, such as faulty tooth-brushing habits, various habits associated with placing hard objects between the teeth, and occasionally from occupational habits.

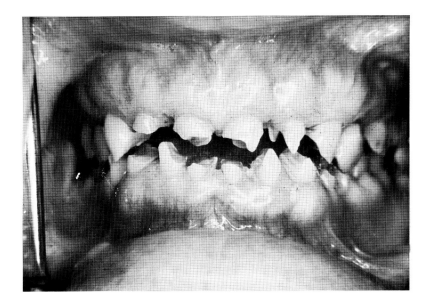

Fig. 17-11. Severe abrasion.

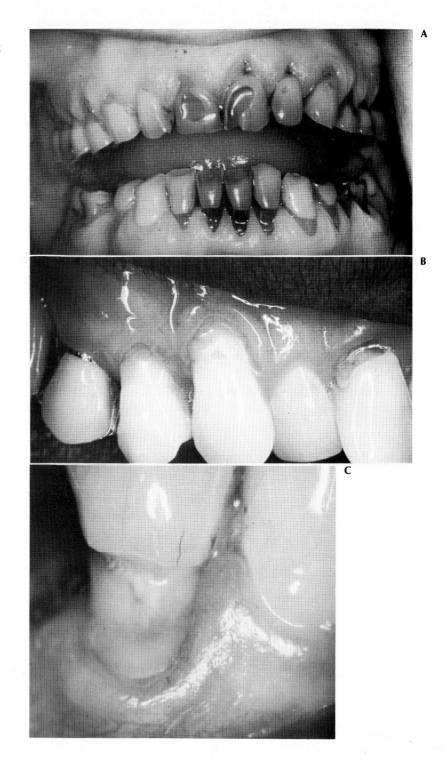

Fig. 17-12. A and **B,** Two examples of cervical erosion. **C,** Close view showing smooth, polished defect.

Erosion is another form of pathologic tooth destruction that is usually caused by a chemical process that at times affects the enamel or involves the cementoenamel juntion (Fig. 17-12, *A*). These defects range from shallow depressions on the labial surfaces of incisors to deep wedge-shaped grooves at the labiocervical area (Fig. 17-12, *B*). In contrast to areas of hypocalcification, which are frequently chalky, rough, and irregular, erosion usually creates smooth, highly polished defects with a hard base (Fig. 17-12, *C*).

It is not unusual to find evidence of various degrees of attrition, abrasion, and erosion in the same mouth, and distinct separation of the entities may be difficult (Fig. 17-13).

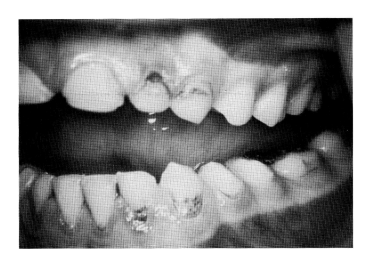

Fig. 17-13. Example of tooth wear that probably indicates attrition, abrasion, and possibly some erosion.

There are a great number of developmental anomalies, many of which have a genetic basis and cause an abnormal number, size, shape, and structure of the dentition. Determining the number of teeth is a routine part of the dental examination. It is not unusual to find an abnormal number of missing teeth or extra (supernumerary) teeth. The terms *anodontia* (total absence) and *hypodontia* (partial absence) refer to the absence of teeth. The third molars, maxillary lateral incisors, and mandibular second premolar are the most common missing teeth. Total anodontia is extremely rare, but in patients with ectodermal dysplasia varying stages of partial anodontia may be found (Fig. 17-14).

Fig. 17-14. A, Sparse hair associated with ectodermal dysplasia. **B,** Dentition consisting of two malformed incisors.

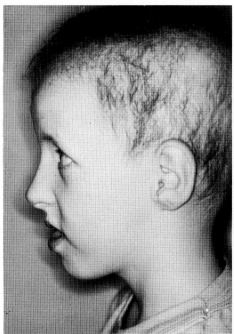

A

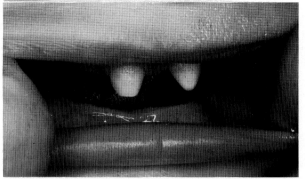

B

Fourth molars represent one of the most common forms of supernumerary teeth (Fig. 17-15). These may range from normal-sized molars to miniature forms or peg-shaped teeth (accessory teeth) (Fig. 17-16). Unerupted supernumerary teeth may prevent the eruption of some of the normal dentition, which may simulate a partial anodontia in the clinical examination. Adult patients with cleidocranial dysostosis may have multiple unerupted supernumerary teeth. The eruption process appears altered in these patients, since even surgical exposure usually fails to help them erupt. In addition to the dentition findings, the clavicles may be totally or partially absent, the skull may have delayed closure of the fontanelles, and there may be other skeletal abnormalities (Fig. 17-17).

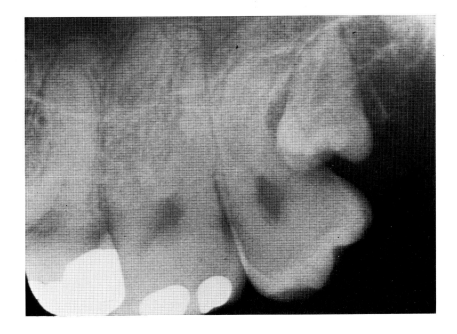

Fig. 17-15. Fourth molar.

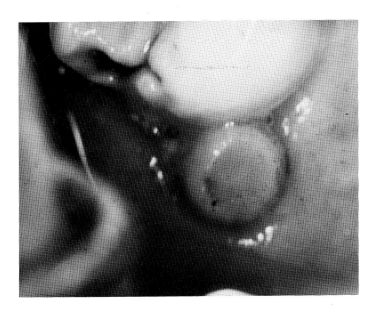

Fig. 17-16. Fourth molar as miniature peg-shaped tooth.

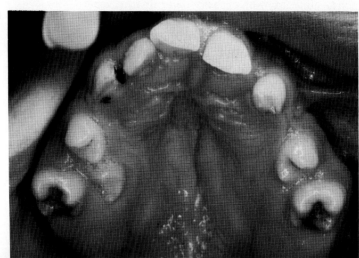

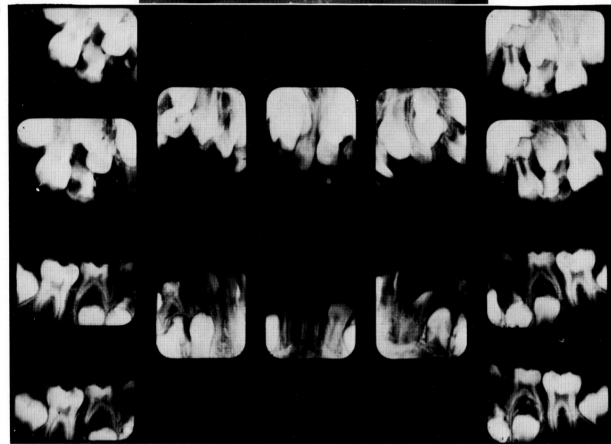

Fig. 17-17. A, Patient with cleidocranial dyostosis showing retained primary teeth and missing teeth as a result of malposed unerupted supernumerary teeth. **B,** Radiographs of same patient.

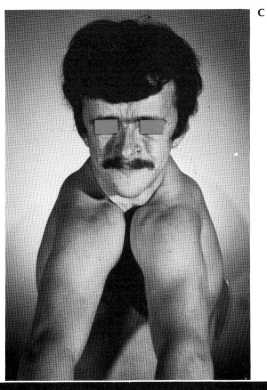

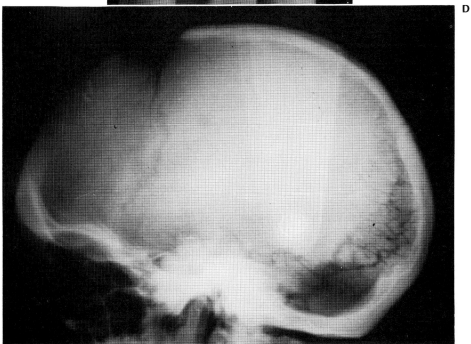

Fig. 17-17, cont'd. C, Absence of clavicles. **D,** Skull radiograph showing open fontanelle.

Abnormal size of teeth is referred to as *microdontia* and *macrodontia*. Complete involvement of the dentition by either condition is extremely rare. More often there appears to be a relative microdontia or macrodontia because of the contrast in jaw size and overall facial features. This is particularly true in the developing child, in whom the size of the newly erupted permanent maxillary central incisors seems out of proportion to the overall growth and development. Third molars and the maxillary lateral incisors show more tendency to develop as microdonts (Fig. 17-18).

Abnormalities of shape or form of the teeth may appear as gemination, fusion, concrescence, dilaceration, dens in dente, taurodontism, supernumerary roots and cusps, enamel pearls, and hypercementosis (Fig. 17-19).

Fig. 17-18. Examples of microdonts (peg laterals).

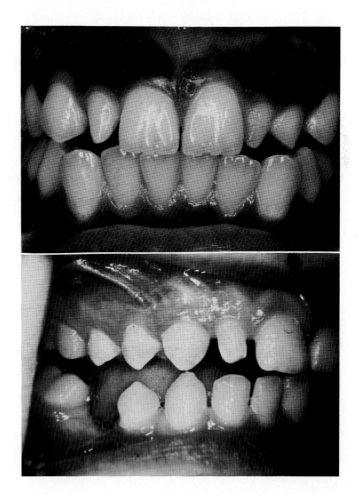

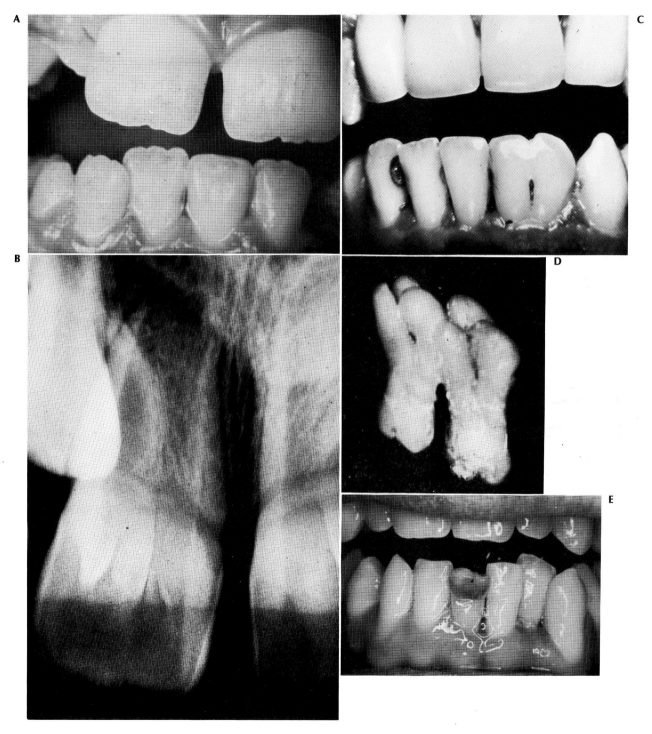

Fig. 17-19. A and **B,** Gemination (twinning of bud). **C,** Fusion (joining by dentin). **D,** Concrescence (joining by cementum). **E,** Dilaceration (sharp bend) of crown.

Continued.

343

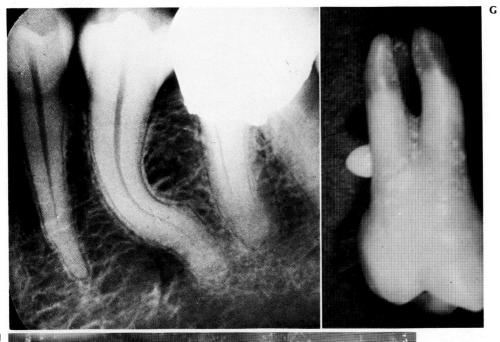

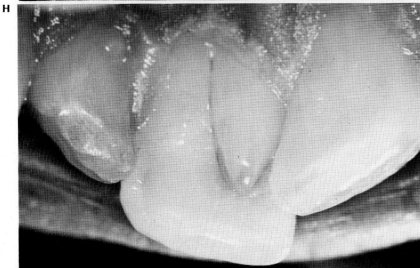

Fig. 17-19, cont'd. F, Dilaceration of root. **G,** Enamel pearl. **H,** Supernumerary cusp. **I,** Supernumerary root.

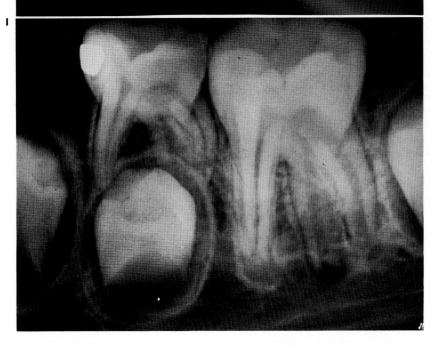

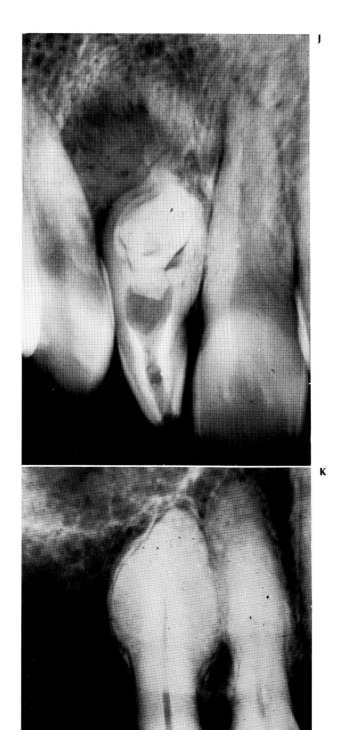

Fig. 17-19, cont'd. J, Den invaginatus (dens in dente). **K,** Hypercementosis.

Most of the abnormalities of number occur during the initial stage of tooth development, those of size during histodifferentiation, and shape abnormalities during the morphodifferentiation stage.

Some of the more common defects in the dentition are structural abnormalities that primarily occur during the apposition and calcification stages of tooth formation. These changes cause defects of enamel, dentin, and cementum. When the enamel matrix formation is affected, enamel hypoplasia results. This results in enamel defects, ranging from tiny pits to vertical grooves to circumferential bands devoid of normal enamel (Fig. 17-20).

Disturbances that interfere with the mineralization of the enamel matrix cause enamel hypocalcification, which usually appears as white chalky spots that are softer than normal enamel. These areas may be stained or pigmented after exposure to the oral cavity.

Enamel hypomaturation is a condition that results from incomplete crystallization in the interrod sheath area. This also appears clinically as opaque white areas, but the surface is harder than areas of hypocalcification and may tend to chip. Collectively, these three enamel conditions may be referred to as *enamel dysplasia*.

These enamel defects may result from local, systemic, or hereditary etiologic factors. There is usually a metabolic disturbance that interrupts normal cellular activity. The clinical enamel defect that results will vary according to the intensity and duration of the disturbance. Frequently enamel hypocalcification and hypoplasia occur in the same dentition.

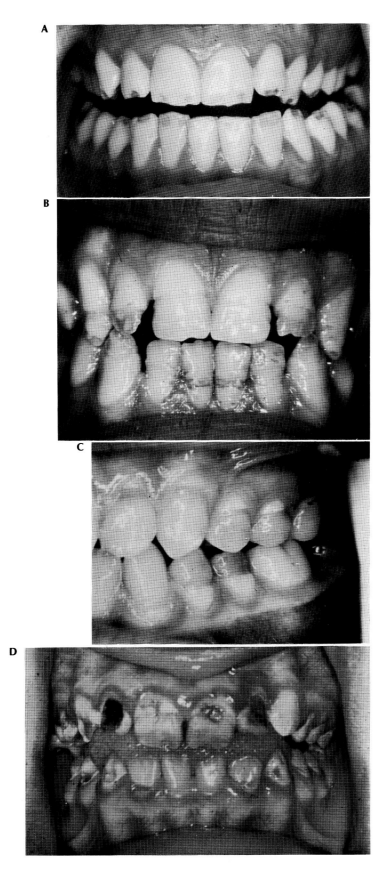

Fig. 17-20. A and **B,** Enamel hypoplasia. **C** and **D,** Enamel hypoplasia and hypocalcification.

There are basically three types of disturbances: (1) those that involve the teeth during a specific stage of development and affect all the teeth at that stage of development; this is referred to as contemporaneous hypoplasia or hypocalcification; (2) hereditary disturbances involving the enamel or dentin independently, usually causing a more generalized type of defect; (3) individual disturbances that affect one or more teeth but not necessarily at a specific zone of development.

The contemporaneous defects have been associated with febrile diseases, endocrine disturbances, vitamin deficiencies, blood dyscrasias, ingestion of chemicals, radiation, and other causes. Dental fluorosis is an excellent example of contemporaneous hypocalcification with or without hypoplasia, depending on the concentration of fluoride ion and duration of ingestion of the excessively fluoridated water supply (Fig. 17-21).

Two conditions that usually have a hereditary basis and involve all the dentition are amelogenesis imperfecta and dentinogenesis imperfecta (Figs. 17-22 and 17-23).

Fig. 17-21. Mottled enamel from endemic fluorosis.

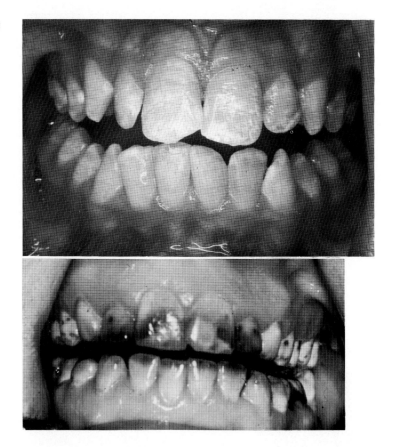

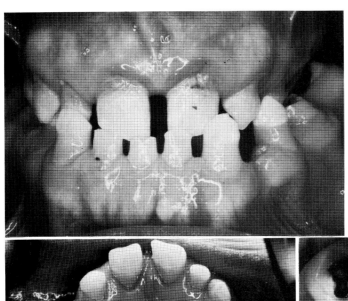

Fig. 17-22. Amelogenesis imperfecta.

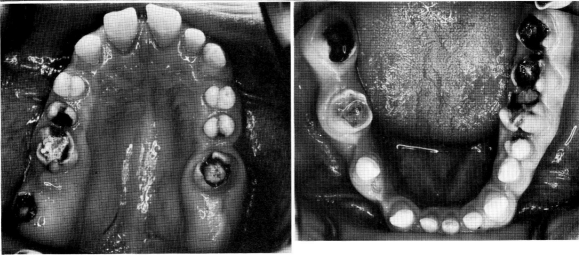

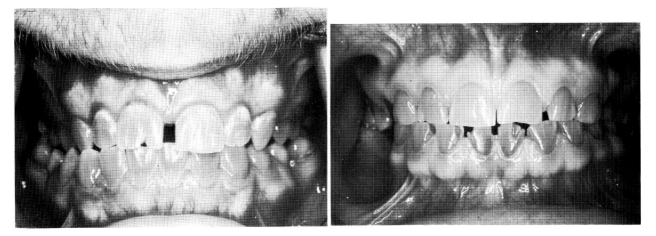

Fig. 17-23. Dentinogenesis imperfecta.

Turner's tooth is an example of an individual disturbance causing a localized hypoplasia (Fig. 17-24). This may be due to localized trauma or periapical inflammation in the primary dentition affecting the underlying developing tooth bud.

Congenital syphilis causes some unique dentition changes that appear to overlap in periods of embryologic development. Hutchinson's incisors and mulberry molars show defects of hypoplasia, but these teeth also have an overall distortion of morphologic form (Fig. 17-25).

Fig. 17-24. Turner's tooth.

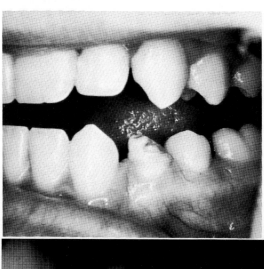

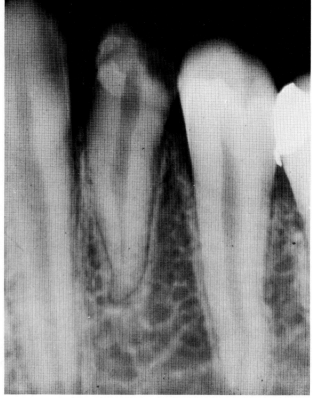

Another gross dentin abnormality is dentinal dysplasia. A significant alteration in the normal dentin tubular architecture will cause an abnormal color in the teeth because of the altered response to transillumination and light refraction.

Generalized cementum disturbances are relatively rare. Hypophosphatasia causes a failure in cementogenesis and hence a lack of normal attachment for the periodontal fibers. The teeth will become mobile and exfoliate spontaneously.

Individual teeth may show hypercementosis, resulting in bulbous roots, which can cause problems when extraction is necessary (see Fig. 17-19, *K*). Involvement of multiple teeth with hypercementosis has been reported in Paget's disease.

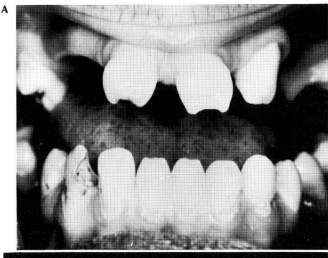

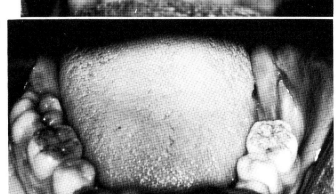

Fig. 17-25. A, Hutchinson's incisors (congenital syphilis). B, Mulberry molars (congenital syphilis).

Discoloration of the teeth other than with the conditions already discussed may result from extrinsic and intrinsic stains. The extrinsic stains result from food dyes, tobacco, some medications, and the reaction of chromogenic bacteria. These stains are often contained in plaque and can be eliminated by prophylaxis with pumice. If enamel defects are present, the stain may be extremely difficult, if not impossible, to remove. Occasionally, staining may be related to an occupational hazard in which metals or salts of metals may be ingested or inhaled.

Intrinsic pigmentation or staining is usually related to blood-borne products or pigments. The most common type of intrinsic staining is the discoloration that occurs in many nonvital teeth. With the loss of normal vascular circulation in the dental pulp, there is usually deposition of hemoglobin breakdown products, as well as decomposition products from the iron and proteins of the pulp tissue (see Chapter 6). Various pigments associated with hemolysis and decomposition cause a wide range of discoloration in the crowns of these teeth.

Teeth subjected to trauma that may cause hemorrhage within the pulp canals or coronal chamber may show extreme shades of dark discoloration.

Other examples of intrinsic pigmentation can be found in tetracycline staining, erythroblastosis fetalis, and porphyrinuria (Fig. 17-26).

Fig. 17-26. A, Intrinsic staining from prolonged tetracyline therapy. **B,** Less severe tetracycline staining.

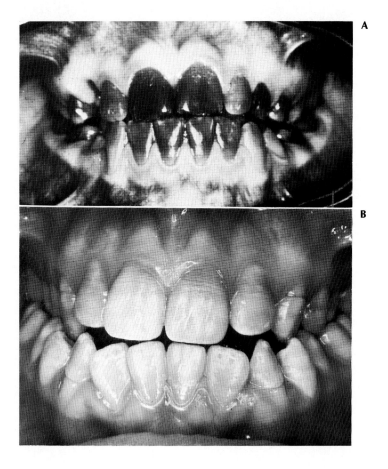

OCCLUSION
Anatomy

The occlusion, or relationship of the teeth to each other is an important part of the stomatognathic system. An examination of the occlusion is part of every complete examination. The information obtained is used both for diagnostic purposes and as a baseline for therapy and reconstruction.

The occlusion is examined from both a static and a functional standpoint. The static evaluation provides information on the jaw-tooth relationships. The functional evaluation provides information on the tooth position in relation to function of the temporomandibular joint.

Examination

Static evaluation. The angle classification of jaw relationships is based on the relationship of the first molars and the canines.[2] The patient is asked to close the teeth together, and the cheeks are retracted so that the first molars and canines can be viewed. The relationship of the anterior teeth is also viewed at this point.

The Angle Class I, or neutrocclusion, is one in which the mesial-buccal cusp of the maxillary first molar lies adjacent to or in the buccal groove of the mandibular first molar (Fig. 17-27). The maxillary canine is in such a position that the cusp tip is just labial to the proximal contact between the mandibular canine and first premolar.

The Angle Class II, or distocclusion, is one in which the mandibular first molar is in a position distal to that of a Class I occlusion (Fig. 17-28). The mesial-buccal cusp of the maxillary first molar is anterior or mesial to the buccal groove of the mandibular first molar. The canine relationship is one in which the mandibular canine is in a position distal to that of a Class I occlusion. The cusp tip of the maxillary canine is labial to the cusp tip of the mandibular canine or in a position anterior to that.

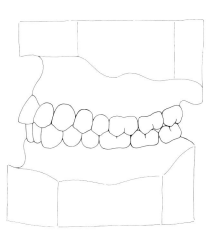

Fig. 17-27. Diagrammatic representation of Angle Class I occlusion.

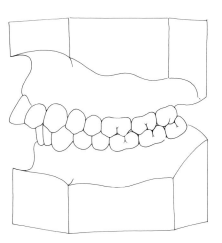

Fig. 17-28. Diagrammatic representation of Angle Class II malocclusion.

A further subdivision of occlusal analysis in the Angle system is the subdivisions of the Class II malocclusions. A subdivision I of a Class II malocclusion indicates that the maxillary teeth are in such a position that they protrude labially, or in labial fashion (Fig. 17-29). In subdivision II the inclination of maxillary anterior teeth, particularly the central incisors, is lingual (Fig. 17-30).

The Angle Class III, or mesiocclusion, is one in which the mandibular first molar is anterior or mesial to the position of a Class I malocclusion (Fig. 17-31). The mesial-buccal cusp of the maxillary first molar occludes in a position distal to the buccal groove of the mandibular first molar. The mandibular canine is anterior or mesial to the normal position in the Class I malocclusion. The maxillary canine will generally be buccal to a mandibular premolar.

The anterior teeth are observed for the overjet-overbite relationship. In the normal overjet relationship, the mandibular teeth lie just lingual to the maxillary teeth (Fig. 17-32). In Class II malocclusions, there is usually excessive overjet (Fig. 17-33). In Class III malocclusions, the overjet is reduced, and in fact frequently there is a prognathic chin in which the mandibular anterior teeth occlude anterior to the maxillary anterior teeth (Fig. 17-34). The overbite relationship is the vertical relationship of the anterior teeth. Overbite may be excessive or deficient. Frequently in Class II malocclusions there is excessive overbite, with the mandibular anterior teeth protruding up into and occluding with the palate or occluding in the middle or gingival one third of the maxillary anterior teeth (Fig. 17-35). The deficit in an overbite will produce the condition of an anterior edge to edge bite or an anterior open bite (Fig. 17-36).

Further evaluation of the occlusion involves the classification of crossbites. The posterior teeth should occlude so that the buccal cusps of the maxillary teeth are in a position facial to the buccal cusps of the mandibular teeth. A crossbite occurs if the buccal cusps of the maxillary tooth are in a position lingual to that of the mandibular tooth (Fig. 17-37). The same holds true for the anterior teeth.

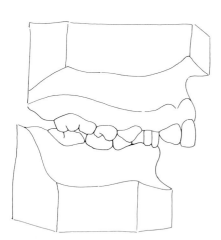

Fig. 17-29. Diagrammatic representation of Angle Class II Subdivision I malocclusion. Incisors have pronounced labial inclination.

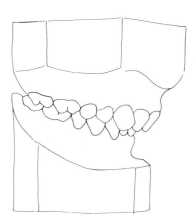

Fig. 17-30. Diagrammatic representation of Angle Class II Subdivision II malocclusion. Incisors are lingually inclined.

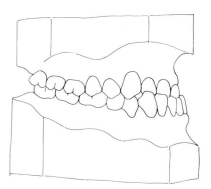

Fig. 17-31. Diagrammatic representation of Angle Class III malocclusion.

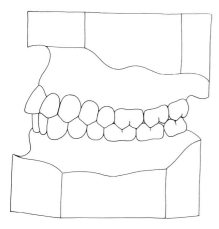

Fig. 17-32. Diagrammatic representation of ideal overjet-overbite relationship.

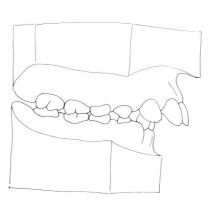

Fig. 17-33. Diagrammatic representation of excessive overjet as frequently seen in Angle Class II malocclusion.

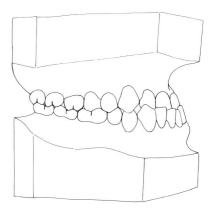

Fig. 17-34. Diagrammatic representation of lack of overjet or prognathic mandible as seen in Angle Class III malocclusion or midface deficiencies.

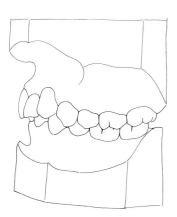

Fig. 17-35. Diagrammatic representation of deep overbite with mandibular incisors impinging on palate.

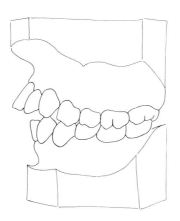

Fig. 17-36. Diagrammatic representation of anterior open bite.

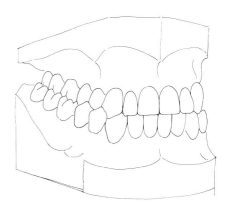

Fig. 17-37. Diagrammatic representation of posterior cross-bite relationship.

Functional evaluation. In addition to the evaluation of the static relationship of the jaws and teeth, an evaluation is made of the functional relationship of the jaws and teeth.

The first step in the functional evaluation is to determine the relationship between centric occlusion and centric relation. *Centric occlusion (CO)* is defined as the most intercuspated (interdigitated) position of the teeth from which lateral movements can be made. This is a tooth-dictated position. *Centric relation (CR)* is defined as the unstrained neutral position of the mandible in which the condyles occupy the most posterior and superior position in the glenoid fossa (joint); this is a muscle-dictated position. The relationship of centric occlusion to centric relation is evaluated by placing condyles in centric relation and then observing the discrepancy between that position and the centric occlusion.

Positioning the jaw in centric relation is a controversial subject, and several methods are practiced. The tooth or teeth in contact in centric relation when there is a discrepancy between centric relation and centric occlusion are called *premature contacts* or *prematurities*. The tooth-guided shift from CO to CR is considered a slide. To examine for this slide an effort is made to get the patient to relax as much as possible. The cranium, via the maxilla, is stabilized with one hand while the mandible is gently manipulated in an up and down arcing movement. Very gentle pressure is applied in a posterior direction in order to guide the mandible toward centric relation. With the thumb on the facial surface of the mandibular incisors, the jaw is first brought up until the examiner's thumbnail touches the maxillary central incisors (Fig. 17-38). This is repeated several times until the examiner feels that the motion is being made with a pure rotary movement of the condyles and until the patient can relax and cooperate to the extent that he or she does not seek

to "find" any particular occlusal contact. Once these conditions have been achieved, the thumb is lowered slightly and the jaw brought upward until the first occlusal contact is made (Fig. 17-39). This is held momentarily as the patient is then asked to "squeeze" the teeth together. As this occurs, the examiner must pay particular attention to the degree and direction of movement of a point on the lower incisors. During the squeeze most patients will slide from centric relation to centric occlusion, and the mandibular incisor point will move forward and upward, the two-dimensional slide. Some patients, however, will move forward, upward, and to the left or right, the three-dimensional slide. Sometimes a very bizarre movement of the incisor point will occur. This procedure is repeated several times to ensure consistency, if possible, and then the cuspal incline planes responsible for the slide are sought.

The "prematurity" in centric relation may be found by using thin carbon paper or a thin sheet of soft wax on the maxillary teeth (Fig. 17-40). The location of this prematurity and the degree and direction of the slide should be noted on the patient's chart. *No attempt* should be made to remove the prematurity at this time. Tracings for sophisticated fully adjustable articulators can be made to determine these positions. These tracings are used primarily for the delicate, accurate mounting of either diagnostic or treatment casts. It is not practical to use this type of sophistication for the everyday evaluation of occlusal discrepancies.

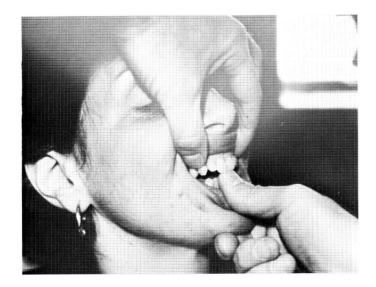

Fig. 17-38. Positioning of hand and thumb with other hand bracing head to obtain centric relation.

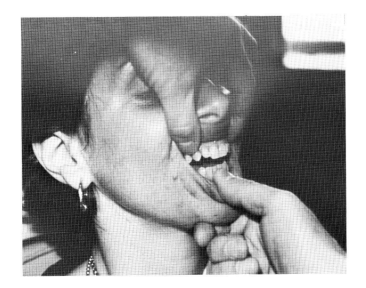

Fig. 17-39. Position of hand and thumb in closing patient into centric relation.

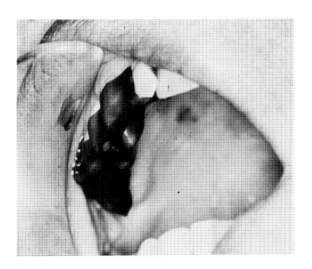

Fig. 17-40. Marking of centric prematurities using occlusal indicator wax.

The guiding or distoccluding tooth on lateral excursions is next determined. This is done by having the patient close in centric occlusion and then move the jaw to one side until the cusp-to-cusp tip relationship of the occluding teeth is obtained (working side). The occlusion on the opposite side of the arch is also evaluated in this position. This occlusion is called the *balancing occlusion*. Balancing contacts are generally considered pathologic.

Often it is difficult to determine whether there is occlusion on the balancing side. This can be further evaluated before the patient's going into the lateral excursion by looping a piece of dental floss around the posterior surface of the last molar so that one end is in the buccal vestibule and the other one in the mouth. In lateral excursion this floss can then be drawn between the teeth to determine whether there is contact (Fig. 17-41).

A thin piece of carbon paper, marking tape, or occlusal wax may also be inserted in the centric occlusion, and as the patient slides into the lateral excursion markings of prematurities will be noted. After one side has been evaluated as to the guidance teeth and the presence or absence of balancing prematurities, the patient is asked to again obtain centric occlusion and slide the jaw to the opposite side, and the same procedure is repeated to determine the guiding tooth or teeth and the presence or absence of balancing prematurities.

The patient then is asked to resume the centric occlusion and to protrude or slide the jaw forward. The patient is again observed to determine which teeth guide the occlusion as the patient slides forward and whether there are posterior teeth or protrusive interferences contacting.

The occlusions on excursions are classified as follows:

1. Mutually protected occlusion (Figs. 17-42 through 17-45): In centric occlusion the molars and premolars are in occlusion. The incisors are close to but not in occlusion. On lateral excursions the canine is the guiding tooth producing the distoclusion. There are no balancing prematurities. In protrusive relation the incisors are the distoccluding teeth with no posterior contact.

2. Unilaterally balanced occlusion or group function (Figs. 17-46 through 17-49): In centric occlusion the molars and premolars occlude, but there is no occlusion on the anterior teeth as in mutually protected occlusion. In lateral excursion there is group function on the working side with no contact on the balancing side. The protrusive occlusion will have guidance on the anterior teeth with no posterior occlusion.

3. Bilaterally balanced occlusion (Figs. 17-50 through 17-53): Centric occlusion includes contact of all teeth, both posterior and anterior. In lateral excursions, there is contact of the posterior teeth on both sides, and of the anterior teeth. In protrusive relation, there is contact of both the anterior teeth and posterior teeth. This type of occlusion is rarely seen in patients with their own dentition. It is basically a denture occlusion.

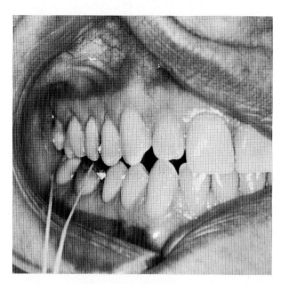

Fig. 17-41. Position of dental floss to identify balancing prematurities.

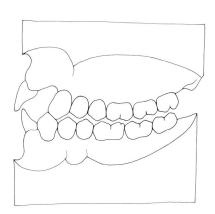

Fig. 17-42. Position of teeth in working side in mutually protected occlusion.

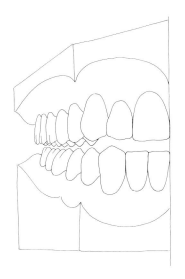

Fig. 17-43. Position of teeth on balancing side in mutually protected occlusion.

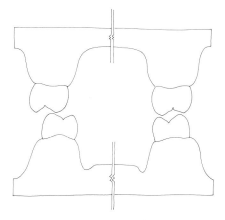

Fig. 17-44. Position of posterior teeth in mutually protected occlusion.

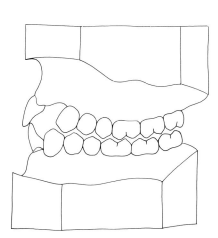

Fig. 17-45. Position of incisors and posterior teeth during protrusive movements in mutually protected occlusion.

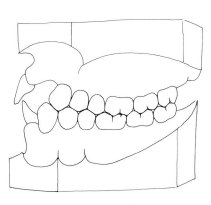

Fig. 17-46. Position of teeth on working side of unilaterally balanced occlusion. Note group function in this position.

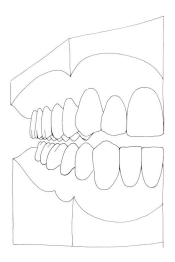

Fig. 17-47. Position of teeth on balancing side of unilaterally balanced occlusion with no balancing prematurities.

359

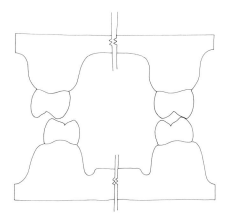

Fig. 17-48. Occlusion of posterior teeth in unilaterally balanced occlusion.

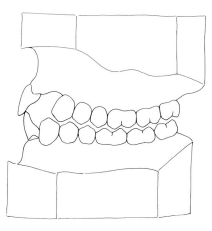

Fig. 17-49. Position of anterior and posterior teeth in unilaterally balanced occlusion on protrusive movements.

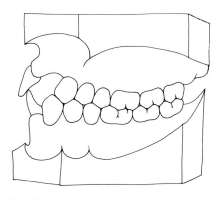

Fig. 17-50. Position of teeth on working side in bilaterally balanced occlusion.

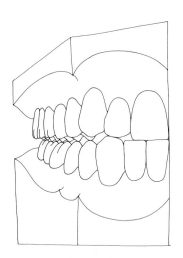

Fig. 17-51. Position of teeth on balancing side of bilaterally balanced occlusion. This can be considered balancing prematurities.

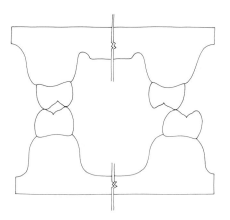

Fig. 17-52. Position of posterior teeth in bilaterally balanced occlusion.

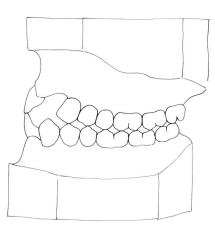

Fig. 17-53. Position of teeth in protrusive movement in bilaterally balanced occlusion.

Particular attention is given to wear facets and other areas of abrasion and attrition on the crowns of the teeth. The amount of tooth wear should coincide with that amount expected for the age of that patient. If wear facets are broad or deep, bruxism must be suspected unless the patient has a particularly abrasive diet. It should be noted, however, that lack of wear does not necessarily indicate the absence of bruxism. The patient may clench the teeth in a fixed mandibular position instead of having the grinding movements that tend to produce wear. Thus, even with little or moderate wear, bruxism may still be present.

One way to assess whether bruxism is present is by using the provocation test. In this test two opposing wear facets are placed in occlusion and the patient is asked to clench hard for 60 seconds. After a short time many patients with bruxism will be able to point to an area on the face that is painful or where pain has been exacerbated.

REFERENCES

1. American Dental Association Council on Dental Research and Council on Dental Therapeutics: Proceedings of the Conference on the Clinical Testing of Cariostatic Agents, Chicago, 1972, The Association.
2. Angle, E.H.: Classification of malocclusion, Dental Cosmos **41**:248-350, 1899.
3. Schluger, S., Yodelis, R.A., and Page, R.C.: Periodontal disease, Philadelphia, 1977, Lea & Febiger.

BIBLIOGRAPHY

Horowitz, H.S.: Clinical trials of preventives for dental caries, J. Public Health Dent. **32**:229, 1972.
Kerr, D.A., Ash, M.M. and Millard, H.D.: Oral diagnosis, ed. 5, St. Louis, 1978, The C.V. Mosby Co.

18   Laboratory examinations

Laboratory examinations can be an important and at times indispensable part of the diagnostic process. Years ago the scope of laboratory studies was rather limited, but now, with our modern technology, a wide range of sophisticated studies is available that can be performed rapidly and at a relatively low cost. Data from these laboratory investigations provide information that often helps to make earlier and more definitive diagnoses that in turn lead to better therapeutic results. These advances have markedly influenced the practice of medicine, but as yet have had only a limited impact on the practice of dentistry.

In the everyday practice of general dentistry, it is rarely necessary for the dentist to obtain special examinations other than radiographs, biopsies, or cultures. Though extensive laboratory investigations are not routinely used by the dentist, this should not imply that the dentist need not be familiar with the indications and interpretations of various basic laboratory examinations. Quite to the contrary, this knowledge is important to the practice of dentistry. It aids in the understanding of medical problems, especially in the assessment of the chronically ill but ambulatory patient who will be seen in the dental office. This type of patient is more likely to be seen in the dental office now than in the past.

There are occasions when a preliminary laboratory evaluation of a patient can be suitably performed by a dentist. This would be warranted for the patient who shows radiographic changes suggestive of hyperparathyroidism (loss of lamina dura, or the ground-glass appearance of bone) or the patient who has signs of a bleeding dyscrasia (petechial hemorrhage or gingival oozing). A knowledge of laboratory medicine is essential so that the appropriate examinations can be requested and correctly interpreted.

Laboratory examinations may be divided into two general categories: screening and diagnostic. Screening studies are intended to identify individuals with disease in the early and asymptomatic stage. Ideally, identification of these patients results in earlier treatment and a better prognosis.

It must be remembered that laboratory examinations provide information that contributes to the diagnostic process. Seldom is this information of value by itself. The results must be interpreted in conjunction with other information that is available about the patient. It should also be noted that a laboratory value outside the normal range does not necessarily indicate disease. That value may represent normal for that specific patient. Usually normal values are determined by testing supposedly healthy people, and these results are used to calculate the mean and normal range. Variables are not considered, and as a consequence the normal ranges are not always valid for all patients. Conversely, if a clinical diagnosis appears valid and is not substantiated by laboratory results, the tests should be repeated to rule out the possibility of laboratory error.

By definition, screening studies must be relatively simple and inexpensive and are useful only when they identify a disease that is relatively frequent (for example, blood glucose, diabetes mellitus; hematocrit, anemia; and VDRL, syphilis). Screening examinations must also be sensitive. *Sensitivity* is defined as the ability of the test to give a positive result when the person tested has the disease being tested for. Ideally this means that the test is 100% positive when a patient has the disease. This quality of sensitivity has the disadvantage of giving positive results when a patient has a disease other than the one for which the screening test is indicated. This results in false-positive reports. For example, the VDRL (a serologic test for syphilis) may give positive results for patients who have had recent vaccinations or acute viral infections. As a consequence, more specific or "diagnostic" tests are necessary to verify the results of the screening studies.

Diagnostic examinations provide more specific information. *Specificity* is defined as the ability of the test to give a negative finding when the person tested does not have the disease being tested for. Ideally in these tests 100% of the normal patients would receive negative results. Usually these tests are more elaborate and expensive. A patient who has a positive VDRL result would require further investigation by more specific tests. In this situation the fluorescent treponemal antibody-absorption (FTA-ABS) test would be used to provide this information.

The distinction between screening and diagnostic laboratory examinations is not always rigid or absolute. For example, the hematocrit may be used to screen for anemia, but when it is used in conjunction with a hemoglobin and red blood cell count, it helps establish the red blood cell indexes (mean corpuscular volume, mean corpuscular hemoglobin, mean corpuscular hemoglobin concentration), which are of diagnostic value. Many laboratory examinations complement each other and are ordered as a group (battery) so that more complete diagnostic information can be obtained.

The facilities for obtaining various laboratory examinations are usually convenient. Most large communities have a number of medical laboratories that are primarily oriented to provide out-patient clinical and pathologic studies. When requested, these laboratories will obtain the appropriate specimens from patients and perform the examinations ordered.

Several different systems have been devised to facilitate laboratory testing of patients in medical and dental offices (for example, rapid urine tests, Chemstrip, and N-Multistix); these systems are usually simple and relatively accurate. It is important that the individuals using these systems be well trained and that a system of quality control be practiced. Random or occasional use of these techniques is discouraged, since proficiency is compromised, and there is an increased risk of inaccurate results. Occasional laboratory examinations of patients are better performed by the established laboratory.

Normal values for all the studies discussed are listed at the end of this chapter. These normal values will not always coincide with those listed in other publications. Variations in laboratory techniques and reagents may produce slightly different normal values. As a consequence it is important that the normal values listed by the laboratory performing the examinations be used to evaluate the reported results.

In 1960 the international organization responsible for units and measurements, the General Conference on Weights and Measures, authorized an international system of units (SI). This system has been adopted by most countries and is being used in most scientific disciplines. The transitional period will be confusing, since both systems will be used at the same time. The base units of SI are listed in Table 6. The unit to designate volume is liter and is written with a small "l." A system of prefixes and symbols is used to designate multiples and submultiples. They are listed in Table 7.

Table 6. Base units of the international system of units (SI)

Quantity	Name	Symbol
Length	Meter	m
Mass	Kilogram	kg
Time	Second	s
Electric current	Ampere	A
Thermodynamic temperature	Kelvin	K
Amount of substance	Mole	mol
Luminous intensity	Candela	cd

Table 7. A system of prefixes used with the international system

Prefix	Symbol	Factor	
Tera	T	10^{12}	= 1,000,000,000,000
Giga	G	10^{9}	= 1,000,000,000
Mega	M	10^{6}	= 1,000,000
Kilo	k	10^{3}	= 1,000
Hecto	h	10^{2}	= 100
Deca	da	10^{1}	= 10
Deci	d	10^{-1}	= 0.1
Centi	c	10^{-2}	= 0.01
Milli	m	10^{-3}	= 0.001
Micro	μ	10^{-6}	= 0.000 001
Nano	n	10^{-9}	= 0.000 000 001
Pico	p	10^{-12}	= 0.000 000 000 001
Femto	f	10^{-15}	= 0.000 000 000 000 0001

BLOOD CHEMISTRY

In recent years the concept of screening studies has been expanded considerably so that groups of studies are conducted during an examination. These tests can be performed rapidly and inexpensively because of automation. As part of a routine physical examination, many patients now receive a "biochemical screening" or "biochemical profile." This is a series of as many as 12 tests that can be performed on as little as 1.8 ml of serum. One of these series is referred to as an SMA (Sequential Multiple Analyzer) 12/60 profile. The value of these profiles in detecting unsuspected disease has not been conclusively documented and is still being reviewed. It has been reported that in routine screening of hospital admissions, these studies have led to significant unexpected diagnoses in about 4% of the patients. Also, these biochemical profiles can lead to early diagnosis of disorders with vague symptoms, for example, hyperparathyroidism, pernicious anemia, and anicteric hepatitis. Another suggested benefit derived from the use of these profiles is the ability to establish "baseline normals" for individual patients.

The SMA 12/60 system is designed to automatically and simultaneously analyze individual serum samples for any 12 of the following tests:

Albumin
Alkaline phosphatase
Calcium
Carbon dioxide
Chloride
Cholesterol
Creatine phosphokinase (CPK)
Creatinine
Direct bilirubin
Glucose
Glutamic oxaloacetic transaminase (SGOT—also aspartate aminotransferase [AST])
Glutamic pyruvic transaminase (SGPT—also alanine aminotransferase [ALT])
Inorganic phosphorus
Lactate dehydrogenase (LDH)
Serum iron
Sodium/potassium
Total bilirubin
Total protein
Triglycerides
Urea nitrogen
Uric acid

The specific tests performed by the system are determined by the requirements of the laboratory. A sample of the type of report prepared by the SMA 12/60 is illustrated in Fig. 18-1. The tests identified in the sample report are those that are used most frequently; those are discussed here.

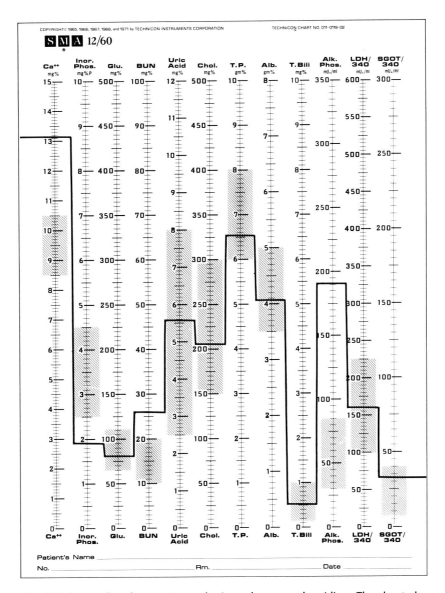

Fig. 18-1. Report that shows pattern of primary hyperparathyroidism. The elevated calcium, decreased phosphorus, and elevated alkaline phosphatase are hallmarks of this disease. Alkaline phosphatase is heat labile and therefore bone in origin. Slight elevation in BUN is due to renal calcinosis.

From Preston, J.A., and Troxel, D.B.: Biochemical profiling in diagnostic medicine, Tarrytown, N.Y., 1971, Technicon Instruments Corp.

Calcium

The calcium present in serum is found either as nondiffusible protein-bound calcium or as diffusible free calcium. Calcium ions are responsible for decreasing neuromuscular excitability and blood coagulation and for activating some enzymes. Serum calcium levels are influenced by the parathyroid hormone and calcitonin. The parathyroid hormone increases serum levels by increasing bone resorption, increasing intestinal absorption of calcium, and increasing resorption in renal tubules.

NORMAL: 9.2 to 11 mg/dl or 2.3 to 2.8 mmol/l

HIGH CALCIUM (hypercalcemia)

Primary hyperparathyroidism
Secondary hyperparathyroidism associated with chronic renal failure
Bony metastases from carcinomas
Sarcoidosis with bone involvement
Bone involvement from lymphoma or multiple myeloma
Carcinoma of the lung and kidney (parathormone production)
Hypervitaminosis D
Long-term use of diuretics
Milk-alkali syndrome
Acidosis

LOW CALCIUM (hypocalcemia)

Low albumin
Hypoparathyroidism (usually surgically induced)
Chronic renal failure
Steatorrhea or malabsorption syndrome
Pancreatitis
Alkalosis

Inorganic phosphorus

There is a reciprocal relationship between calcium and phosphorus. Generally when the level of one increases, the level of the other decreases. The kidney helps regulate phosphorus levels by excreting it. The parathyroid hormone inhibits renal tubular reabsorption of phosphate.

NORMAL: 2.3 to 4.7 mg/dl or 0.78 to 1.52 mmol/l

HIGH PHOSPHORUS (hyperphosphatemia)

Renal failure
Healing bone fractures
Diabetic ketosis
Hypoparathyroidism
Hypervitaminosis D
Acromegaly (early sign)

LOW PHOSPHORUS (hypophosphatemia)

Rickets
Hyperparathyroidism
Hepatic disease
Osteomalacia
Fanconi's syndrome
Ingestion of antacids

Glucose

Glucose is the principal form of energy for cellular function. Normally the blood concentration is maintained within fairly narrow limits. Several hormones can influence glucose metabolism; insulin causes the blood glucose level to fall, whereas the blood glucose level is raised by glucagon, which stimulates glycogenolysis and gluconeogenesis. Epinephrine promotes liver glycogenolysis and an increase in plasma glucose. The glucocorticoids, primarily cortisol, stimulate gluconeogenesis in the liver.

Blood glucose values will vary in relation to meals. To obtain meaningful results specimens must be obtained at specific times. Blood for fasting blood glucose values is obtained after an 8- to 12-hour fast.

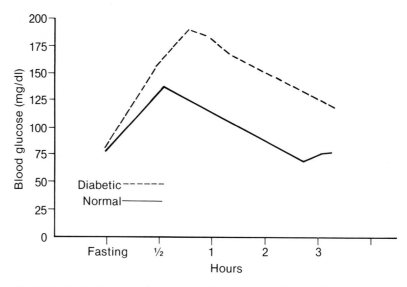

Fig. 18-2. Graph showing values obtained in normal subject and diabetic subject during glucose tolerance test.

The glucose tolerance test (GTT) measures the rise and fall of the blood glucose level after a large dose of glucose. It is assumed that this change in blood glucose level is due primarily to the production of insulin in response to hyperglycemia. In the test a patient is challenged with a 100 gm dose of glucose. A fasting blood specimen is taken before the glucose challenge and then $1/2$ hour, 1, 2, and 3 hours after ingestion. The blood glucose level rises to a peak usually in 15 to 60 minutes. In a normal curve the peak must be reached in 1 hour and must not exceed 160 to 170 mg/dl blood glucose. Subsequently the curve falls steadily but slowly, reaching a level of 120 mg/dl or less within 2 hours. Higher values at this time are abnormal. The criteria for interpreting the test are not uniform. Usually if two of the values on the curve are abnormal (fasting, 1, 2, or 3 hours) a diagnosis of diabetes is made (Fig. 18-2).

The 2-hour postprandial blood glucose test is a good screening test, since it challenges the body's homeostatic mechanisms as the GTT does. A patient is given a 100 gm dose of glucose, and then blood is drawn after 2 hours. If the blood glucose level has not returned to 120 mg/dl then diabetes is suspected. In essence, this method tests an isolated segment of the GTT and circumvents the necessity of multiple blood glucose determinations.

NORMAL FASTING: 70 to 110 mg/dl.

HIGH GLUCOSE (hyperglycemia)

Diabetes mellitus
Cushing's disease
Pheochromocytoma
Brain trauma

LOW GLUCOSE (hypoglycemia)

Excess insulin administered to a diabetic patient
Addison's disease
Bacterial sepsis
Islet cell adenoma of the pancreas
Massive hepatic necrosis
Psychogenic conditions

Blood urea nitrogen (BUN)

Urea is the end product of protein metabolism and is synthesized in the liver through the deamination of amino acids. Since urea is excreted by the kidneys, blood urea nitrogen is a useful screening test for kidney function.

NORMAL: 8 to 23 mg/dl

HIGH BUN

Dehydration (mild to moderate elevation)
Gastrointestinal hemorrhage
Acute glomerulonephritis
Chronic nephritis
Obstruction of urinary tract

LOW BUN

Liver failure
Negative nitrogen balance

Uric acid

Uric acid is the end product of purine metabolism. It is derived from endogenous sources, reflecting nucleic acid turnover, and from dietary nucleic acid. The major route of excretion is the kidney. The relative insolubility of urate predisposes it to precipitation in all tissues if there is hyperuricemia.

NORMAL: 2.5 to 8 mg/dl

HIGH URIC ACID (hyperuricemia)

Renal failure
Gout
Eclampsia of pregnancy with hepatic necrosis
Leukemias or lymphomas
Metabolic acidosis
Starvation
Thiazide diuretics, salicylates, ethanol, and other drugs
Lead poisoning
Infectious mononucleosis
Chemotherapy for cancer

Cholesterol

Almost all cells in the body can synthesize cholesterol, but the liver forms most of the cholesterol produced by the body. Only a small amount is derived from dietary sources. Cholesterol is used by the body to form bile salts, steroid hormones, and cell membranes.

NORMAL: 150 to 250 mg/dl or 3.9 to 6.5 mmol/l

HIGH CHOLESTEROL (hypercholesterolemia)

Cardiovascular disease
Obstructive jaundice
Hypothyroidism
Nephrosis
Uncontrolled diabetes
Pregnancy

LOW CHOLESTEROL (hypocholesterolemia)

Malabsorption
Severe liver disease
Hyperthyroidism
Anemia
Sepsis
Stress and drug therapy

Total protein

The proteins make up approximately 7% of the plasma volume. Most of them are synthesized in the liver. Their principal functions are transport, maintenance of osmotic pressure, buffer for acid-base balance, defense reaction, and coagulation. They also serve as a source of protein nutrition for tissues during protein deprivation. If levels of the total proteins are elevated, this invariably occurs because of increased globulin levels (hyperglobulinemia) and not albumin. Hyperalbuminemia does not occur.

NORMAL: 6 to 7.8 g/dl

HIGH PROTEIN (hyperproteinemia— hyperglobulinemia)

Lupus erythematosus
Rheumatoid arthritis
Other collagen diseases
Chronic infections
Multiple myeloma (and other malignant tumors)
Acute liver disease

Albumin

More than half the protein found in plasma is made up of albumin. The other major protein is globulin. A ratio (A/G) exists between the two proteins, with the normal range being 1.5 to 2.5. Albumin helps maintain the osmotic pressure. It also has a widespread binding capacity that is useful for transport and serves as a pool of resource protein. Because the albumin molecule is small, it is usually the protein that is found in the urine of patients with renal disease.

NORMAL: 3.8 to 5 g/dl

LOW ALBUMIN (Hypoalbuminemia)

Inadequate protein intake
Severe liver disease
Malabsorption
Diarrhea
Nephrosis
Exfoliative dermatitis
Burns
Represents uncontrolled IV

Bilirubin

Approximately 80% of the bilirubin formed each day comes from the degradation of hemoglobin. The remaining amount arises from other substances, such as myoglobin, catalases, and cytochromes. The heme portion is separated from the globin in the reticuloendothelial system. Then iron is removed from the cyclic porphyrin ring, which is opened to form a linear tetrapyrrol (bilirubin). This bilirubin is insoluble in water but is transported in plasma by protein binding. In the liver cell the bilirubin is made water soluble by enzymatic conjugation (direct bilirubin). Unconjugated bilirubin (indirect) is the type that is found in the blood before being carried to the liver. The bilirubin is then secreted into bile. Determining whether the increased amounts of bilirubin are unconjugated or conjugated is useful in identifying the nature of the problem producing elevated levels of bilirubin. Clinical jaundice usually becomes apparent when the plasma bilirubin level exceeds 2 to 2.5 mg/dl.

NORMAL: 0.1 to 1.2 mg/dl (total)

HIGH BILIRUBIN (hyperbilirubinemia)

Hemolytic anemia
Trauma with the presence of a large hematoma
Hemorrhagic pulmonary infarct
Hepatic metastases
Hepatitis
Lymphoma
Cholestasis secondary to drugs
Decompensated cirrhosis
Carcinoma of the head of the pancreas
Choledocholithiasis
Dubin-Johnson syndrome

Alkaline phosphatase

There are several different isoenzyme forms that have optimal activity in an alkaline pH range. This enzyme is present in practically all tissues of the body and occurs in high levels in the intestine, bone, liver, and placenta. The normal levels of alkaline phosphatase in adults are derived primarily from the liver. Increased osteoblastic activity in children is responsible for the higher normal levels of enzyme found at this age. Serum alkaline phosphatase determinations are useful in evaluating hepatobiliary disease and bone disease.

NORMAL:
Children
  20 to 150 IU/l
  20 to 150 U/l
Adults
  20 to 90 IU/l
  20 to 90 U/l

HIGH ALKALINE PHOSPHATASE
(hyperphosphatasia)

Metastatic carcinoma involving the bones
Primary malignant neoplasms
Healing fractures
Obstructive liver disease
Hyperparathyroidism, primary or secondary
Paget's disease of the bone
Pulmonary infarct
Acute or chronic liver disease
Osteomalacia
Cholestasis

LOW ALKALINE PHOSPHATASE
(hypophosphatasia)

Arrested bone growth
Hereditary hypophosphatasia

Acid phosphatase

An entirely different enzyme that may be a source of confusion is acid phosphatase. Like alkaline phosphatase, the activity of this enzyme depends on pH. It exhibits its greatest activity in an acidic pH range. Acid phosphatase is present in large amounts in adult human prostatic tissue and in much smaller concentrations in bone, liver, kidney, and red cells. An elevated acid phosphatase level strongly suggests metastatic prostatic carcinoma.

Lactic dehydrogenase (LDH) or Lactate dehydrogenase (LD)

Lactate dehydrogenase is an intracellular enzyme that is present in all tissues, with high concentrations found in the heart, liver, kidney, skeletal muscle, and red blood cells. Increases in the serum levels usually indicate cellular death and leakage of the enzyme from the cell. Increased levels also occur when neoplastic cells proliferate.

NORMAL: 25 to 100 IU/l

HIGH LDH

Acute myocardial infarction
Acute leukemia
Hemolytic anemia of any type
Acute pulmonary infarction
Metabolic acidosis
Acute renal infarction
Hepatic disease
Skeletal muscle necrosis
Sprue

Serum glutamic oxaloacetic transaminase (SGOT) or aspartate aminotransferase (AST)

Like LDH, this enzyme is present in most tissues, especially skeletal and cardiac muscle, the liver, and the kidney. Elevated levels indicate tissue damage. Enzyme levels are of value in investigating myocardial and liver damage.

NORMAL: 8 to 29 U/l

HIGH SGOT

Acute hepatitis
Acute myocardial infarction
Active cirrhosis
Hepatic necrosis (chemically and drug induced)
Hepatic metastases
Acute pancreatitis
Trauma to skeletal muscle; irradiation of skeletal muscle
Pseudohypertrophic muscular dystrophy
Dermatomyositis
Acute hemolytic anemia
Acute renal disease
Severe burns

A chart listing the more common diseases and their patterns of abnormal test results can be found in Fig. 18-3.

Diseases and their patterns of abnormal test results

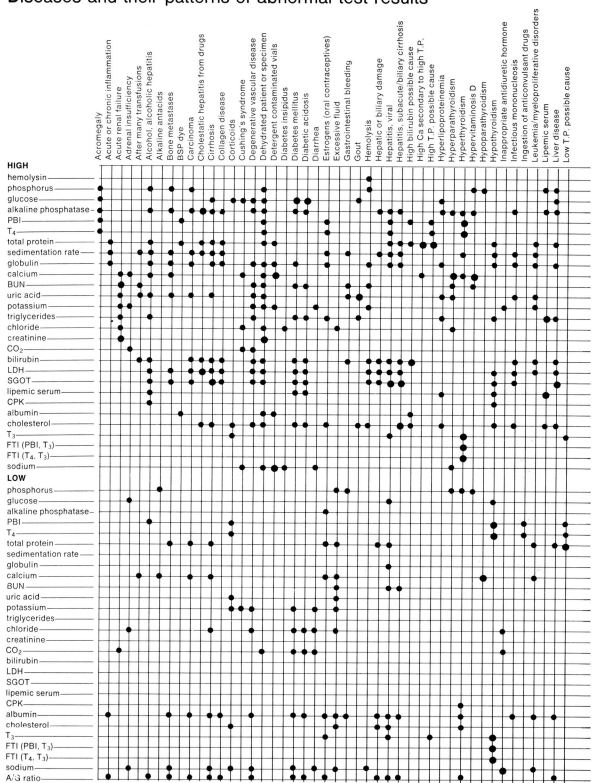

Fig. 18-3. Small dot at intersection of vertical and horizontal guideline means that corresponding value for that test

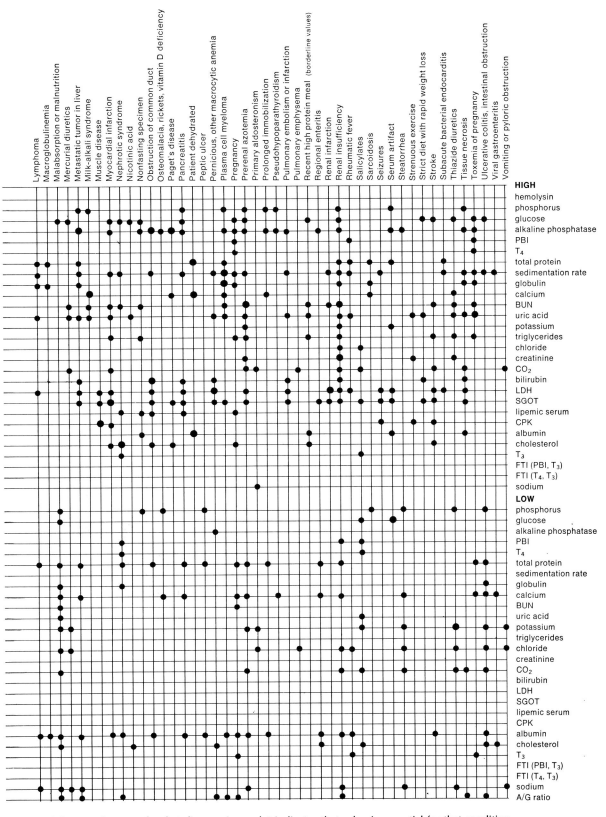

result is part of pattern for that disease. Large dot indicates that value is essential for that condition.

COMPLETE BLOOD COUNT

A wide range of studies can be performed on blood. In fact, this area is so complex that hematology laboratories are divided into sections to deal with specific tests. When the blood is examined, usually a group of tests is ordered at the same time. This provides information that is more meaningful. A complete blood count (CBC) usually includes a white blood cell count (WBC), red blood cell count (RBC), hemoglobin (Hb), hematocrit (Hct), the red blood cell indexes, and a microscopic examination of the RBC morphology. A differential WBC count may or may not be a routine part of the examination.

White blood cell count (WBC)

The WBC count provides an overview of the total number of circulating white blood cells. Variations from the normal range indicate disease.

NORMAL: 5,000 to 10,000/mm^3 or 5 to 10 $\times$ 10^9/l

When the WBC count goes above normal, the condition is referred to as *leukocytosis*. This term is used without consideration of the specific cell types that may be increased. If a total count reaches the level of 30,000 per mm^3 or more, the condition is referred to as a leukemoid reaction. Reasons for leukocytosis are considered under the specific cell types. A decrease in the total WBC count below normal is referred to as *leukopenia*. One or all cellular elements in the WBC series may be decreased. Reasons for leukopenia are also considered under the specific cell types.

There are also qualitative deficiencies, in addition to the quantitative problems that can involve white blood cells. Defects in chemotaxis have been described in the lazy-leukocyte syndrome. The neutrophils in patients with chronic granulomatous disease and the Chédiak-Higashi syndrome have an impaired ability to kill microorganisms. Phagocytosis is normal, but the ingested bacteria remain viable. Special tests are necessary to identify the qualitative defects in these cells.

The following are normal values for the various white blood cells found in a total count:

Band neutrophils	0% to 5%
Segmented neutrophils	50% to 70%
Lymphocytes	25% to 40%
Monocytes	4% to 8%
Eosinophils	1% to 4%
Basophils	0% to 1%

Band neutrophils. These are immature neutrophils. An increase in their number indicates an inflammatory process and is referred to as a shift to the left.* It has been reported that a leftward shift is found more consistently than a leukocytosis in an inflammatory process.

---

*Schilling classified neutrophil counts according to the maturity of cells. In his method of counting, the immature cells were listed on the left side of the report and the more mature forms on the right. As a consequence, an increase in the proportion of younger cells was called a "shift to the left."

Segmented neutrophils. The primary function of neutrophils is phagocytosis, the killing and digestion of microorganisms. Neutrophils usually degenerate after the phagocytized material is digested.

INCREASED NEUTROPHILS (neutrophilia)

Infections, bacterial and fungal
Burns
Tissue necrosis
Hypersensitivity states
Acute renal failure
Myelocytic leukemia
Polycythemia vera
Metastatic carcinoma
Acute hemorrhage or hemolysis

DECREASED NEUTROPHILS (neutropenia)

Idiopathic neutropenia
Cyclic neutropenia
Acute leukemia
Aplastic anemia
Hematotoxic drugs
Typhoid
Infectious mononucleosis
Infectious hepatitis
Measles
Overwhelming sepsis

The term *granulocytopenia* is used to describe the condition in which there is a decrease in all granulocytic cells, that is, neutrophils, eosinophils, and basophils. At times the term is also used to describe only a decrease in the number of neutrophils.

Lymphocytes. The lymphocytes are responsible for humoral and cellular immunity. One cell type (B-lymphocyte) is responsible for the production of immunoglobulins. Another cell type (T-lymphocyte) is involved in cell-mediated immunity.

INCREASED LYMPHOCYTES (lymphocytosis)

Infectious mononucleosis
Infectious hepatitis
Pertussis
Brucellosis
Syphilis
Lymphocytic leukemia

DECREASED LYMPHOCYTES (lymphopenia)

Acute stressful illnesses
Uremia
Congestive heart failure
Lymphomas
Aplastic anemia
Lupus erythematosus
Immunologic deficiency syndromes

Monocytes. Monocytes are phagocytic cells with functions similar to those of neutrophils. After leaving the bone marrow they circulate for only a few days and then move into the tissue. There they are transformed into macrophages and are frequently found in areas of chronic inflammation. As macrophages they help process antigens for the immune system.

INCREASED MONOCYTES (monocytosis)

Tuberculosis
Subacute bacterial endocarditis
Brucellosis
Malaria
Sarcoidosis
Malignancies
Leukemia
Lymphoma

DECREASED MONOCYTES (monocytopenia)

Acute stressful illnesses
Aplastic anemia
Acute leukemia

Eosinophils. The exact functions of eosinophils are not known. They are capable of phagocytosis and become active in the later stages of inflammation. Eosinophils are also active in allergic reactions and parasitic infections. They contain significant amounts of histamine.

INCREASED EOSINOPHILS (eosinophilia)

Drug reactions
Parasitic infections
Allergic diseases
Collagen vascular diseases
Hodgkin's disease
Chronic myelogenous leukemia
Mycosis fungoides

DECREASED EOSINOPHILS (eosinopenia)

Acute stress
Corticosteroids

Basophils. These cells are believed to be involved in certain acute allergic responses. Their distinctive granules are rich in histamine.

INCREASED BASOPHILS (basophilia)

Chronic myelogenous leukemia
Myelofibrosis
Polycythemia vera

Red blood cell count

The primary functions of the red blood cell are transport of oxygen and carbon dioxide and the control of blood pH. The red blood cells make up the largest portion of the formed elements of the blood.

NORMAL:

Men
   4,600,000 to 6,200,000/mm^3 or
   4.6 to 6.2 $\times$ 10^{12}/l
Women
   4,200,000 to 5,400,000/mm^3 or
   4.2 to 5.4 $\times$ 10^{12}/l

INCREASED RED BLOOD CELLS (erythrocytosis)

Polycythemia, secondary
Polycythemia vera
Pulmonary arteriovenous fistulas
Congenital heart disease
Cushing's syndrome
Renal tumors

REDUCED RED BLOOD CELLS (erythrocytopenia)

Leukemia
Aplastic anemia
Renal disease
Hypothyroidism
Hemorrhage
Sickle cell anemia

Hemoglobin

Hemoglobin makes up approximately 95% of the dry weight of the red blood cell. Its primary functions are the uptake and unloading of oxygen. Abnormal hemoglobin may result because of combination with certain substances (carboxyhemoglobin, carbon monoxide) or because of genetic disease. The most common example of the latter is hemoglobin S, which produces either the sickle cell trait or sickle cell anemia.

NORMAL:
   Men   13.5 to 18 g/dl
   Women   12 to 16 g/dl

Hematocrit

The hematocrit (packed cell volume) indicates the percentage of a given volume of whole blood that is made up of red blood cells.

NORMAL:
   Men   40% to 54%
   Women   37% to 47%

Low hemoglobin concentrations and hematocrit values usually mean that there is anemia as a result of blood loss, hemolysis, or underproduction of red blood cells.

Red blood cell indexes

The indexes are used to define the size and hemoglobin content of the red blood cell. These measurements are calculated using the red blood cell count, hemoglobin, and hematocrit, and are extremely useful in evaluating anemias.

MEAN CORPUSCULAR HEMOGLOBIN (MCH)

The MCH determines the mass of hemoglobin in the average erythrocyte.

$$MCH = \frac{hemoglobin \times 10}{red\ blood\ cell\ count} picogram\ (pg)$$

NORMAL: 27 to 31 pg

MEAN CORPUSCULAR VOLUME (MCV)

The MCV indicates the average volume of the red blood cells.

$$MCV = \frac{hematocrit \times 10}{red\ blood\ cell\ count} cubic\ micrometers\ (\mu m^3)$$

NORMAL: 80 to 96 μm^3

MEAN CORPUSCULAR HEMOGLOBIN CONCENTRATION (MCHC)

This index gives the average concentration of hemoglobin in the red blood cells.

$$MCHC = \frac{hemoglobin \times 100}{hematocrit} percent$$

NORMAL: 32% to 36%

Microscopic examination

A blood smear is prepared at the time of examination so that the size, shape, and color of red blood cells can be examined. Red blood cells may show significant changes in morphologic type in various anemias. *Anisocytosis* and *poikilocytosis* are general terms used to describe changes in size and shape. Anisocytosis means unequal and is used to indicate variations in size. Poikilocytosis means varied and is used to indicate variations in shape.

In addition, there are many terms used to describe more specific changes. *Macrocytes* are enlarged red blood cells and are found in megaloblastic and aplastic anemia. Cells decreased in size are referred to as *microcytes*. They are found in microcytic anemia, iron deficiency anemia, and thalassemia. *Spherocytes* are not biconcave and lack a central area of pallor. They are found in hereditary spherocytosis and autoimmune hemolytic anemias. *Hypochromia* refers to cells that have decreased hemoglobin concentrations and a large central area of pallor. This may be seen in iron deficiency anemia and thalassemia.

Target cells are red blood cells that have a centrally stained area. They are seen in varying numbers in iron deficiency anemia, thalassemia, and certain hemoglobinopathies. Cells that are shaped like a sickle or crescent are referred to as *sickle cells* and are present in sickle cell anemia. Howell-Jolly bodies are round, purple-staining nuclear fragments found in red blood cells. They are usually seen after splenectomy and in cases of splenic atrophy, hemolytic anemia, pernicious anemia, and thalassemia. These are just a few of the more common changes.

BLEEDING

Problems relating to hemostasis are relatively infrequent in the dental office, but when present can pose a serious problem. Since congenital defects will usually have been identified early in the course of the patient's life, the acquired bleeding problems are those that will be encountered most frequently. A good history usually will identify the patient with a bleeding problem. When bleeding problems are readily apparent, the patient should be referred to a physician for a complete evaluation. In those situations in which there is some question as to a defect in hemostasis, screening studies should be ordered. The studies should resolve the question as to whether a problem exists.

Bleeding problems can be attributed to defects in one of three systems: vascular, platelet, and coagulation (Fig. 18-4). Specific procedures or tests can identify defects in these systems. Frequently the history or physical examination will provide some evidence as to the nature of the problem. When a bleeding problem is suspected, the following four studies should be ordered to screen for defects: bleeding time, platelet count, partial thromboplastin time, and prothrombin time. A nonspecific but useful test is the tourniquet test. It can be used in the office as a preliminary screening technique.

Tourniquet test (Rumpel-Leede test or capillary fragility test)

The tourniquet test is a technique of testing the integrity of the capillary walls by obstructing venous flow. If the capillary wall is abnormal, blood will escape and produce petechial hemorrhage. Also, if there is a qualitative or quantitative defect in the platelets, there may be petechial hemorrhage. The tourniquet test is performed by using a sphygmomanometer as if blood pressure were being recorded. The cuff should be inflated to a point halfway between the patient's diastolic and systolic pressures, but never over 100 mm Hg. The pressure is maintained for 5 minutes, and then the cuff is deflated. After the cuff is removed, the antecubital fossa and the lower arm should be examined for petechial hemorrhage. Usually a few petechiae will be seen. In patients who have vascular or platelet defects, numerous petechiae will be found. The results of this test have also been positive in some patients who have had coagulation defects.

NORMAL: Fewer than 10 petechiae

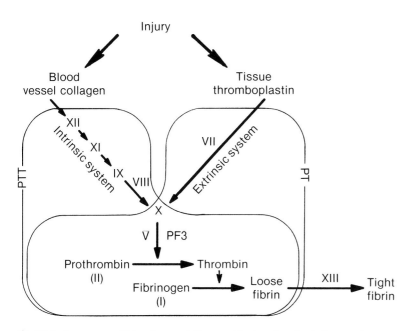

Fig. 18-4. Sequence of blood coagulation and factors involved. Segments of coagulation process tested by prothrombin time (PT) and partial thromboplastin time (PTT) are indicated by circled areas.

Bleeding time

The bleeding time is a measure of vascular and platelet function. A standardized wound is produced on the forearm, and the time required for the wound to stop bleeding is determined. This tests the ability of the vessels to contract and produce hemostasis. It also tests the ability of the platelets to aggregate and produce a hemostatic plug in the wound. Individuals who have coagulation defects but normal platelet counts will have a normal bleeding time.

NORMAL: 1 to 7 minutes

Platelet count

Platelets are formed in the bone marrow and removed from the circulation primarily by the spleen. They have a life span of about 10 days. Platelets promote hemostasis by forming plugs and contributing to thrombin formation. The platelet count determines the number of platelets (thrombocytes) per cubic millimeter. Bleeding usually does not occur until the platelet count is below 50,000.

NORMAL: 150,000 to 400,000/mm^3 or 0.15 to 0.4 × 10^{12}/l

THROMBOCYTOPENIA

Drug toxicity
Leukemia
Idiopathic thrombocytopenic purpura (ITP)
Hypersplenism
Disseminated intravascular coagulation

There are hereditary and acquired disorders of platelet function. In these cases the count may be normal, but there is a qualitative defect. Special tests are necessary to identify these problems.

Partial thromboplastin time

The partial thromboplastin time test measures all clotting factors except factor VII. The entire coagulation system is tested by adding a constant amount of platelet substitute to the patient's plasma before it is recalcified.

NORMAL: 60 to 70 seconds

The test will be prolonged if there is a deficiency in any of the factors except VII.

Prothrombin time

The prothrombin time test depends on factors VII, X, V, prothrombin (II), and fibrinogen (I). Adding tissue extract (usually brain) before recalcification bypasses intrinsic clotting through factors XII, XI, IX, and VIII. This test is used to monitor anticoagulation therapy.

NORMAL: 12 to 14 seconds

The test time is prolonged if factor VII (extrinsic) is deficient or if the factors in the common pathway (X and V) are deficient. It is also prolonged if there are abnormalities of prothrombin or fibrinogen.

SEROLOGIC TEST FOR SYPHILIS

Several tests are used to screen for syphilis. It should be noted that these are screening studies and are nonspecific. When *Treponema pallidum* invades tissue, two basic types of antibodies are formed: antibodies to the treponema itself and antibodies known as reagins that develop in response to lipoidal antigens of the treponema or as a result of the interaction of the treponema with tissue. Tests for antibodies of the second type, which are called nontreponemal tests, are used for screening.

The VDRL (Venereal Disease Research Laboratory) is a sensitive test that will detect patients with syphilis in the late primary stage, secondary stage, or tertiary stage. Unfortunately, the test is so sensitive that it gives a positive (false-positive) result for patients who have other diseases and for narcotic addicts. Whenever results of a serologic test for syphilis are positive, it should be repeated. If results of the second test are positive, the patient must be referred for more specific testing. Patients who have had syphilis and have been adequately treated may continue to give positive test results (serofast). A test that is just as useful as the VDRL is the RPR (rapid plasma reagin).

HEPATITIS B TEST

In past years viral hepatitis has been divided into infectious hepatitis (A) and serum hepatitis (B) on the basis of history. Now laboratory studies are available that help distinguish the two types. Of significance is the fact that patients who have had hepatitis B may become carriers and have the capacity to infect others. This not only poses a health problem to the dentist, but also may jeopardize his or her ability to practice. It has been suggested that patients who have had hepatitis that has not been identified as to type should be tested to exclude the possibility that they might still be infectious.

The test that should be ordered is the hepatitis B surface antigen (HB_sAg) test, which in the past has also been referred to as the Australian antigen test. Patients with positive test results must be managed carefully to avoid the possibility of infecting the dentist, the staff, or others.

URINALYSIS

Examination of urine specimens is usually performed as a screening procedure. Specific diagnostic studies are necessary at times but require special preparation. Special techniques and materials have been developed so that multiple analyses can be performed on urine specimens obtained in the office (Chemstrip, N-Multistix). The standard urinalysis includes information as to appearance, specific gravity, pH, glucose, protein, ketones, bilirubin, and microscopic examination of the sediment.

Appearance

Urine usually appears amber, clear, and transparent. It may be turbid shortly after a meal. Pus produces a white appearance and hemorrhage a red, smoky appearance. As it becomes concentrated, urine takes on a reddish color.

Specific gravity

The specific gravity of the urine indicates the ability of the kidney to concentrate urine. A diseased kidney loses this ability. The normal specific gravity of urine usually ranges between 1.001 and 1.035.

pH

A freshly voided specimen is acid, and the pH may range from 4.8 to 7.0. The urine becomes more acidic in diabetic acidosis, fevers, diarrhea, and dehydration. An increase in pH is noted in chronic cystitis, certain genitourinary tract infections, pyloric obstruction, acute and chronic renal failure, and renal tubular acidosis.

Glucose

Glucose is normally reabsorbed in the kidney by the tubules after it has passed the glomerular filter. If the blood concentration exceeds the renal threshold, which is about 160 mg/dl, then glucose is found in the urine (glycosuria). The most common reason for glucose in the urine is diabetes mellitus. It may also occur in patients who have Cushing's disease, pheochromocytoma, increased intracranial pressure, and liver damage, and in those who are pregnant.

Protein

Normally protein is not found in the urine. On occasion it may be found in the urine of normal individuals who have had excessive muscular exertion or exposure to cold. Protein is also found in individuals who have orthostatic proteinuria. Urinary protein, usually albumin, is found most frequently in patients with renal disease that produces increased glomerular permeability. Proteinuria is usually found in acute glomerulonephritis, pyelonephritis, or malignant hypertension. At times proteinuria is also seen in pregnancy, disseminated lupus erythematosus, congestive heart failure, and benign hypertension.

Ketones

Ketone bodies, including acetone, diacetic acid, and betahydroxybutyric acid may appear in normal urine following carbohydrate-deficient states. If glucose is not available, the body uses fat stores for energy. These are then reduced to ketone bodies. Ketonuria may occur in uncontrolled diabetes, renal glycosuria, and starvation.

Bilirubin

Normally bilirubin is not found in the urine. Bilirubin can be excreted in urine only after it has been conjugated. Urine bilirubin is found in liver disease, biliary obstruction, cirrhosis, and carcinoma of the head of the pancreas.

Microscopic examination

Examination of the urinary sediment can provide extremely useful information. Red blood cells in the urine (hematuria) may be the result of kidney or bladder tumors, cystitis, hypertension, glomerulonephritis, or trauma. White blood cells (pyuria) indicate an infection involving the kidney, ·bladder, urethra, or prostate gland. When proteinuria occurs, some of the protein is precipitated in the renal tubules. This protein may be mixed with epithelial cells or other debris, and it may gel in the shape of the tubule. As fragments are dislodged, they pass through the genitourinary tract and become part of the urinary sediment that is referred to as "casts." Many different types of casts can be formed, depending on the material that is incorporated. All casts reflect some type of disease.

TISSUE EXAMINATION

Tissue from a lesion may be obtained by two different techniques: biopsy and cytology. In general, more definitive diagnostic information can be obtained by biopsy. Oral cytology is less involved and produces less discomfort to the patient, but has an extremely limited diagnostic value.

The technique of oral cytology obtains cells from the surface of the lesion. As a consequence, changes deep in the tissue are frequently missed. A cytologic diagnosis is based on individual cell changes without the benefit of seeing the tissue architecture, as is possible with a biopsy. Cytology has proved useful in investigating lesions of herpes, candidiasis, and pemphigus. It should not be used when a lesion is suspected of being a carcinoma. In these situations a biopsy is mandatory.

When a lesion is to be biopsied, the selection of the site to be sampled is important. The area should represent a recent manifestation of disease so that the changes are more likely to be diagnostic. The tissue should be near a margin and viable, since necrotic tissue provides little useful information. An adequate sample of the lesion should be taken so that there is sufficient material to examine. If the lesion is small, then an excisional biopsy should be considered. In those situations in which the tissue specimen is small or there is a possible problem in orientation, it is helpful to place the specimen on a small piece of cardboard before placing it in the fixative. This allows the specimen to retain its shape and helps the pathologist with the orientation of the lesion and its mucosal surface. Notes can be made on the cardboard in pencil by the surgeon to further help orientation. Specimens should be handled carefully to avoid tears and compression artifacts. It is extremely important that the specimen be fixed in an ample amount of fixative immediately after removal to avoid degenerative changes.

The materials necessary for fixing and mailing both cytologic and biopsy specimens can be obtained from oral pathology departments at dental schools or local pathology laboratories. On request these laboratories will forward specimen bottles with fixative, mailing containers, and appropriate history forms. If there are questions as to the correct sampling or management of the specimen, the laboratory should be consulted to ensure that diagnostic material is submitted.

MICROBIOLOGIC EXAMINATION

An infrequently used but important technique is the culturing of inflammatory lesions that are suspected to be infectious. Clinicians tend to become complacent in the management of these oral infections because some are self-limited, whereas most others readily respond to either penicillin or erythromycin.

Ideally, whenever an infection is suspected, the lesion should be cultured so that the responsible microorganism can be identified and the most appropriate antimicrobial agent selected for treatment. Few individuals will be prepared to obtain a culture unless they are practicing in a clinic setting or have a special interest in microbiology. The procedures are not very involved, and the information and materials necessary for taking a culture will be provided by the laboratory.

In obtaining a specimen it is important that sufficient material be acquired and that the specimen be transported to the laboratory as rapidly as possible. The latter is extremely important, since some microorganisms are quite susceptible to drying and to temperature changes. To facilitate the transport of specimens, individually packaged disposable containers are available (Fig. 18-5). The diagnostic laboratories will usually provide a supply of transport medium containers on request.

It is also important that appropriate information be given with the specimen so that the laboratory knows how to manage it. Information such as the nature of the material, location where it was taken, and suspected diagnosis should be listed. The clinician should also indicate the type of information that is desired. Most frequently the identification and sensitivity of the microorganisms are requested. If specific microorganisms are suspected, then the laboratory should be advised, since special techniques may be necessary to identify them.

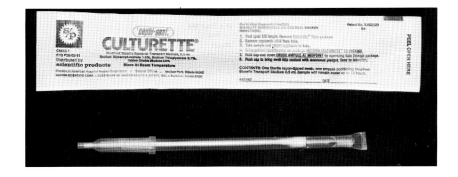

Fig. 18-5. Example of self-contained, disposable system for collection and transport of microorganisms. Packet contains swab and transport medium.

Table 8. Normal values—blood chemistry

Test	Present units	SI units
Albumin	3.8-5.0 g/dl	38-50 g/l
Bilirubin		
Direct	<0.3 mg/dl	<5.1 μmol/l
Indirect	0.1-1.0 mg/dl	1.7-17.1 μmol/l
Total	0.1-1.2 mg/dl	1.7-20.5 μmol/l
Calcium	9.2-11.0 mg/dl	2.3-2.8 mmol/l
	4.6-5.5 mEq/l	
Cholesterol	150-250 mg/dl	3.90-6.50 mmol/l
Creatinine	0.6-1.2 mg/dl	53-106 μmol/l
Globulins	2.3-3.5 g/dl	23-35 g/l
Glucose	70-110 mg/dl	3.85-6.05 mmol/l
Lactate dehydrogenase	25-100 IU/l	0.4-1.7 μmol/l
Phosphatase, alkaline		
Child	20-150 IU/l at 30° C	20-150 U/l at 30° C
Adult	20-90 IU/l at 30° C	20-90 U/l at 30° C
Phosphorus	2.3-4.7 mg/dl	0.78-1.52 mmol/l
Protein, total	6.0-7.8 g/dl	60-78 g/l
Transferases		
Aspartate amino (SGOT)	16-60 U/ml at 30° C	8-29 U/l at 30° C
Alanine amino (SGPT)	8-50 U/ml at 30° C	4-24 U/l at 30° C
Urea nitrogen	8-23 mg/dl	2.9-8.2 mmol/l
Uric acid		
Male	2.5-8.0 mg/dl	0.15-0.48 mmol/l
Female	1.5-6.0 mg/dl	0.09-0.36 mmol/l

Table 9. Normal values—hematology

Test	Present units	SI units
Leukocyte count (WBC)	5000-10,000/mm^3	5-10 × 10^9/l
	5-10 × 10^3/μl	
Neutrophils		
Segmented	50%-70%	
Band	0%-5%	
Lymphocytes	25%-40%	
Monocytes	4%-8%	
Eosinophils	1%-4%	
Basophils	0%-1%	
Erythrocyte count (RBC)		
Male	4.6-6.2 million/mm^3	
	4.6-6.2 × 10^6/μl	4.6-6.2 × 10^{12}/l
Female	4.2-5.4 million/mm^3	
	4.2-5.4 × 10^6/μl	4.2-5.4 × 10^{12}/l
Hemoglobin		
Male	13.5-18.0 g/dl	2.09-2.79 mmol/l
Female	12.0-16.0 g/dl	1.86-2.48 mmol/l
Hematocrit		
Male	40%-54%	0.40-0.54
Female	37%-47%	0.37-0.47
RBC indexes		
Mean corpuscular hemoglobin	27-31 pg	0.42-0.48 fmol
Mean corpuscular volume	80-96 μm^3	80-96 fl
Mean corpuscular hemoglobin concentration	32%-36%	0.32-0.36 g/dl
Platelet count	150,000-400,000/mm^3	0.15-0.4 × 10^{12}/l
	150-400 × 10^3/μl	
Bleeding time (Ivy)	1-7 min	1-7 min
Partial thromboplastin time	60-70 sec	60-70 sec
Prothrombin time	12-14 sec	12-14 sec

SUMMARY

As can be noted from the above brief review, a wide array of diagnostic studies is available to help in the evaluation and diagnosis of disease. These studies are constantly being augmented by refining old techniques and developing new ones. Individuals who are not routinely using the laboratory for diagnostic purposes may find it difficult to remain well versed as to the most appropriate studies to request and their interpretation. Whenever there are questions, the laboratory staff should be consulted. It must also be emphasized that laboratory results by themselves do not make a diagnosis. The "doctor" is responsible for assimilating and analyzing all of the information pertinent to the problem and then for making a diagnosis.

BIBLIOGRAPHY

Koepke, J.A.: Guide to clinical laboratory diagnosis, ed. 2, New York, 1979, Appleton-Century-Crofts.

Lehmann, H.P.: Metrication of clinical laboratory data in SI units, Am. J. Clin. Pathol. **65**:2, 1976.

Massachusetts General Hospital: Normal reference laboratory values, N. Engl. J. Med. **298**:34, 1978.

Sabes, W.R.: The dentist and clinical laboratory procedures, St. Louis, 1979, The C.V. Mosby Co.

Sonnenwirth, A.C., and Jarett, L.: Gradwohl's clinical laboratory methods and diagnosis, ed. 8, St. Louis, 1980, The C.V. Mosby Co.

Steven, J.H., and Cole, G.W.: Reference values based on hospital admission laboratory data, J.A.M.A. **240**:279, 1978.

19 Consultation and communication

Most dental problems encountered during the everyday practice of dentistry are rather straightforward. Likewise, most of the patients are essentially healthy and without problems that require special precautions during dental treatment. Without question, though, there will be those occasions in every dentist's practice when the dental problem is not straightforward and the patient is not without complicating systemic disease. In these situations it may be appropriate to seek the advice or opinion of a colleague—a consultation. The patient's well-being is the chief consideration, and if there is a question as to the accuracy of the diagnosis or the appropriateness of the treatment, then a consultation is mandated.

Though infrequent, many different situations may dictate the necessity for requesting a consultation. The reasons for consultations by dentists can be divided into two principal groups: dental and medical. The dental group can be further subdivided into those related to diagnostic and to therapeutic problems. Medical consultations can be conveniently divided into three categories: those relating to more detailed information about a patient's known medical problems, recommendations as to the medical management of a patient with systemic disease during dental care, and evaluation of a patient who has evidence suggestive of systemic disease, which was detected during the dentist's examination.

DENTAL CONSULTATION
Diagnostic

Infrequent or rare lesions of the oral mucosa, peculiar changes in radiographs and occasional cases of orofacial pain are the types of problems that can prompt a consultation. Inexperience or lack of the appropriate facilities may make a clinician less than confident in establishing a diagnosis. The dental and medical professions have established specialty areas of practice that can help provide assistance in situations such as these. The clinician should freely use both dental and medical specialists, since they can contribute to the best management of the patient and can also provide a learning experience by their response. The specialty areas of practice recognized by the American Dental Association and by the American Medical Association are as follows:

DENTAL SPECIALTIES

Dental public health
Endodontics
Oral pathology
Oral and maxillofacial surgery
Orthodontics
Pedodontics
Periodontics
Prosthodontics

MEDICAL SPECIALTIES

Allergy and immunology
Anesthesiology
Colon and rectal surgery
Dermatology
Emergency medicine
Family practice
Internal medicine
    Cardiovascular disease
    Critical care medicine
    Endocrinology and metabolism
    Gastroenterology
    Hematology
    Infectious disease
    Medical oncology
    Nephrology
    Pulmonary disease
    Rheumatology
Neurologic surgery
Nuclear medicine
Obstretrics and gynecology
    Gynecologic oncology
    Maternal and fetal medicine
    Reproductive endocrinology
Ophthalmology
Orthopedic surgery
Otolaryngology
Pathology
    Anatomic and clinical pathology
    Anatomic pathology
    Clinical pathology
    Forensic pathology
    Hematology
    Neuropathology
    Chemical pathology
    Medical microbiology
    Blood banking
    Radioisotopic pathology
    Dermatopathology

Pediatrics
    Cardiology
    Critical care medicine
    Endocrinology
    Hematology and oncology
    Neonatal and perinatal medicine
    Nephrology
Physical medicine and rehabilitation
Plastic surgery
Preventive medicine
Psychiatry and neurology
    Child neurology
    Child psychiatry
    Neurology
    Psychiatry
Radiology
    Diagnostic radiology
    Nuclear radiology
    Therapeutic radiology
Surgery
    Pediatric
Thoracic surgery
Urology

The dentist should never be reluctant to request a consultation to help make a diagnosis. The most essential step in the diagnostic process, detection of disease, without which there would be no diagnosis, has been achieved. The detection of disease is a significant service in itself and can lead to early and successful treatment if the patient is managed properly.

Therapeutic

In some situations a diagnosis is not difficult to achieve, but the proper treatment of the problem may be in question or unknown. Assistance in determining the appropriate treatment becomes important. It may range from identifying the currently most useful form of palliative care for dentistry's bane, aphthous ulcers, to evolving an elaborate dental treatment plan for a patient with ectodermal dysplasia. Again, specialists can provide support and should be used whenever necessary.

By requesting a consultation, the clinician does not necessarily renounce the privilege of participating in the patient's care. In the consultation request, the clinician can indicate that he or she only desires an opinion and will provide the care. The clinician also has other options: that the responsibility for care be shared or that the consultant provide total care. The interests and capabilities of the clinician should dictate the degree of participation in patient management.

MEDICAL CONSULTATION
Acquisition of information

A complete and accurate medical history is essential before one proceeds with dental care. On occasion a patient may be vague or elusive in providing data. This may be due to a patient's lack of knowledge or recall, or it may be an attempt to avoid disclosure of something that would result in a "hassle" during dental care. Patients with serious systemic disease have been known to deny illness to avoid taking antibiotics or exercising certain precautions that *they* believe are unnecessary. Whenever there is any question in regard to a past or current medical history, a request for additional information must be forwarded to the patient's physician. To obtain this information legally a release signed by the patient must accompany the consultation.

Vague comments by patients about problems such as heart murmurs or hepatitis must be resolved. With a history of hepatitis, for instance, it must be determined whether the patient had infectious hepatitis or serum hepatitis and, if it was serum hepatitis, whether the patient was tested for HB_sAg (hepatitis B surface antigen). Dental treatment can be a hazard to the patient in the first example and the dentist in the second example without this type of information.

At times, instead of being vague, patients provide more information than necessary and tend to embellish their histories. The consultation illustrated in Fig. 19-1 is an example of such a situation, in which the patient's history suggests that she is in rather poor health. The response by the physician, which is quite complete, indicates that the patient has more of a functional problem, rather than serious organic disease. Probably the most frequent use of a consultation will be to resolve questions about the patient's medical history.

CONSULTATION REQUEST

Name—Last—First

TO Dr. M.A. Cantab   DATE November 3, 1981

REASON FOR CONSULTATION

Mrs. Hall states that she is currently under your care. During a review
of her medical history, she indicated that there has been a previous or
current history of: hypertension, abnormal bleeding following the removal
of a tooth, penicillin allergy, hepatitis, thyroid disease, renal disease,
and the removal of a tumor.

This patient will require routine restorative dental care (fillings) to be
done under local anesthesia, and the fabrication of a lower partial denture.

Would you please provide a brief medical history and list her current
medications? Thank you.

George Gordon   D.D.S.

REPORT OF CONSULTANT

Mrs. Hall has been under my care and follow-up for the past 8 years. I
feel that the following diagnoses have been established: 1) irritable bowel
syndrome, 2) hemorrhoids (small with minimal recurrent symptomatoloty),
3) exogenous obesity, 4) recurrent (although infrequent) urinary cystitis,
5) chronic anxiety state (mild), 6) early menopausal syndrome with
menometrorrhagia and water retention associated with menses (mild to
moderate), and 7) mild hypothyroidism or "hypometabolic" state.

In my opinion she has no liver or kidney disease, and is normotensive rather
than hypertensive. There has been no evidence of a bleeding problem and
the prothrombin time was 80% last November. She is presently on no medication except Synthroid 0.1 gm/d and Equanil 400 mg q 6-8 h prn (which she
takes infrequently). Except to be alert to "faintness" on a psychophysiologic
basis, I see no other precautions which need to be taken and see no
contraindications.

M. A. Cantab, M.D.

Form 8082 C1-13—Rev. 5/69

Fig. 19-1. Consultation pertaining to patient who identified multiple systemic problems. It represents rather complete response, other than replying to inquiry about tumor that patient mentioned. Response is brief but provides information necessary to adequately manage patient during dental care.

Evaluation and management

Often a complete and comprehensive medical history will be available, but because of the nature of the systemic problem, there is a question of the patient's ability to cope with prolonged or stressful procedures. This is especially true now, with the increased number of chronically ill individuals who are ambulatory as a result of newer drugs and improved management. They will also be seeking routine dental care.

When a patient with an extensive or complicated health history is seen, a consultation for medical evaluation is essential. As an example, consider a 46-year-old man who has had two myocardial infarctions, the most recent being 1 year ago, who had a cerebral vascular accident at approximately the same time, who currently has mild hypertension, and who is taking dicumarol. Before dental care for this patient is begun, it would be prudent to determine how well he would tolerate any dental procedures. In these consultations, the physician should be informed as to the dental treatment proposed in terms that convey some idea of the duration and stress involved in the procedures. The health status of the patient may be marginal, and modification or curtailment of the proposed treatment plan may be necessary. Occasionally a patient's prognosis may be so poor that extensive dental care is contraindicated or unwarranted. In these situations only emergency or maintenance treatment should be provided.

The medical management of a patient during dental treatment is another important consideration. Though medical evaluation and medical management are frequently interrelated and considered together, they can pose different problems. At times the patient's health status may be quite apparent, and the only question may pertain to the appropriate management of the patient.

Our 46-year-old man serves as a good illustration again. The patient may be considered a reasonable risk, but if dental treatment is to be performed for this patient, what precautions should be taken to control anxiety? Furthermore, if surgery is required, how will the anticoagulation therapy be modified, and who will monitor its level?

Questions such as these are best resolved through a cooperative effort between the dentist and physician. The health status of some patients may be so marginal and management so complex that outpatient treatment is inappropriate and hospitalization is required. Though the dentist's primary concern is dental care, he is responsible for the adequate assessment of a patient's health status and for identifying those patients who require a consultation for medical evaluation and management before proceeding with dental treatment. The axiom *primum non nocere* (in the first place do no harm) is most appropriate in conveying the dentist's responsibility in these situations.

Evidence of systemic disease

The dentist can and frequently does provide a health screening service during the evaluation of his or her patients. Evidence that suggests systemic disease may be noted during the systems review segment of the history or during the physical examination. Conditions such as a persistent sore throat or shortness of breath suggest the possibility of serious disease. A slowly enlarging, noduloulcerative lesion of the skin, a generalized lymphadenopathy, or multiple areas of mucous membrane pigmentation, all of which may be signs of serious disease, may be found during a physical examination.

When these signs and symptoms of disease are detected, the patient must be referred for a careful investigation so that the significance of these changes can be determined. A consultation request in this situation should identify the problem that is the source of concern (referral) and that requires investigation. Whenever possible, the consultation request should be sent to the family physician. If the physician is not available or the patient does not have a family physician, then a direct referral to an appropriate specialist is in order.

At times some of the patients who have relatively asymptomatic but signigicant signs of disease (such as a painless, enlarging ulcer or an enlarged, nontender lymph node) tend to minimize or deny their problems. They are prone to discount the seriousness of the problem, since it does not ''bother'' them. It is important that every effort be taken to ensure that these individuals are seen by a physician. If necessary, the dentist should call and schedule an appointment for the patient immediately. Though the patient cannot be forced to see someone in consultation, persistent, gentle persuasion can be effective.

385

CONSULTATION FORMAT

Generally, consultations comprise written requests and responses. Information may be obtained by telephone, but this is discouraged unless the urgency of the situation requires it. Written records help avoid misunderstandings and provide a permanent source of information. Consultations are probably used most frequently in hospitals, and specific forms are used for this purpose. Usually these forms follow a similar format at most hospitals and institutions. A typical form is illustrated in Fig. 19-2. A special form is not necessary to request a consultation; a formal letter or short note may be appropriate. In a busy practice, there is a tendency to be less formal and to expedite the process. Frequently, information will be provided in short phrases or in outline form. Regardless of the form, certain basic information must be included with the request. The following information is necessary and should be included in a consultation request.

Identification of patient

Sufficient information to identify the patient must be provided to avoid confusion. It must include the full name and at least the birth date. Additional information, such as a hospital number, Social Security number, or address is also helpful.

Identification of consultant

The name of the individual who is to see the patient and respond to the request should be listed. At times this may be a clinic or group practice and should be identified as such.

Date

The date that the consultation is requested and also the date that the reply is written should be listed.

Brief summary of information and reason for consultation

If appropriate, a short, succinct statement providing background information should be included. When laboratory results or other data are pertinent, they should be included or appended, and then the specific reason for the consultation should be stated. If specific information is desired, it needs to be requested. The following are abbreviated examples of the types of information that might be requested:

Diagnostic: This patient had an acute onset of ulcerative stomatitis. I am uncertain as to the diagnosis. Please evaluate and treat.

Therapeutic: This patient has recurrent episodes of erythema multiforme that is confined to the oral cavity. Please provide symptomatic relief and management.

Acquisition of information: This patient states that you have detected a heart murmur but is uncertain as to its nature. Please indicate whether the murmur is functional or organic.

Evaluation: This patient has congestive heart failure and requires the removal of five grossly decayed teeth. Please evaluate as to risk for outpatient surgery under local anesthesia (specify anesthetic agent and epinephrine content.).

Management: This patient has severe hypertension and requires endodontic treatment for two teeth. The procedure will require approximately 2 hours and be somewhat uncomfortable. Do you have any recommendations as to the management of the patient during dental treatment?

The consultation should be signed and a return address provided. It may be sent with the patient or through the mail. A more detailed and prompt reply is usually obtained if the patient takes the request to the consultant.

GENERAL CONSULTATION REQUEST

TO _____Hematology_____ DATE _October 18, 1981_____
(PHYSICIAN AND/OR SERVICE)

☐ OUTPATIENT   ☐ INPATIENT

PROVISIONAL DIAGNOSIS:

REASON FOR REFERRAL:

This patient was seen in the Dental Clinic for routine care. During his
physical examination it was noted that his occipital, submandibular, cervical
and axillary lymph nodes were markedly enlarged. Other than a sore throat
for the past 4 days, the patient feels well. He was advised that a medical
evaluation would be appropriate and will be calling for an appointment.

(Use Reverse Side if Necessary)___*George Gordon DDS*___

REPORT AND OPINION OF CONSULTANT

DATE _____November 3, 1981_____

This 21 year old man was seen in the Clinic today for evaluation of generalized
lymphadenopathy. Mr. Lucy states that except for an episode of urethritis 1 1/2 years
ago, he felt well until October, 1981. Apparently he had a diagnosis of venereal
disease confirmed with "blood tests" one and a half years ago, treated with antibiotics.
He is reported to have a positive RPR recently. In October, he did have several episodes
of night sweats. He has had fatigue over the past 2 months, and an intermittent sore
throat. He denies weight loss.

On physical examination, he does have impressive lymphadenopathy including: small occipital
nodes, a 2 x 3 cm right posterior cervical node, other smaller but multiple R and L anterior
cervical nodes, a 1 x 1 cm R supraclavicular node, 1 x 1 cm R and L axillary nodes, small
bilateral epitrochlear nodes, and multiple inguinal, femoral, and iliac nodes. The remainder
of his physical examination was normal except for an erythematous posterior pharynx
associated with tonsillar enlargement.

Assessment: The lymphadenopathy is indeed impressive. The most likely diagnostic
possibilities include: 1) Non-Hodgkin's lymphoma, 2) Hodgkin's Disease, 3) infectious
mononucleosis, 4) histoplasmosis, and 5) tuberculosis. Number 1 is most likely.
Will proceed with lymph node biopsy and obtain baseline studies. Will inform you of
the results.

(Use Reverse Side if Necessary ___*M.A. Catmal,*___ _____M.D.

FORM - #24004

1-4 \ CONSULTS

Fig. 19-2. This consultation was prepared because physical examination revealed evidence suggestive of systemic disease.
Before proceeding with dental care patient was referred for medical evaluation. Reply indicates physician's initial impression
and planned course of action. In cases such as this there should be follow-up letter informing clinician of final diagnosis and
proposed treatment.

CASE PRESENTATION

An important, though not strongly emphasized, aspect of undergraduate and especially graduate training is the presentation of patient cases as a part of clinic or seminar programs such as clinicopathologic conferences. Through patient or case presentations, the student learns to prepare and deliver information that is organized, concise, and confined to the salient features. The appropriate selection and use of cases also offer the students increased exposure to a wide range of interesting and challenging material that otherwise would not be experienced. Also, the subsequent discussion by "experts" of the diagnostic features and therapeutic considerations provides all the participants with knowledge and experience that is not always found in textbooks or journals.

The quality of presentations improves with experience and reaches some degree of sophistication when students reach the senior level of advanced specialty education programs. Though many different factors can influence the quality of the presentation, the most important is careful and thorough preparation. A rambling, extremely detailed, and prolonged report will lose its value and the audience's attention. There is a logical sequence that should be followed in a presentation. It should be concise, without dwelling for prolonged periods on specific items. Only the important and pertinent information should be included. The use of illustrative material, if available, enhances the presentation immensely.

The organization and content of a presentation should follow or be similar to the outline used for the accumulation of information when making a diagnosis:

ORGANIZATION AND CONTENT OF THE PRESENTATION

Orienting statement
Present illness
Past dental history
Past medical history
Physical examination
Laboratory data
Diagnosis
Treatment

The *orienting statement* provides background information about the patient. This includes the biographic data (age, race, sex, and occupation) and the presenting problem (chief complaint). The history of the *present illness* should give a brief narrative account in a chronologic order of the signs and symptoms that pertain to the patient's problem. The *past dental history* should contain only information that might bear on the patient's current problem or that in some way characterizes traits that might be pertinent to the analysis of the problem.

The *past medical history* should contain information about the patient's previous medical problems and also include information regarding the patient's current medical status. This presentation should be selective, limited to information that may have a bearing on the diagnosis or dental treatment. The presentation of the results of the *physical examination* should not be restricted to the positive findings, since negative findings may also be pertinent; when they are, they should be included.

The results of all *laboratory data* should be reported. If it is possible, these data should be prepared for projection, since it is easier to review and analyze them in this fashion. Abnormal results should be identified and normal values noted for comparison. Radiographs pertinent to a diagnosis or to the management of the patient should be included. When it is possible, they should be prepared for general viewing or projection. Abnormalities should be identified and described.

When the *diagnosis* is presented, the evidence that supports the diagnosis should be noted. When several diseases occur concurrently, then the one that pertains to the presenting problem or chief complaint should be listed first and the others listed in the order of their significance. The last item to be presented is the management or *treatment* plan pertaining to the patient's problem. In cases in which a diagnosis is not conclusive and further studies are necessary to establish a diagnosis, the procedures that are to be performed should be listed. The rationale for these additional studies should be explained. When patients have a therapeutic problem, the proposed management or treatment should be identified and the anticipated results discussed.

The patient presentation should be as spontaneous as possible. Notes are frequently necessary, but they should be abbreviated. A patient presentation that is read from a prepared manuscript loses its impact. The individual presenting the case should have a clear understanding of the entire problem so that he or she can respond to inquiries for information in addition to that presented. If it is possible, the complete history and other source material should be available, so that if there are requests for detailed information it can be provided. A well-prepared and well-delivered case presentation can be a unique and stimulating learning experience.

THE PATIENT WITH SERIOUS DISEASE

On rare occasions the dentist may be confronted with the initial management of a patient with a serious disease, such as leukemia or cancer. This might be a patient who believes that a problem such as persistent gingival hemorrhage or a slowly enlarging ulcer indicates some type of dental disease. The dentist, on recognizing that these are manifestations of potentially serious problems, may elect to proceed with initial diagnostic studies, such as a CBC and platelet count or a biopsy. Conversely, he or she may elect to refer the patient to someone else for evaluation. Regardless of the course of action, there are two points that are critical to the proper management of the patient. First, the patient must be managed in a positive fashion; and second, a specific diagnosis should not be mentioned until there is good supporting evidence.

If it is suspected that a patient has a serious disease, a definitive course of action must be followed. When a patient is to be referred, the specialist who is to be consulted should be identified, and, if it is possible, an appointment should be scheduled for the patient. Sending a consultation request will tend to force the patient to comply, and its reply will acknowledge that the patient was seen. A casual remark such as "you should see someone about this problem" may have little impact on the patient and may be interpreted as suggesting that the problem is not serious. As a consequence, he or she may defer or neglect further consideration of the problem. The number of patients who tend to minimize or deny serious disease if given the opportunity is surprising and somewhat disappointing.

Some patients respond in an opposite fashion, interpreting any evidence of disease as ominous. In addition, a request for a consultation or laboratory studies may be considered foreboding. These patients may also be extremely inquisitive, which probably reflects their anxiety to some degree. Caution must be exercised in the amount of information that is provided. Even though a serious problem is strongly suspected, the diagnosis should not be mentioned until it has been proven. If a patient is persistent, an honest but noncommittal statement such as "your problem is rather unusual, and we will have to do some tests to better understand it," may serve to allay some of the apprehension. Informing the patient of the suspected diagnosis can have serious consequences. Reportedly, a patient was informed that a tongue lesion appeared to represent a carcinoma, and a biopsy was performed. Before the biopsy report was available, the patient committed suicide in anticipation of the assumed treatment. Unfortunately, the clinical impression was incorrect and the patient needlessly frightened—the biopsy was reported as a benign lesion!

Once a diagnosis is established, if it identifies serious disease the patient must be referred as soon as possible to the specialist who will provide the treatment. Again, some caution must be exercised as to the extent of the information that is provided to the patient. It is best to refer inquiries for detailed information about the disease and treatment to the individual responsible for treatment. This helps ensure that the patient receives the most correct and appropriate information.

Communication between the dentist and his or her colleagues can be extremely important in helping establish a diagnosis and in influencing therapy or the management of the patient. To be valid and beneficial, this exchange of information should follow the basic principles previously discussed. The most significant point is that consultation between colleagues about patients almost invariably leads to improved health care and should always be encouraged.

BIBLIOGRAPHY

Brasher, W.J., and Rees, T.D.: The medical consultation: its role in dentistry, J. Am. Dent. Assoc. **95:**961, 1977.

Drinnan, A.J., and Fischman, S.L.: Medical-dental relationships, Dent. Clin. North Am., March 1968, pp. 31-41.

Morgan, W.L., and Engel, G.L.: The clinical approach to the patient, Philadelphia, 1969, W.B. Saunders Co.

Peck, A.: Emotional reactions to having cancer, Am. J. Roentgenol. Radium Ther. Nucl. Med. **114:**591, 1972.

Webb, B.W.: Medical evaluation for outpatient dental procedures, J. Fam. Pract. **6:**971, 1978.

20 Examination of the unconscious patient

Although the chances of a dental patient's collapsing fatally in a dental office are very small, such deaths have been reported. Apart from the emotional effects that such a happening might have on the dentist, the staff, and the relatives of the deceased person, there may also be legal repercussions if the death were considered to be a result of dental malpractice or if it were felt that sufficient resuscitative measures had not been instituted.

All people working in the dental office should be trained and regularly retrained in the procedures that each should follow in an emergency. Each person should know his or her role, and the dental office should always be prepared for an emergency by having available adequate resuscitative equipment, emergency drugs, and a list of telephone numbers of a hospital emergency room, an ambulance or rescue service, and a competent physician.

There are several conditions that can lead to unconsciousness in the dental office; fortunately, they are nearly all reversible and nonfatal. The dentist must know how to evaluate the signs and symptoms of any patient who is in distress or who has collapsed.

The first portion of this chapter is devoted to some aspects of the state of consciousness and is followed by a section devoted to the underlying physiologic or pathologic nature of each of several conditions that might lead to the loss of consciousness. The chapter concludes with a review of the signs and symptoms of those conditions that the dentist is more likely to see and to be called on to diagnose and treat in dental practice.

For a more detailed discussion of this subject, the reader is referred to a definitive text, such as that by Malamed.[2]

CONSCIOUSNESS AND UNCONSCIOUSNESS

The precise physiologic nature of the state of consciousness is not fully understood. Several factors are important in determining whether a person will remain conscious or not, and the more significant of these are discussed below.

Oxygen

The central nervous system depends on an adequate supply of oxygen. The blood circulation of the brain is especially rich, and the brain enjoys a high blood flow to weight ratio. Any cessation of oxygenated blood flow to the brain will lead to loss of consciousness in a very short time, and continued oxygen lack will lead to irreversible brain cell damage in a few minutes.

The delivery of oxygen to the brain depends on adequate blood pressure to pump the blood through the cerebral blood vessels (reduced in syncope, shock, and certain forms of heart disease), satisfactory oxygen-carrying capacity of the blood (impaired in severe anemia and carbon monoxide poisoning), and adequate oxygenation of the blood as it flows through the respiratory system (deficient in chronic respiratory disease, bronchitis, and emphysema).

The most probable of these factors to result in the loss of consciousness in the dental office is a diminution in blood flow in the cerebral vessels.

Glucose

Optimal function of the brain requires an adequate supply of glucose. Brain cells have little capacity to store glucose, and if the blood glucose level falls, there may be a deterioration in brain cell function that may lead to a loss of consciousness. There are several complex mechanisms by which blood sugar levels are maintained. These include, but are not limited to, hormones from the pancreas (insulin and glucagon) and adrenal gland (glucocorticoids). Glucose levels are maintained in the range of 70 to 100 mg of glucose per 100 ml of blood in the fasting state and normally rise after the ingestion of food. If the serum glucose should fall to the 40 mg/100 ml level or lower, the patient may begin to feel "light-headed" and may lose consciousness. Details of those patients likely to develop hypoglycemia in the dental office are discussed later in this chapter under the heading Coma in a Diabetic Patient.

pH

The pH of the blood may influence the state of consciousness. Small changes in the normal hydrogen ion concentration may cause significant alterations in the metabolism of tissues. The regulation of body pH is therefore one of the body's most important functions. A lowering of pH generally leads to central nervous system depression, disorientation, and coma. An increase of pH results in an overexcitability of the nervous system with perhaps the development of tetany (spasm of muscles). In very severe cases tetany may involve the muscles of respiration and lead to anoxia and death. There are several conditions in which the blood pH may change. For example, in uncontrolled diabetes a patient may accumulate ketones, acetoacetic acid, and other acidic byproducts in the bloodstream that lower pH and produce a diabetic acidosis. With sufficient change in the blood pH a patient may lapse into unconsciousness.

Continued rapid breathing (hyperventilation) can expel more carbon dioxide than is usual, with the result that the blood pH is less acidic, the pH rises, and the patient develops respiratory alkalosis. Such a situation may occur in the dental office when an especially nervous patient hyperventilates for a long period of time.

There are, of course, other reasons for loss of consciousness, such as the presence of an anesthetic agent in the bloodstream or the "electrical brainstorm" that occurs in some types of epilepsy.

The various conditions mentioned above provide a useful basis for the following discussion, as they are the more usual causes of untoward events that occur in the dental office.

CLINICAL CONDITIONS ASSOCIATED WITH LOSS OF CONSCIOUSNESS
Syncope

Syncope has been defined as "loss of consciousness resulting from a sudden diminution in cerebral blood flow." This generic term is used to denote unconsciousness occurring from several different mechanisms. These include:

Cardiac syncope

Fainting (a vasovagal or vasodepressor syncope)

Obstructive carotid, vertebral, or cerebral artery disease

Orthostatic hypotension

Miscellaneous causes, including carotid sinus syncope and cough syncope

Cardiac syncope. This occurs when the primary problem arises in the heart itself. Reduced cardiac output with decreased cerebral flow may result from a heart that beats too slowly, too fast for the chambers to fill adequately, or does not beat at all! The commonest causes of these irregularities are heart block and cardiac arrhythmia. The term *Adams-Stokes syndrome* has been applied to syncope arising from some form of heart block.

The onset of paroxysmal (sudden recurrence of symptoms) tachycardia may also provoke a syncopal attack. The rapidly contracting heart muscle does not permit adequate heart filling, and consequently the cardiac output falls. Certain forms of organic heart and lung disease may also affect the efficiency of the heart and limit its output. Valvular damage, such as aortic stenosis or pulmonary hypertension, may produce syncope, particularly after some increased call on the heart to perform, for example, after exercise.

Fainting (vasovagal or vasodepressor syncope). Some people have suggested that a distinction should be made between "faint" and "syncope." The generic term *syncope* indicates unconsciousness occurring in a wide variety of conditions, whereas a faint has been defined as "just another condition which may progress to syncope." Bourne[1] has defined the faint as "a reflex peculiar to man, characterized by a sudden decrease in blood pressure and heart rate with pallor, sweating, and when fully developed, loss of consciousness and muscle tone." Fainting is certainly the most common untoward reaction likely to occur in dental practice. However, because it appears so similar to the early stages of syncope resulting from other, much more serious conditions, the dentist should be able to recognize it and to distinguish it from the other conditions. The precise mechanisms of a faint are not known. It is assumed that the normal balance between cardiac output and peripheral vascular resistance, which normally determine blood pressure, is disturbed. There is a drop in cardiac output and a dilatation of blood vessels. The patient who faints has been described as "bleeding into his own blood vessels." The resultant "loss of blood" leads to a decreased venous return to the heart with a consequent reduction in cardiac output, lowered blood pressure, and decreased cerebral flow. The body, presumably attempting to rectify this disturbance, produces adrenaline, which accounts for the paleness and sweating seen in the fainting patient. The body is presumably reacting to the disturbance with a "fear, flight, or fright reaction."

In a study of 9513 patients seeking minor oral surgical treatment, Mc-Gimpsey[3] reported that 100 (1.1%) fainted. This figure agreed with similar studies that have reported a fainting frequency of 2% in dental patients and 3% to 6% in blood donors.

The condition is usually self-limiting, and the normal balance is soon restored. Signs, symptoms, and treatment are discussed later.

Obstructive carotid, vertebral, and cerebral artery disease. Obstruction of one or more of the vessels that carry the blood to the brain, such as occurs in atherosclerosis, may produce cerebral ischemia, which is sufficient to produce syncope. Obstruction of one carotid artery will not normally cause fainting unless the contralateral artery is also compressed. However, the presence of atherosclerosis in the other vessels carrying blood to the brain, with a resultant narrowing of their lumina, may prejudice their ability to compensate for a lack of "carotid" blood.

Occasionally, the act of turning the head may be sufficient to produce some "kinking" of one of these important blood vessels with the result that the brain is deprived of adequate oxygen.

Although they are rare, it must be remembered that cases have been reported in which excessive palpation of the neck has dislodged a fragment of atheromatous plaque from the carotid artery. This plaque, acting as an embolus, then travels through the cerebral circulation and may produce blockage of cerebral vessels with resultant brain cell damage.

Orthostatic (postural) hypotension. The normal maintenance of an adequate blood pressure and therefore adequate cerebral blood flow during positional changes is mediated through several mechanisms. These include baroceptors (pressoreceptors—neurologic end organs that respond to pressure changes) located in the aortic arch and the carotid sinuses, and nerves that control heart function and affect the diameter of peripheral blood vessels.

An increase in the number of baroceptor impulses reaching the central nervous system resulting from an increase in blood pressure will affect the central nervous system, producing the net effects of (1) vasodilatation of peripheral vessels and (2) excitation of the vagal center with decreased heart rate and force of contraction. These combine to lower blood pressure. Conversely, low blood pressure will reflexively cause the blood pressure to rise.

When a person moves from a supine or sitting position to a more erect position, there is a tendency for the blood to pool in the blood vessels of the lower extremities. The decreased venous return that this produces results in a reduction in cardiac output and lower pressure in the aortic and carotid arteries. Aortic and carotid sinus mechanisms normally compensate for these blood pressure variations produced by position changes. In some people the compensatory mechanisms may be sluggish, and a transitory period of "light-headedness" may be experienced during sudden changes of position. This is particularly likely to occur in a person who suddenly stands up after lying in the sun for a long time. The heat of the sun causes dilatation of peripheral skin blood vessels, and these vessels "sponge" the blood as the person stands up and gravity pulls the blood down.

Orthostatic (pertaining to or caused by standing erect) hypotension may also occur in patients who have diseases, such as diabetes and tabes dorsalis, in which neuropathies develop. Some patients have orthostatic hypotension as a side effect of certain drugs. These may be drugs that alter the functions of the nerves (such as ganglion-blocking drugs) or reduce blood volume (such as diuretics).

Miscellaneous causes. In some patients the carotid sinus mechanisms are particularly sensitive, and pressure over the carotid sinuses may lead to a considerable bradycardia and a fall in blood pressure. (It is as if the carotid sinus were interpreting the external pressure on it as being due to a marked elevation in blood pressure—the effect would be to reduce an elevation of blood pressure).

A violent bout of coughing may lead to a feeling of "blacking out" or of actual syncope. Presumably one of the reasons that this occurs is that the increased intrathoracic pressure developed during coughing interferes with normal hemodynamics and affects cardiac output.

Shock

Shock is an abnormal condition in which the cardiac output is reduced so much that the tissues of the body begin to deteriorate for lack of nutrition.

Shock has been regarded as a more profound and lasting condition than syncope that normally indicates a transient loss of consciousness. Shock may be progressive in that its effects (diminished tissue circulation and poor nutrition) on the cardiovascular system further depress that system, so that the "shock" state gets worse. Fortunately, this vicious cycle does not always develop. Nonprogressive shock describes a condition in which the cardiac output is decreased, but not enough to cause significant cardiovascular depression.

The causes of shock are many and various and may be grouped as hypovolemic, cardiogenic, obstructive, neuropathic, anaphylactic, and miscellaneous.

Hypovolemic. The maintenance of an adequate blood pressure depends not only on an adequate cardiac output but also on an appropriate peripheral vascular resistance. A reduction in cardiac output as a result of hypovolemia (an abnormally decreased volume of circulating fluid [plasma]) may develop from several conditions and lead to shock. The severity and speed of development of the shock syndrome depend on whether the hypovolemia occurs suddenly or slowly. Loss of fluid from the body by hemorrhage, severe vomiting or diarrhea, or excessive urination (diabetes mellitus or insipidus) or from the skin (excessive exudation of serum from burned or eroded skin surfaces, such as develops in pemphigus) may be so profound that adequate hemodynamic mechanisms cannot be maintained. In some cases blood or other body fluids may still be retained within the body but "lost" from the cardiovascular system. The net effect—low blood volume—is the same as if the fluid had been lost from the body. Such sequestration of body fluids may occur in ascites or intestinal obstruction, or following severe bleeding into the abdomen (hemoperitoneum) or thorax (hemothorax). Fortunately, shock arising from hypovolemia is not likely to be a diagnostic problem in the dental office.

Cardiogenic. A severe disturbance of cardiac function, such as occurs in an abnormal rhythm or following a myocardial infarction, may lead to a prolonged state of circulatory collapse. The signs and symptoms of cardiogenic shock and its management are discussed later in this chapter.

Obstructive. Any sudden mechanical obstruction of the normal circulatory system may lead to shock. Perhaps the best example of such a condition is pulmonary embolism. The sudden movement of a large blood clot from the pelvic or lower limb regions may produce significant obstruction of the circulatory system when the embolus is trapped in the lung. Such a disturbance may be fatal or may lead to severe shock.

Neuropathic. There are several conditions that produce severe impairment of the central nervous system, the net effect of which is to "suppress" the various cardiovascular regulatory mechanisms.

The administration of an anesthetic agent produces a depression of the central nervous system, and in some cases excessive administration of or hypersensitivity to an anesthetic agent may result in shock.

Anaphylactic. Anaphylaxis refers to an abnormal response of the body to some exogenous agent. The actual cellular mechanisms by which anaphylaxis is produced are not discussed here, but it is important to remember the net effects—marked depression of the cardiovascular system resulting in low blood pressure, profound sweating, and a rapid pulse rate. The recognition and management of an anaphylactic shock are discussed later.

Miscellaneous. Severe infections producing septicemias may lead to the development of the shock state. A marked deficiency in or absence of certain endocrines may also lead to a collapse of the cardiovascular system, for example, Addison's disease or profound myxedema.

Cerebral vascular accidents

Cerebral vascular accidents may be classified as cerebral hemorrhage, cerebral thrombosis, and cerebral embolism.

Hemorrhage. Intracranial bleeding may arise from arteries, veins, or capillaries. It is usually associated with a weakness of vessel walls and with hypertension. The vessels may be weakened as a result of a developmental defect, such as an aneurysm, or may arise from diseases of the blood vessels themselves, such as atherosclerosis. Bleeding may also arise in disorders of the blood or clotting mechanisms.

Thrombosis. Most cases of cerebral thrombosis arise in vessels already damaged by disease or are caused by primary disorders of the blood. Certain blood diseases, such as polycythemia, leukemia, or sickle cell disease, predispose to intravascular clotting, and this may occur in the cerebral vessels.

Embolism. Cerebral emboli may be portions of blood clots, atheromatous plaques, tumor, air, fat, or heart valve vegetations. They may originate in the heart, aorta, or vessels of the neck. The commonest origin of cerebral emboli is the heart. The effects of the emboli depend on their size and their final resting place.

Coma in a diabetic patient

Generally, the diabetic patient can become unconscious as a result of the diabetes (or its treatment) in two ways. Uncontrolled diabetes that permits the accumulation of β-hydroxybutyric acid, acetone, and acetoacetic acid in the blood is characterized by a reduction in blood pH, compensatory changes in the respiratory system, a high blood glucose level, and slow onset. A drop in body fluid pH to 6.9 may result in a coma. It is extremely unlikely that anyone would lapse into unconsciousness in the dental office as a result of a diabetic coma (acidotic or hyperglycemic). It is much more likely that a relatively rapid onset of loss of consciousness arising in a diabetic patient is an insulin reaction producing hypoglycemia. Such a reaction occurs as a result of an overdose of insulin. This may be because more than the usual amount was given or because the patient received the usual dose but had an inadequate diet.

The dentist must always identify those diabetic patients who are likely to develop hypoglycemia, and such patients should be identified during the history-taking phase of the evaluation. It is not sufficient to establish only whether a patient is or is not diabetic. Details of the type of diabetes, age at onset, and the method by which it is treated are most important. Of course, it should always be remembered that a diabetic patient who is unconscious is not necessarily so because of the diabetes. Diabetics are also prone to the other conditions (such as epilepsy, cardiovascular accidents, and syncope) that can lead to a loss of consciousness. Occasionally a patient who has *not* been diagnosed as being diabetic may suffer from hypoglycemic attacks. Such patients would normally be detected by a determination of the blood glucose level during an attack and the finding of an abnormal glucose tolerance test.

Epilepsy

Epilepsy has been defined as an episodic, transient disorder of the brain. The attacks tend to recur and follow the same pattern each time. The precise nature of the epileptic process remains unknown. It can be considered an uncontrolled disorderly excessive discharge of nerve energy. Various types of epilepsy are recognized clinically. Some of these are extremely mild and may appear to be no more than short attacks of "daydreaming" (petit mal). The more dramatic attack, or grand mal seizure, can lead to a loss of consciousness that may last several minutes. Only very rarely will an attack of epilepsy progress to *status epilepticus,* in which recurring attacks of grand mal follow so closely that consciousness is never regained in the intervals between. Status epilepticus must be regarded as a medical emergency, and appropriate treatment must begin immediately. The signs and symptoms of epilepsy are discussed later in this chapter.

Changes in pH of the blood

Reference has already been made to the fact that marked disturbances in the pH of the blood may be associated with changes of consciousness. Such changes in acidity or alkalinity may arise from many conditions involving several body systems, including the respiratory and metabolic systems.

Mention has been made of the acidosis that may arise in the untreated diabetic patient. It is unlikely that diabetic acidosis will appear as a diagnostic problem for the dentist. It is much more likely that a pH variation resulting in the alteration of a patient's consciousness will originate from the respiratory system. Hyperventilation syncope is a not uncommon condition seen in dental practice. Patients who are extremely anxious or nervous, especially if kept waiting unduly long for a dental appointment, may begin to hyperventilate. Excessive breathing causes a "washing out" of carbon dioxide from their blood and produces the condition of respiratory alkalosis. This is associated with such neurologic phenomena as numbness, tingling, light-headedness, and at times tetany. The diagnosis is usually straightforward, as the patient's hyperventilation can be readily appreciated.

395

Myocardial infarction

No chapter on the unconscious dental patient would be complete without a reference to myocardial infarction. Fortunately, the incidence of such attacks in the dental office is very low, but the possibility must always be considered when evaluating an unconscious patient. Coronary arterial thrombosis does not necessarily lead to a loss of consciousness. Many cases of coronary arterial thrombosis produce no symptoms or some that are so minimal that they are not recognized. Indeed, the fact that one may have occurred may be detected, as it were, by accident, when a routine electrocardiogram is recorded at a later date. In some patients coronary thrombosis produces tissue damage that severely interferes with the function of the heart. The heart may continue to beat regularly but inefficiently, may develop ventricular fibrillation, or may simply arrest—that is, not beat at all. The net effect of these alterations in cardiac function is to reduce blood pressure, with a resultant diminution of cerebral blood flow. Signs and symptoms of myocardial infarction are described later.

DIAGNOSIS OF THE UNCONSCIOUS DENTAL PATIENT

A dentist must assume the responsibility for the well-being of dental patients and must be prepared to diagnose and treat those patients who develop untoward reactions. Perhaps the most important aspect of diagnosing an unconscious patient is to be aware of those conditions that can lead to unconsciousness and to appreciate their underlying pathologic and physiologic nature. The most important conditions have been summarized briefly above, and it is now necessary to deal in detail with the signs and symptoms and with methods of managing the more common conditions that are likely to arise in dental practice.

Fortunately, not all of the conditions referred to occur with great frequency, and for some of them, the circumstances preceding them are usually quite dramatic and can be recognized easily. For example, a cough syncope will be preceded by a severe bout of coughing and a hyperventilation syncope by a prolonged period of hyperventilation. An important objective of the dentist is to *prevent* the onset of problems in "high risk" patients. A knowledge of each dental patient obtained from a searching medical history will permit the dentist to recognize the "high risk" patients; for example, those with epilepsy, or diabetic patients prone to hypoglycemic episodes. The hypertensive patient with a history of prolonged high blood pressure is naturally more likely to be a candidate for a cerebral vascular accident than the normotensive individual. *To be forewarned is to be forearmed.*

The most likely causes of unconsciousness that the dentist will be called on to diagnose in the office are fainting, shock, hypoglycemia, hyperventilation, epileptic seizures, and myocardial infarction (cardiovascular collapse). For each of these conditions details are given of the unusual circumstances preceding an episode, the symptoms, the signs, and treatment.

Fainting (vasovagal collapse)

Features preceding an attack. Attacks of fainting are often precipitated by emotional shock, pain, anxiety, fever, or a hot, stuffy atmosphere. Most faints that occur outside the dental office occur when a patient is standing. In the dental office it is important to determine details of any previous episodes of fainting. A patient may report fainting "every time I get an injection," "whenever I see blood," or "when the dentist has finished his treatment." Obviously, knowing when a particular patient is *likely* to faint is of special value in dental practice.

Symptoms. Patients may complain of feeling weak for a minute or two before blacking out. They may have sensations of heat or cold, have nausea, begin to perspire, feel lightheaded, and have blurred vision.

Signs. The patient looks anxious. The eyes may roll and the skin may be pale, particularly around the mouth (circumoral pallor). There is usually marked sweating of the hands and around the lips. Just before passing out, the patient may have a series of mild muscle spasms that are probably initiated by cerebral anoxia. Care should be taken that these spasms are not misinterpreted as an epileptic seizure.

Treatment. The most important point to remember is that, if a faint is recognized early, it may be possible to abort the unconsciousness through restoring cerebral flow by placing the patient supine with the head down. In the dental chair this is relatively easy to do. Care must be taken to ensure that the patient's airway is open and that there are no loose foreign objects in the mouth. Placing the patient in a position in which the legs are higher than the heart aids the venous return and in most cases quickly restores cerebral blood flow with a resultant regaining of consciousness. During unconsciousness the patient's blood pressure will be found to be low. In practice, however, by the time a blood pressure cuff can be obtained and the blood pressure measured, the patient is recovering from the faint. The pulse should always be monitored. During the attack it is likely to be slow, but the dentist must be certain that it can be detected and be confident that the patient has not had a cardiac arrest. The pulse also gives an indication as to whether there may be some cardiac syncope occurring as a result of abnormal heart rhythm, for example, heart block. The patient, when recovered from the faint, may usually feel a little nauseous, but drowsiness or mental confusion is very uncommon. The use of oxygen is of questionable value during the actual faint. It should be remembered that the primary problem is a lack of cerebral blood flow, rather than poor oxygenation of the blood itself. In our experience oxygen provides more of a psychologic lift than a physiologic one.

Anaphylactic shock

The causes of shock are many and were discussed earlier in this chapter. Not all these conditions are likely to occur with equal frequency in the dental office. The two most likely to appear as diagnostic challenges to the dentist are anaphylactic shock and myocardial shock. The latter is discussed later.

Features preceding an attack. An attack usually occurs after the administration of a medication, although it can occur after such insults as a bee sting or other insect bite. Generally, an anaphylactic reaction to a drug will occur in someone who has a preexisting history of allergic disease or a previous drug reaction. It should be remembered, however, that very occasionally a person may develop a severe anaphylactic reaction following the first dose of a medication. Fortunately, severe anaphylactic reactions in the dental office are relatively uncommon and especially so following the administration of local anesthetic agents. The most likely drug to cause an anaphylactic reaction in the dental office is penicillin.

Symptoms. The patient may feel light-headed, and feel waves of hot or cold, have blurring of vision and some difficulty in breathing, black out, or remain conscious but feel very strange.

Signs. The patient appears very nervous and pale and perspires copiously. The blood pressure is low. The pulse may be fast, rather difficult to detect at the wrist, and may be weak or "thready." There may be difficulty in breathing, and in an extreme case an abrupt cessation of respiratory and circulatory function may develop.

Treatment. The best treatment of anaphylactic shock is to prevent its occurring. This can be achieved in many cases by the dentist's being meticulous about taking histories of previous allergic reactions to various substances, including medications. A patient who appears to be in shock should be placed in the supine or semireclining position. The patient should have a patent airway and be given oxygen. If there is evidence of continuing respiratory or circulatory depression, then it may be necessary to use epinephrine. This medication, which should always be included in a dental office emergency kit, is administered by a 0.5 ml injection of a $^1/_{1000}$ solution intramuscularly or in severe cases intravenously. Fortunately, most cases can be managed by the administration of oxygen and the placing of the patient in a supine position, but it should be remembered that a severe case may call for the administration of cardiopulmonary resuscitation procedures.

Hypoglycemia

Features preceding an attack. Most diabetic patients who experience insulin reactions will report them as occurring at approximately the same time each day. This, of course, will be valuable information for the dentist to have. A missed meal, excessive physical exertion, or an overdose of insulin may also precede an attack.

Symptoms. The patient experiences irritability, sweating, inability to concentrate, and headache. The patient may notice light-headedness for some time before lapsing into unconsciousness. Some patients may recognize their need for sugar and ask for some food that contains it.

Signs. The patient's behavior may be somewhat irrational. The skin may be pale, warm, and sweaty. The pulse is of full volume and at normal rate. Convulsions before lapsing into unconsciousness are infrequent but may occur in very profound hypoglycemia.

Treatment. Ideally, incidents of hypoglycemia in the dental office should be very rare. A dentist should recognize those patients likely to develop hypoglycemia and either arrange to attend to them when it is most unlikely that an episode will occur or arrange for them to be given glucose *before* the start of a dental procedure. Glucose may be provided by giving the patient a candy bar, orange juice, or another source. A small amount of sugar is extremely unlikely to harm the diabetic patient but will almost certainly prevent the occurrence of a hypoglycemic episode. If the patient does become unconscious, no attempt should be made to give anything by mouth. The patient may be given glucose intravenously or may be given an intramuscular injection of glucagon. As soon as the patient's glucose levels are elevated, the patient will have a rapid return of consciousness with very few aftereffects. It has been said that as soon as a patient wakens from a hypoglycemic episode, he or she should be given some sugar to drink.

Hyperventilation

Features preceding an attack. Hyperventilation is likely to occur in those anxious or nervous patients who are very frightened about the prospect of receiving dental treatment. It may occur in the dental chair during treatment or in the dental office waiting room, especially if the patient has been kept waiting for an unreasonable length of time. Patients may report having had episodes of hyperventilation during previous dental visits, and any report of untoward reactions occurring during dental treatment should be evaluated most carefully.

Symptoms. The patient feels peculiar and may be completely unaware of breathing too rapidly. It is unusual for a patient to hyperventilate into unconsciousness. The patient is more likely to complain first of feeling dizzy and peculiar. Some numbness and tingling of the extremities may be reported. This sensation is very likely to increase anxiety, and often the patient breathes even faster.

Signs. The patient is clearly hyperventilating. The rapid breathing may not appear particularly labored and may be overlooked by the dentist. The patient may have some muscular twitching, suggesting a change in the neuromuscular sensitivity as a result of the pH change occurring as the patient exhales excessive amounts of carbon dioxide. The patient may not respond readily to questions or commands.

Treatment. The rate of breathing must be reduced. Sometimes it is possible to persuade the patient to do this by asking the patient to hold the breath while the dentist counts, say, for 30 seconds. The patient is then asked to take a deep breath and to once again hold the breath for a time. This maneuver is repeated until there is a buildup of blood carbon dioxide tension, which reduces the signs and symptoms. In those cases in which the patient cannot voluntarily hold the breath, it may be an advantage to have the patient rebreathe the self-expired air. This can be done by asking the patient to breathe into and out of a paper bag. The patient under these circumstances will be inhaling a significant amount of carbon dioxide from the exhaled air, which will permit the carbon dioxide level to be restored to normal. In some severe cases in which patients cannot seem to be controlled easily, it may be necessary to give intramuscular sedative preparations, although such measures seldom need to be taken in the dental office.

Epilepsy

Features preceding an attack. Most epileptic seizures are of abrupt onset. An attack may be precipitated by external stimuli, such as flashing lights, certain colors or patterns, or some incident that startles a person or promotes emotional shock. It has been noted that attacks may be more common in periods of relaxation than during activity. Some patients experience a vague feeling of "not being well" some hours or even days before an attack.

Symptoms. An epileptic seizure may be preceded by an "aura" that warns that an attack is imminent. This warning may be motor, sensory, visceral, or emotional. Occasionally the aura may not be obvious to the patient but may be perceived by an observant witness. Most patients have the same type of aura before each attack.

Signs. There are a variety of signs that may be seen in an epileptic attack. They may be "local," that is, limited to one part of the body (focal epilepsy), or they may start as a local disturbance that then gradually progresses to a wider area and eventually leads to loss of consciousness. The generalized convulsion (grand mal) is very dramatic. The muscle spasms, which are usually heralded by a cry, are generally first of tonic type (characterized by continuous tension) and may involve muscles from the head to the foot. Respiratory movements stop, and the patient may become cyanotic. The tonic spasms break and are followed by intermittent spasms (clonic phase), during which the patient may bite the tongue, and the sputum becomes blood tinged and frothy as a result of the forceful respirations. The bladder and the anal sphincters may relax, and there may be urinary and fecal incontinence. After the clonic phase the patient lies flaccid in a coma that may last a few minutes to hours. During this stage the pulse and respirations may be difficult to detect, and the corneal and light reflexes are lost. Most comas last for less than 2 minutes, and the patient will emerge from the coma with a gradual return of normal pulse, respiration, and reflexes. The patient will begin to move spontaneously and recognize people but may be unaware of the episode itself. During this phase the patient may perform quite complicated maneuvers which he or she subsequently forgets making (postepileptic automatism).

The patient will usually fall into a deep sleep and may waken with a headache, nausea, and aching in the limbs and muscles. The grand mal attack is variable and may differ in intensity from patient to patient and even differ from attack to attack in a particular patient.

Treatment. There is little that can be done during the actual muscle spasm phase except to prevent the patient from injury against furniture or other sharp objects. It may be possible to prevent tongue biting by forcing the teeth apart with a tongue blade around which gauze has been taped. (Such a prepared tongue blade should be ready and available at the dental chairside for all epileptic patients.) It should be remembered that, contrary to popular belief, there is *no* danger that an epileptic can choke by "swallowing one's own tongue." The patient, when recovered from the postepileptic sleep, should be permitted to go home. Whether the patient needs to be accompanied will obviously depend on the mental status and on the dentist's assessment of the patient's ability for self-care.

Continuing bouts of grand mal seizures during which the patient does not appear to regain consciousness suggest status epilepticus. This should be regarded as a medical emergency and the patient referred for definitive care as soon as possible. The dentist's responsibilities during this phase are to be certain that the airway remains open and to prevent the inhalation of vomit or any other foreign material.

Myocardial infarction

Features preceding an attack. A myocardial infarction may occasionally arise without any obvious preepisode stimuli. More usually, however, there are precipitating factors, such as sudden emotional excitement, a painful stimulus or injury, or some unusual physical effort.

Symptoms. The classic myocardial infarction produces a sudden onset of severe retrosternal chest pain, which is described as a feeling of tightness or pressure. This tightness may radiate into the arms, jaws, neck, or through to the back. The patient may feel nauseous and may vomit, sweat, and feel as if about to black out. The pain is usually persistent (compare this with the pain of angina pectoris, which normally "comes with effort—goes with rest"). If the left ventricle is badly damaged by the infarction, then there may be failure with resultant back pressure of blood into the respiratory system, producing severe breathlessness.

Signs. The signs of the condition will depend on the severity of the infarction. There may be nothing more to see than a patient in some discomfort, who may be pale, sweating, and looking anxious. The blood pressure and pulse may be within normal limits, although, of course, if there has been severe cardiac damage with lowered cardiac output, then the blood pressure may be low, and the patient may be in shock, having pallor, moist extremities, and a weak, thready, fast pulse. In some early stages of myocardial infarction the blood pressure may even be higher than usual. This is presumably a response to the severe pain.

Treatment. The most important aspect of management is for the dentist to recognize the need for immediate definitive treatment. This may require the services of trained medical emergency technicians and hospital personnel. The patient's pulse must be continuously monitored, for if there is evidence that the heart has developed a severe arrhythmia or ventricular fibrillation, then steps must be taken to initiate cardiopulmonary resuscitation. These steps can be summarized as:

1. *Airway*
2. *Breathing*
3. *Circulation*
4. *Definitive steps*

As soon as unconsciousness is recognized, the patient should be placed in the optimal position (approximately horizontal, perhaps with the brain at a slightly lower level than the heart), and attention must be paid to the *airway*. Any objects in the mouth (blood clots or other debris) should be cleared away and the head tilted back. This maneuver elevates the tongue and establishes maximal patency of the airway. Spontaneous respiratory movements should be looked for; if there are none, then the next step, *breathing* for the patient, should be started. The carotid pulse should be evaluated, and if it is not detectable then attention should be paid to *circulation*. The administration of cardiopulmonary resuscitation (CPR) has been well defined; the precise technique of CPR depends on whether there are one, two, or more rescuers. For a complete account of the various methods of CPR, the reader is referred to Malamed's text.[2] When the airway, breathing, and circulation steps have been taken, then *definitive steps* may be commenced. These steps may involve intramuscular, intravenous, or intracardiac injections of substances to combat acidosis, stimulate the circulation by producing constriction of blood vessels, and combat cardiac arrhythmias, among other purposes.

The extent to which CPR is applied in the dental office, particularly as far as definitive steps are concerned, will depend on the training, experience, and readiness of the dentist.

SUMMARY

There are many conditions that may lead to the loss of consciousness in the dental patient. Most of these conditions can be determined before the provision of dental treatment by taking a good medical history. As far as possible, every step should be taken to *prevent* the occurrence of an untoward event in the dental office. For example, patients with a known tendency to hypoglycemic episodes should be given glucose before dental treatment is begun or be seen at times when episodes are unlikely to occur. The evaluation of the unconscious state in the dental patient depends on the dentists':

1. Knowing the basic pathophysiologic nature of the most important conditions that could lead to unconsciousness.
2. Knowing the circumstances immediately preceding the incident.
3. Evaluating the physical signs of the patient, noting blood pressure, pulse characteristics, and respiratory movements.
4. Differentiating those conditions that may be managed in the dental office from those that require emergency medical care.

REFERENCES

1. Bourne, J.G.: Studies in anaesthetics including intravenous dental anaesthesia, London, 1967, Lloyd-Luke.
2. Malamed, S.F.: Handbook of medical emergencies in the dental office, St. Louis, 1978, The C.V. Mosby Co.
3. McGimpsey, J.G.: Fainting in the dental surgery, Br. Dent. J. **143:**53, 1977.

21   Special diagnostic problems

Usually changes in sensation, appearance, or function are perceived by patients as evidence of disease. Cultural background, education, and emotional status all influence the patient's interpretation of the significance of these changes and dictate their course of action. These changes may be related to a normal physiologic process or to a life-threatening disease, but help will be sought only when the patient perceives them as serious. Then the clinician will be challenged to evaluate the signs and symptoms that the patient has identified.

This chapter deals with the analysis and interpretation of signs and symptoms of diseases that represent a potpourri of problems that may be encountered in the dental office. Some are relatively common, whereas others are infrequent and unusual, but represent types of problems that will occasionally confront the dentist. There is no intent to provide detailed information about these problems but only to include sufficient discussion that will allow for the recognition and understanding of these problems and provide a basis for further investigation.

ABNORMALITIES OF TASTE

A variety of circumstances can produce various degrees of taste abnormality. This may range from a decrease in taste acuity *(hypogeusia)* to a complete loss of taste *(ageusia)* or may appear as a distorted taste sensation *(dysgeusia)*.[8] *Cacogeusia* is a term used to describe an abhorrent or obnoxious taste. The mechanisms responsible for these alterations in taste are not known. Much of the information that is cited is based on empirical evidence. Convincing evidence is not always available to prove a cause and effect relationship for all the factors identified as producing abnormalities of taste.

When patients complain of taste abnormalities, local factors should be considered first. The tongue and palate contain the taste receptors in the oral cavity. Lesions of the tongue, such as atrophy, leukoplakia, or hairy tongue, can be responsible for a diminished taste acuity. Patients who wear complete upper dentures may complain of hypogeusia. A salty or bad taste may be described by patients who have acute necrotizing ulcerative gingivitis, suppurative periodontitis, chronic parotitis, tonsillitis, or sinusitis.

A decrease in salivary flow has been associated with taste abnormalities. Diminished taste acuity occurs during radiation therapy for head and neck cancer and in patients with Sjögren's syndrome. Hypogeusia in these patients apparently occurs for other unknown reasons, in addition to the xerstomia.

Lesions of the facial nerve central to the origin of the chorda tympani and injury to the chorda itself can cause taste abnormalities. Food may be tasteless for patients with Bell's palsy or the Ramsay Hunt syndrome. Dysgeusia, sometimes described as a metallic taste, may occur following injury to the chorda tympani during stapedectomy. Taste loss may also be early evidence of an intracranial tumor.

Taste abnormalities that usually appear as a decrease in taste acuity have been associated with dysautonomia, hypothyroidism, pseudohyperparathyroidism, adrenal cortical insufficiency, and diabetes. Hypogeusia has also been reported as occurring during the acute phase of upper respiratory tract illness and then persisting for indefinite periods of time after the illness resolves.

Increasing numbers of drugs have been implicated in producing taste alterations. Usually patients complain of a decreased ability to taste, but dysgeusia has also been reported. The drugs that have been most frequently identified as causing these symptoms are penicillamine, carbimazole, clofibrate, griseofulvin, lincomycin, tetracycline, imipramine, and lithium carbonate. Taste is not consistently abnormal with the use of these drugs and usually returns to normal when the drugs are discontinued.

Though taste abnormalities are attributed to psychogenic factors less frequently now, some of the patients who appear with bizarre taste symptoms have mental illness, frequently depression. A careful evaluation is necessary to identify these patients. Some patients with dysgeusia on a presumed emotional basis have had relief with zinc therapy, suggesting a zinc deficiency. A good history and a means of testing the taste sense are necessary to adequately resolve complaints of taste abnormalities.

XEROSTOMIA

Dryness of the mouth may occur as the result of many different causes.[6] Usually it is transient and does not pose a serious problem. These transient episodes may be the result of anxiety, dehydration, acute sialadenitis, or current medications.

A long-term or permanent decrease in the flow of saliva may predispose a patient to a low-grade mucositis, increased caries activity, and abnormalities of taste, as mentioned previously. Edentulous patients will have difficulty in wearing their dentures. Xerostomia occurring as the result of radiation therapy for head and neck cancer is usually the most profound and dramatic seen. These individuals have a relatively abrupt decrease in secretions near the midpoint of therapy, with little if any return of salivary gland function after therapy has been completed.

Infiltrative disease of the salivary glands will result in a diminished flow of saliva. As more of the gland is replaced, less saliva will be produced, and xerostomia will become more profound. The diseases that involve the glands in this fashion are Mikulicz's disease, Sjögren's syndrome, and Heerfordt's disease. Salivary gland enlargement may be a feature of these problems, but need not be present.

A wide range of drugs are used now in the everyday practice of medicine. Many of these, such as the antihypertensive and antidepressant agents, have marked effects on the production of saliva. With prolonged use, which is usually the case, changes similar to those seen following radiation occur.

With aging there is some atrophy and fatty replacement of salivary gland tissue. If this is superimposed on fibrosis caused by previous disease, then a cumulative effect may be seen. This could result in a rather profound xerostomia.

A crude assessment of the quantity of saliva produced by a gland can be made during the examination of the mouth. The duct orifice of a salivary gland should be exposed and observed as the gland is compressed. Normally a small quantity of saliva can be expressed. It should be serous and clear. A more critical evaluation of saliva production by a gland can be made either by collection at timed intervals or by doing secretory sialography.

TRISMUS

Spasm of the masticatory muscles results in trismus. Clinically this is manifested as a limitation in the opening of the jaws. Normally an individual can open to a minimum of 40 mm, as measured between the incisal edges of the upper and lower anterior teeth. Patients with trismus frequently cannot open beyond 20 mm.

Trismus following an inferior alveolar nerve block is not an uncommon problem.[2] Typically these patients will have a normal postoperative period with a sudden onset of trismus occurring 1 to 3 days after the block. Intervals as long as 2 weeks have been reported. There is no swelling or tenderness, and the condition is remarkably painless unless the patient attempts a forced opening. The limiting sensation is described as if some type of mechanical restriction were present.

One of the signs of progressive pericoronitis is limited opening. The associated findings of an operculum, tenderness around the unerupted tooth, and regional lymphadenitis should offer sufficient evidence for the diagnosis. Any inflammatory disease that involves the muscles of mastication can produce trismus. Trauma of the head and neck region can also be responsible for trismus. This may be caused by a fracture, muscle spasm, or direct injury to the temporomandibular joint. Radiographs are necessary to rule out a fracture, but otherwise the history and physical examination should identify the problem. Tenderness will be noted in the area of muscle or joint injury.

Infiltrating tumors in the region of the jaws will produce trismus. Usually they are far advanced and readily apparent clinically or radiographically. Subsequent treatment for these tumors, whether it be surgery or radiation, will usually result in some degree of limited opening.

Jaw stiffness followed by trismus may be the first symptom of tetanus (lockjaw). This may be associated with or followed by neck stiffness, spasm of the facial muscles, or rigidity of the muscles of the abdomen, neck, and back. The muscle spasms, which last only a few seconds, are very painful and are provoked by physical stimulation. On occasion, strychnine poisoning can produce spasms of the jaw muscles that are similar to tetanus. These patients are also restless and apprehensive and have simultaneous contraction of all muscles. Rarely, severe tetany may produce trismus, but this is always preceded by sharp flexion of the wrist and ankle joints, which is referred to as *carpopedal spasm*.

The inability to open the mouth to its full extent is also found in patients who have TMJ arthritis or the myofascial pain dysfunction syndrome (see Chapter 15).[3] Patients with arthritis will have joint disease, which is usually apparent on radiographic examination. It has a slow onset and will have been present for some time. Patients who have the myofascial pain dysfunction syndrome may have trismus as the initial and only manifestation of the disease, or it may be present in addition to clicking of the joint and muscle tenderness. This trismus is presumably related to muscle spasm and disappears once the spasm is resolved.

403

NUMBNESS

Sensory loss can occur because of cold, hysteria, tetany, tissue hypoxia, and neurologic disease. Numbness of the face or oral tissues is an infrequent problem, but when present it must be investigated carefully, since it usually protends serious disease. Numbness of this region may be the result of tumor, multiple sclerosis, or cerebral ischemia. The first symptom of an intracranial tumor or jaw tumor may be a decrease in sensation, which slowly progresses to a total loss of sensation. Central lesions produce symptoms in all branches of the trigeminal nerve, whereas local lesions involve isolated areas. Leukemic infiltrates of the mandible have produced anesthesia of the lower lip.

Transient episodes of localized numbness and tingling may occur in the early stages of multiple sclerosis. Patients may describe numbness involving the trigeminal region without any other evidence of disease. Infrequently, transient ischemia of the basilar arterial system has been reported as producing numbness in the face.

Undoubtedly the most common reason for prolonged anesthesia of the face or oral tissues is traumatic injury to one of the branches of the trigeminal nerve. Numbness of the lip or tongue is a not uncommon sequela that follows an inferior alveolar nerve block injection or the removal of a difficult mandibular impaction. Usually there is some improvement of the symptoms but not complete recovery of sensation.

FACIAL PARALYSIS

Paralysis of the facial muscles is a situation that is rarely encountered in the dental office as a diagnostic problem; however, it may occur as a complication of giving local anesthesia. If the anesthetic solution is placed too far posteriorly and near the parotid gland while giving an inferior alveolar nerve block, the facial nerve will be affected. The resulting facial paralysis is somewhat disconcerting, but is transient and without any sequelae.

Patients may be seen with varying degrees of paralysis. Total loss of motor function (paralysis or palsy) frequently is preceded by a partial loss of motor function or muscle weakness (paresis). This is especially true in patients who have tumor involvement of the nerve. Intracranial tumors, particularly in the cerebellopontine angle, can produce a progressive facial palsy. In fact, tumors anywhere along the course of the facial nerve have the capacity to produce a loss of motor function. One of the hallmarks of a malignant tumor of the parotid gland is facial paralysis.

Bell's palsy is the most common form of facial paralysis. It produces a unilateral paralysis of relatively rapid onset and pain or discomfort in the mastoid region. If a patient attempts to close the lid on the affected side, there is a restricted movement of the orbicular muscle of the eye, and the eye on the paralyzed side will roll upward (Bell's phenomenon).

Approximately 20% of patients with the Melkersson-Rosenthal syndrome will have facial paralysis. They will also have swelling of the face or lips and a fissured tongue. A herpes zoster infection of the geniculate ganglion, Ramsay Hunt syndrome, will result in a facial paralysis that is preceded by a severe earache.

Facial paralysis may also occur in patients who have acute or chronic otitis media, uveoparotid fever (Heerfordt's disease), or the Guillain-Barré syndrome or who have had trauma to the facial nerve.

HALITOSIS

Bad breath, or oral malodor, is related to local factors in more than 80% of the cases. It is part of a normal physiologic process that is markedly influenced by personal hygiene and local disease.[9] Experimental evidence attributes these odors primarily to hydrogen sulfide and methyl mercaptan, which are produced by microbial putrefaction of sulfur-containing proteinaceous substrates. The normal physiologic pH of the oral cavity, anaerobic conditions, and a low carbohydrate environment favor putrefactive activity. Exfoliated epithelial cells, leukocytes, food debris, saliva, and blood are considered to be the prime substrates. Local conditions that predispose to increasing the intensity of mouth odors are poor oral hygiene, gingivitis, periodontitis, acute necrotizing ulcerative gingivitis (Vincent's disease), coated tongue, caries, healing extraction and surgical wounds, and tissue necrosis from any cause (such as leukemia, malignant tumors, and ulcerations). Factors that tend to decrease the intensity are toothbrushing, dental prophylaxis, tongue brushing, rinsing with antiseptic mouthwash, and eating.

Any situation that increases the trapping of saliva and food debris or decreases the ability of the mouth to cleanse itself promotes halitosis. During sleep there is decreased salivary flow and stagnation, which optimize conditions for putrefaction and contribute to early morning halitosis. Any patient with reduced salivary gland function will have increased difficulty with bad breath. The handicapped or semiconscious patient who cannot practice reasonable oral hygiene provides an optimal environment for putrefaction and is legend for having halitosis.

The upper and lower respiratory passages also can be the cause of malodor. Infections such as sinusitis, tonsillitis, or pharyngitis and necrosis of nasopharyngeal tumors are some of the diseases that contribute to the problem. Infrequently, halitosis may be noted with pulmonary diseases, such as infections, abscesses, bronchiectasis, or malignant tumors.

Though pyloric stenosis has been reported as producing a fetid breath, in general gastrointestinal problems are not a major contributing factor in halitosis. Belching (eructation) can cause a transient halitosis and dysgeusia. Odorous substances in the blood may pass into the lungs and upon expiration become evident in the breath. Various foods, beverages, and drugs produce halitosis in this manner. The classic offender is garlic. Alcohol and compounds containing chloral hydrate or iodine also have been reported to reach the breath via the systemic route. The sublingual use of isosorbide dinitrate has been reported as causing halitosis.

With kidney failure the breath takes on an ammonia odor because of the buildup of waste products in the blood. The acetone or fruity breath of the diabetic patient is due to the abnormal accumulation of ketones in the blood and their excretion by way of the lungs. This same odor may be noted in patients who are on high protein diets or who are starving. There is also evidence that the fat in the diet may be related to halitosis. It is thought that volatile fatty acids produced in the intestine are absorbed into the blood and eventually excreted in the breath.

PAIN

During the practice of dentistry many diagnostic problems are encountered, but none are as perplexing or frustrating as those seen in some patients with pain. They can pose the ultimate challenge. These pain problems may be the result of oral, paraoral, or systemic disease and simulate a dental problem. Almost without exception, a good history will be necessary to make a diagnosis. It may be the only source of diagnostic information or may be important in directing the diagnostic investigation. The techniques for obtaining an appropriate and complete history were discussed in Chapters 4 and 5.

The following material highlights the clinical features of the more common pain problems that might find their way to a dental office. The entities are grouped and discussed in the following order: odontogenic, neurologic, vascular, and other.

Toothache can be a devastating pain that at times is extremely difficult to localize. Unless information such as a history of a recent restoration or radiographic evidence of caries, a deep restoration, or apical change is available, it may prove frustrating to identify the responsible tooth. When pain is the result of pulpitis without apical involvement, the symptom of tenderness to either percussion or palpation of the apical tissue is not present. The selective use of local anesthesia can be extremely helpful in localizing tooth pain when it is diffuse or referred. Thermal pulp testing can be useful in identifying involved teeth by either initiating pulp pain or intensifying it. Though the problem of pulpitis is still controversial, it is generally believed that a reversible pulpitis can usually be distinguished from one with irreversible changes by the pain characteristics.

Reversible pulpitis produces infrequent episodes of pain of short duration. It occurs after thermal stimulus, usually cold, and stops seconds after the stimulus is removed. There is not a long-standing history of pain, and the pain does not occur spontaneously.

Irreversible pulpitis is characterized by pain that occurs either spontaneously or after thermal stimulus and persists for prolonged periods. The pain is more diffuse, radiating, and throbbing. Not infrequently, pulpitis in one jaw may refer pain to the opposite jaw.

The *cracked tooth syndrome* has rather characteristic pain symptoms, though it may be responsible for a wide range of bizarre symptoms.[4] Patients complain of a sharp pain while masticating food. It can be localized to an area but usually not to a specific tooth. Occasionally patients will experience a dull ache for prolonged periods or increased sensitivity to thermal change, especially cold. If the pulp is involved, any of the symptoms of pulpitis can occur. The involved tooth, usually a posterior tooth with a large proximal restoration, can be identified by one of the following procedures: percussing the individual cusp tips, wedging with an explorer between tooth substance and the restoration, having the patient bite on an object to transmit force to individual cusps, and staining with iodine.

Infrequently, *pericoronitis* may be responsible for a dull ache without showing other evidence of disease. The typical signs and symptoms of swelling, redness, trismus, tenderness, and purulent exudate from underneath the operculum may be absent or extremely subtle. Local tenderness to palpation is the most constant finding in these instances.

405

An intermittent or persistent dull ache may be caused by isolated areas of *periodontal disease*. The severity of symptoms at times is not consistent with the extent of disease that is present. A similar problem may also be seen in patients with early *acute necrotizing ulcerative gingivitis*. The severity of pain described may simulate that experienced with pulpitis.

Trigeminal neuralgia (tic douloureux) is characterized by a severe lancinating pain that lasts only seconds to minutes.[1] It is frequently precipitated by sensory stimuli, such as touching the face during shaving or washing, or by facial movements, such as yawning, talking, chewing, or swallowing. The patient may be without pain during the interval between attacks or have a mild dull ache. The trigger zone is usually in the second or third division and is found on the right side more often than on the left. Trigeminal neuralgia usually begins after age 40 and occurs more commonly in women. It is important to note that trigeminal neuralgia occurs in a signigicantly larger number of patients with multiple sclerosis than would be expected. Multiple sclerosis should be suspected whenever trigeminal neuralgia occurs in a patient under 40 years, since pain may be the first symptom.

Glossopharyngeal neuralgia (vagoglossopharyngeal neuralgia) is considered the "trigeminal neuralgia" of the glossopharyngeal nerve but occurs far less frequently. The pain can also radiate into the auricular and pharyngeal branches of the vagus nerve; hence the alternate term, vagoglossopharyngeal neuralgia. The pain is described as burning or sharp and lasts from seconds to minutes. It usually occurs on the left side after age 40 and has no sex predilection. The most common means of provoking the pain is swallowing. It may also be provoked by talking, eating, yawning, coughing, laughing, nose blowing, head turning, or touching the mucosa of the posterior tongue, soft palate, tonsil, or pharynx. The pain can radiate to the posterior tongue, tonsils, pharynx, middle ear, and external auditory canal.

Geniculate neuralgia is a complication of the Ramsay Hunt syndrome. Patients describe the pain as sharp, shooting, or burning and persisting for hours. There may be episodes of short duration. The pain is located deep within the ear or in the auditory canal or pinna. The neuralgia occurs in young or middle-aged adults and has been reported in women more often.

An infrequent but serious sequela of herpes zoster infections is *postherpetic neuralgia*. It is a constant burning ache with occasional paroxysms of stabbing pain. The pain may be provoked by peripheral stimulation. This condition rarely occurs before the age of 45 years.

In *cluster headache* (Horton's headache, periodic migrainous neuralgia) the typical patient will complain of a severe boring or throbbing pain that has had a sudden onset and builds to a peak during the first hour. The pain spreads to the temporal, periorbital, or maxillary region. It has frequently been confused with toothache. The pain will last from 30 minutes to 4 hours and will occur daily for a period of 2 to 6 weeks; hence, the name cluster. The pain tends to occur at approximately the same time each day and favors the early morning hours. It subsides as rapidly as it occurs. After a "cluster" of attacks, there is an interval of remission that might continue for years. In addition to pain, flushing, lacrimation, rhinorrhea, nasal congestion, and conjunctival congestion are frequently associated manifestations. The disease is more prevalent in middle-aged men.

Carotid arteritis or carotidynia appears as carotid tenderness and a constant dull ache that may involve the neck, jaw, or temporal area. The patient frequently complains of a stiff neck or sore throat. The most constant finding is a carotid tenderness detected by gentle pressure near the bifurcation. The pain may be aggravated by lateral rotation of the head, mastication, or swallowing. Spontaneous remission may occur after a few days or weeks. At times it persists for longer intervals and requires treatment.

The pain of *temporal arteritis* is variable and may be described as mild and aching or severe and lancinating. Usually the pain is of recent onset and is of a severe throbbing nature. It may radiate to the jaw. The involved temporal artery is thickened, firm, tender, nodular, and usually pulseless. Malaise, anorexia, weight loss, joint pain, and musculoskeletal aching have been associated with the problem. The most serious consequence of the disease is that some degree of permanent vision loss occurs in almost half the patients. The disease is rare in patients under 60 years of age.

Cardiac pain can be referred to the jaws, especially the lower posterior teeth. This jaw pain may be the only evidence of an anginal attack, or it may occur coincidentally with chest pain. The pain is described as a constant dull ache that is intensified with physical activity. The onset may be spontaneous and rapid. Associated pain may be noted in the neck, shoulder, or arm. Obviously, if cardiac disease is suspected the patient must be referred for medical evaluation immediately.

Acute *maxillary sinusitis* can appear as symptoms of dental disease. Patients will complain that their posterior teeth ache and are tender. The teeth may also feel elongated. The pain, a constant dull ache, is localized in the cheek and often exacerbated by coughing or a dependent position. Characteristically, the pain increases during the course of the day. Tenderness can be elicited with pressure over the sinus region (see Fig. 9-23). Swelling is seen infrequently. Radiographs will show a cloudy sinus.

Earache or pain in the region of the ear may be the result of many different problems. Since the sensory innervation of the ear is derived from the third division of the fifth, seventh, ninth, and tenth cranial nerves, pain can be referred from many areas. Inflammatory or neoplastic lesions of the nasopharynx, pharynx, larynx, tongue, tonsil, teeth, and temporomandibular joint have been reported as producing pain in the ear region. As a consequence, complaints of earache must be carefully evaluated if evidence of local disease is not apparent.

Patients with *Eagle's syndrome* may complain of a vague discomfort in the throat, difficulty in swallowing, glossodynia, or facial pain. The symtoms can mimic those found in glossopharyngeal neuralgia and are produced by an elongated styloid process. The styloid process in these cases frequently can be palpated intraorally in the tonsillar region. Palpation of the process will usually reproduce the symptoms that the patient has experienced. Lateral jaw radiographs or a panograph will show the elongated process.

Facial pain that occurs as a result of *intracranial tumor* may be variable in characteristics and duration. At the onset it is of short duration and described as a steady nonthrobbing dull ache. The pain becomes more intense with time, and the duration increases from minutes to hours. Some patients have described a pain that is brief, sharp, and lancinating, similar to that of tic douloureux. Usually as the symptoms become progressively more severe the patient will have some sensory loss. Whenever there is pain of an uncertain nature, the possibility of intracranial or extracranial tumor must be suspected and investigated.

A poorly defined and often abused diagnosis is *atypical facial pain*.[7] In recent years it has been used to identify patients who complain of pain that is burning, knife-like, or boring. The pain is usually constant and described as unbearable or incapacitating, even though the patient appears quite comfortable while describing symptoms of ongoing pain. The pain may not follow a neurologic distribution and at times crosses the midline. Typically, local anesthesia does not provide relief of the pain. The pain is frequently aggravated by fatigue, worry, nervousness, and tension. This problem is seen more often in young or middle-aged women and is thought to be a manifestation of conversion hysteria, hypochondriasis, or depression.

LOCALIZED FACIAL SWELLING

The initial assessment of an area of swelling should be directed to determining whether it is produced by bone or soft tissue. If bone is involved, radiographs are necessary for a complete evaluation. The changes seen in the radiographs will dictate the nature and extent of other necessary diagnostic studies.

With soft tissue swellings, cellulitis or abscess is encountered most often; cellulitis appears as a diffuse enlargement and an abscess is more localized and better defined. These swellings are warm, tender, and somewhat tense. Invariably they are caused by a nonvital tooth or advanced periodontal disease. The tooth responsible for the problem is usually quite easily identified because of its tenderness. Other than major salivary gland lesions or lymphadenitis, nonodontogenic reasons for inflammatory swellings are extremely infrequent.

Epidermal cysts are found most frequently around the ears but can occur anywhere on the face. Their size and duration are quite variable. When not inflamed, the cysts are firm, well defined, freely movable, close to the surface of the epidermis, and at times appear tethered to the epidermis.

Any component of the underlying connective tissue may develop into a glandular or mesenchymal tumor that may be either benign or malignant. Clinical features such as growth rate, tissue consistency, and outline may provide some indication as to a diagnosis, but these lesions cannot be adequately assessed without a biopsy. They occur infrequently.

Angioedema may produce a localized swelling anywhere on the face but involves the lips most frequently. The patient will have a marked swelling that appears very similar to that produced by a dentoalveolar abscess. In contrast to an abscess, the swelling of angioedema is neither warm nor tender. The patient is relatively asymptomatic and may complain only of a pressure or tense feeling. The swelling has a rapid onset and will usually resolve in 1 or 2 days.

A lip swelling similar to that produced by angioedema will occur with the Melkersson-Rosenthal syndrome.[5] With repeated episodes of swelling, the lip becomes firmer and stays swollen for longer periods. In time it remains swollen. Lip swelling in association with facial palsy is referred to as Melkersson's syndrome. If a fissured tongue is also part of the symptom complex, then it becomes the Melkersson-Rosenthal syndrome. The disease cheilitis granulomatosa (Miescher's disease) is thought to be a singular or incomplete manifestation of the Melkersson-Rosenthal syndrome, with only the lip swelling being present.

A chronic swelling of the lower lip is seen in cheilitis glandularis apostematosa. The enlarged lip is usually quite obvious and will have been present for many years. The lip feels firm and nodular. It may be tender, and the patient may complain of occasional discomfort. The most striking feature of the disease is the appearance of minor salivary gland orifices on the everted and exposed portion of the lip.

REFERENCES

1. Baker, A.B., and Baker, L.H.: Clinical neurology, New York, 1976, Harper & Row, Publishers, Inc.
2. Brown, A.E.: Persistent limitation of opening following inferior alveolar nerve block injections, Br. Dent. J. **141**:186, 1976.
3. Butler, J.H., Folke, L.E.A., and Bandt, C.L.: A descriptive survey of signs and symptoms associated with the myofascial pain-dysfunction syndrome, J. Am. Dent. Assoc. **90**:635, 1975.
4. Cameron, C.E.: The cracked tooth syndrome: additional findings, J. Am. Dent. Assoc. **93**:971, 1976.
5. Gorlin, R.J., Pindborg, J.J., and Cohen, M.M., Jr.: Syndromes of the head and neck, ed. 2, New York, 1976, McGraw-Hill Book Co.
6. Hausler, R.J., and others: Differential diagnosis of xerostomia by quantitative salivary gland scintigraphy. Ann. Otol. Rhinol. Laryngol. **86** (3 Pt 1):333, 1977.
7. Paulson, G.W.: Atypical facial pain, Oral. Surg. **43**:338, 1977.
8. Thawley, S.E.: Disorders of taste and smell, South. Med. J. **71**:267, 1978.
9. Tonzetich, J.: Production and origin of oral malodor: a review of mechanisms and methods of analysis, J. Periodontol. **48**:13, 1977.

Index

Page numbers in *italics* indicate illustrations.
Page numbers followed by *t* indicate tables.

Ecthyma, 137
Ectomorph, evaluation of, *16,* 17
Ectropion of eyelid, 101
Eczema, nummular, 148
Eczema herpeticum, 140
Eczema vaccinatum, 140
Eczematous dermatitis, allergic, 147
Educational goal for teaching physical evaluation, 5
"Ejection" systolic murmurs in aortic stenosis, 162
Electrocardiogram (ECG), 163-164
Elevated lesions of skin and oral mucosa, 47-49
Embolism, cerebral, loss of consciousness in, 394
Emergency, patient interview in, 37
Empathy
  in facilitating patient dialogue, 38-39
  importance of, 13-14
Emphysema
  chest shape in, 167
  palpation of heartbeat in, 157
  respiratory changes in, 80
Enamel, tooth
  dysplasia of, 346, *347*
  hypocalcification of, 346, *347*
  hypomaturation of, 346
  remineralization of, promotion of, 333
Enamel pearls, *344*
Encephalotrigeminal angiomatosis, 132
Endocrine disorders, hair changes in, 85
Endomorph, *16,* 17
Enema, barium, for gastrointestinal tract evaluation, 181
Entropion of eyelid, 101
Eosinopenia, causes of, 373
Eosinophilia, causes of, 373
Eosinophils in white blood cell count, 373
Ephelis, *69,* 134
Epidermal cysts
  in cheek, 87
  localized facial swelling in, 408
  in neck, 96
Epidermis, anatomy of, 120
Epidermoid cyst, 142
Epidermolysis bullosa, 150
Epilepsy
  diagnosis and treatment of, 399
  loss of consciousness in, 395
Epiphora from ectropion of eyelid, 101
Epithelial cyst, 142
Epithelial nevus, 143
Epithelioma
  basal cell, of skin, 145-146
  calcifying, of Malherbe, 146
Erosion
  definition of, 73
  of teeth, *336,* 337
Erysipelas, 138
Erythema
  acute infectious, 139
  of skin and oral mucosa, 61
Erythema gyratum, systemic significance of, 153

Erythema migrans oralis, 302
Erythema multiforme, *70, 71,* 149
  lips in, 242
Erythrocytopenia, causes of, 373
Erythrocytosis, causes of, 373
Eschar, definition of, 73
Evaluation, definition of, 15
Exanthems, 139
Excoriation, definition of, 126
Exophthalmos in hyperthyroidism, 86
Exostoses, gingival, 272
Extracapsular disorders of temporomandibular joint, 226
Extravasation of blood into skin and oral mucosa, 62
Eye(s), 98-109
  diseases of, and dental infections, 109
  examination of, 98-108
    color vision in, 100
    conjunctiva in, 102-105
    cornea in, 106
    external ocular structures in, 100
    iris in, *106,* 107
    lens in, 107-108
    lids in, 101-102
    movements in, 100
    pupil in, 107
    retina, 107-108
    sclera in, 102
    tonometry in, 100
    visual acuity in, 98
    visual fields in, 100
  injuries to, in dental office, 109
  movements of
    in cranial nerve evaluation, 190
    evaluation of, 100
  pressure in, measurement of, 100
  structures of, *99*
Eyelashes, turned in, 101
Eyelids, examination of, 101-102

F

Face, 85-89
  abnormalities of, 86-89
  anatomy of, 85
  clefts involving, 87
  examination of, 86
  numbness of, evaluation of, 404
  paralysis of, 86
    evaluation of, 404
  swelling of, localized, 408
Facial nerve (VII)
  damage to, facial paralysis in, 404
  examination of, 193-195
Facial surface of teeth, 326
Faculty for teaching physical evaluation, 7
Fainting, 392
  diagnosis and treatment of, 397
Fat, accumulation of, yellow lesions from, *71, 72*
Fauces, 289-292
  abnormalities of, 292
  anatomy of, 289-290
  examination of, 291
  pillars of, 289

Federation Dentaire International (FDI) system
  for designating teeth, 328, *329*
Fever, dental causes of, 80
Fibrillation, atrial, 78
Fibrocartilage in temporomandibular joint, 200
Fibroepithelial polyps on labial mucosa, 248
Fibroma(s), *58, 66*
  irritation, *49*
    on labial mucosa, 248, *249*
  peripheral ossifying, *49*
  of tongue, 303
Fibromatosis, idiopathic, of gingiva, 273
Fibrous skin tumors, 146
Fields, visual, examination of, 100
Fifth disease, 139
Filiform papillae of tongue, 295
Final diagnosis, definition of, 11
Fingernails, evaluation of, 22
Fingers, clubbing of, significance of, 21-22
Fissure, definition of, *73,* 124
Flat lesions of skin and oral mucosa, *52, 53*
Fluctuance, evaluation of, by palpation, 24
Fluid, accumulation of, in skin and oral mucosa, 58, *60*
  white lesions from, *64, 65*
Fluid wave in ascites, 177
Fluoride, topical, in promoting remineralization of enamel, 333
Fluoroscopy for gastrointestinal tract evaluation, 181
Fluorosis, dental, 348
Foliate papillae of tongue, 296, *297*
Folliculitis, 138
Fontanelles, lack of closure of, 84
Foramen cecum of tongue, 292
Fordyce's granules
  of buccal mucosa, 256
  of lips, 238, *239*
Forensic odontology, data for, health record as, 28
Forgetting, inaccurate observation due to, 15
Format for consultation, 386, *387*
Fovea palatinae, 280
Fractures, TMJ disorders due to, 226
Freckles, 134
Friction rubs, 171
  abdominal, 177
Fundus, examination of, 108
Fungiform papillae of tongue, 295
Furuncle, 138
Fusion of teeth, *343*

G

Gait, evaluation of, 18
Gallbladder, enlarged, palpation of, 179
Gangrene of skin and oral mucosa, 70
Gemination of teeth, *343*
Generalized elevated lesions of skin and oral mucosa, 47
Geniculate neuralgia, pain in, 406
Genioglossus muscles in floor of mouth, 310
Geniohyoid muscles in floor of mouth, 310
Genitalia, examination of
  in female, 183
  in male, 182

Mean corpuscular volume (MCV), 374
Measles, 139
  German, 139
Median rhomboid glossitis, 302
Medical consultation, 383-385
Medical management of patient, medical consultation for, 385
Megalencephaly, definition of, 84
Melanin
  accumulation of, in skin and oral mucosa, 68, 69
  increased, causes of, 122
  in oral pigmentation, 54, 55
    distribution of, 56-57
Melanoma(s), 70, 135-136
  juvenile, 136
  lentigo maligna, 134
Melanosomes of skin and oral mucosa, 68, 69
Melanotic freckle of Hutchinson, 134
Melasma, causes of, 134
Melkersson-Rosenthal syndrome
  facial paralysis in, 404
  localized facial swelling in, 408
Membrane, tympanic, examination of, 112
Memory in mental status examination, 42
Mental disorders of dental patients, 42-43
Mental status examination in psychologic assessment, 40, 41-42
Mercury gravity manometer for blood pressure determination, 76
Mesial surface of teeth, 326
Mesiocclusion, evaluation of, 354
Mesomorph, 16, 17
Metals, heavy, poisoning from, gingiva in, 278
Microbiologic examination of cultures, 379
Microcephaly, definition of, 84
Microcytes, 374
Microdontia, 342
Miescher's disease, localized facial swelling in, 408
Migrainous neuralgia, periodic, pain in, 406
Migratory glossitis, 302, 303
Migratory stomatitis, benign, 302
Mikulicz's disease, 89
Mikulicz's syndrome, 89
Milia, 142
Milroy's disease, 133
Mitral area of precordium, 158, 159
Mitral regurgitation, 161
Mitral stenosis, 161
  thrills of, 157
Mobility, evaluation of, 18-19
Moles, 135-137
Molluscum contagiosum, 141
Mongolism, facial abnormalities in, 86
Monocytes in white blood cell count, 373
Monocytopenia, causes of, 373
Monocytosis, causes of, 373
Mood in mental status examination, 42
Morbilli, 139
Moriscatio labiorum, 246
Motor activity in mental status examination, 42
Motor power, testing of, 187
Mouth, 229, 316; see also Oral cavity

Mucobuccal fold, 252
Mucocele(s), 49, 60
  of floor of mouth, 315
  of labial mucosa, 248
  of maxillary sinus, 115
Mucogingival junction, 264, 265
Mucosa
  alveolar, 264-279; see also Alveolar mucosa
  buccal, 251-263; see also Buccal mucosa
  labial, 245-250; see also Labial mucosa
  oral
    lesions of, characteristics of, 45-73; see also Lesions of skin and oral mucosa
    and skin, comparison of, 119
Mucous membrane pemphigoid, 65
Mucous retention cyst in floor of mouth, 315
Mucous retention phenomenon, 49, 60
  in floor of mouth, 315
Multiple sclerosis
  description of, 199
  numbness in, 404
Murmurs, heart, 160
  in aortic regurgitation, 162
  in aortic stenosis, 162
  "ejection" systolic, 162
  flow, 160
  functional, 162
  in mitral regurgitation, 161
  in mitral stenosis, 161
Muscle(s)
  of back, palpation of, in TMJ examination, 218
  digastric, 202
    palpation of, in TMJ examination, 216, 217
  facial, paralysis of, evaluation of, 404
  genioglossus, in floor of mouth, 310
  geniohyoid, in floor of mouth, 310
  masseter, 202, 203
    palpation of, in TMJ examination, 214, 215
  of mastication, tenderness in, in TMJ pain-dysfunction syndrome, 227
  orbicular, testing of, 193
  pterygoid
    lateral, 202
      palpation of, in TMJ examination, 218-219
    medial, 202, 203
      palpation of, in TMJ examination, 214, 215
  sternocleidomastoid, 90
    palpation of, in TMJ examination, 212
  temporal, 202, 203
    palpation of, in TMJ examination, 213
  trapezius, 90
Myasthenia gravis, facial paralysis in, 86
Myocardial infarction
  diagnosis and treatment of, 400
  loss of consciousness in, 396
Myofascial pain-dysfunction syndrome (MPD), 226, 227-228
  depression and, 42-43
  trismus in, 403
Myxedema, facial abnormalities in, 86

Nails
  abnormalities of, 130
  evaluation of, 121
Nasal polyp, 113
Nasopharynx, 289
Neck, 90-97
  abnormalities of, 94-97
  anatomy of, 90-92
  examination of, 92-93
  lymph nodes of, 90, 91-92
    enlarged, 94-95
    palpation of, 92-93
Necrobiosis lipoidica diabeticorum, systemic significance of, 153
Necrosis of skin and oral mucosa
  black lesions from, 70
  white lesions from, 64, 65
Necrotizing ulcerative gingivitis, acute, pain in, 406
Neoplasia of skin and oral mucosa, 58, 59
Neoplasm(s)
  involving floor of mouth, 316
  temporomandibular joint disorders due to, 226
Nerve(s)
  abducent (VI), examination of, 190
  accessory (XI), examination of, 198
  acoustic (VIII), examination of, 196-197
  chorda tympani, examination of, 195
  cranial, examination of, 188-198
  facial (VII)
    damage to, facial paralysis in, 404
    examination of, 193-195
  glossopharyngeal (IX), examination of, 198
  hypoglossal (XII), examination of, 198
  oculomotor (III), examination of, 190
  olfactory (I), examination of, 188
  optic (II), examination of, 188-189
  trigeminal (V)
    damage to, numbness in, 404
    examination of, 192
  trochlear (IV), examination of, 190
  vagus (X), examination of, 198
Nervous system, 185-199; see also Nerve(s)
  examination of, basic principles of, 185-187
Neuralgia
  geniculate, pain in, 406
  glossopharyngeal, pain in, 406
  migrainous, periodic, pain in, 406
  postherpetic, pain in, 406
  trigeminal, 192
    pain in, 406
  vasoglossopharyngeal, pain in, 406
Neurodermatitis, 148
Neuropathic shock, loss of consciousness in, 394
Neutrocclusion, evaluation of, 353
Neutropenia, causes of, 372
Neutrophilia, causes of, 372
Neutrophils
  band, in white blood cell count, 372
  segmented, in white blood cell count, 372
Nevoid basal cell carcinoma syndrome, 146